CARDIOPULMONARY SYSTEM

Cardiopulmonary System

Daniel R. Richardson, Ph.D.

Professor of Physiology

Department of Physiology

University of Kentucky College of Medicine

Lexington, Kentucky

David C. Randall, Ph.D.

Professor of Physiology

Department of Physiology

University of Kentucky College of Medicine

Lexington, Kentucky

Dexter F. Speck, Ph.D.

Associate Professor of Physiology

Department of Physiology

University of Kentucky College of Medicine

Lexington, Kentucky

**Fence Creek
Publishing**

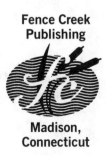

**Madison,
Connecticut**

Typesetter: Pagesetters, Brattleboro, VT
Printer: Port City Press, Baltimore, MD
Illustrations by Visible Productions, Fort Collins, CO
Distributors:

United States and Canada
Blackwell Science, Inc.
Commerce Place
350 Main Street
Malden, MA 02148
Telephone orders: 800-215-1000 or 781-388-8250
Fax orders: 781-388-8270

Australia
Blackwell Science, PTY LTD.
54 University Street
Carlton, Victoria 3053
Telephone orders: 61-39-347-0300
Fax orders: 61-39-347-5001

Outside North America and Australia
Blackwell Science, LTD.
c/o Marston Book Service, LTD.
P.O. Box 269
Abingdon Oxon, OX 14 4XN England
Telephone orders: 44-1-235-465500
Fax orders: 44-1-235-465555

2 3 4 5 6 7 8 9 10

TABLE OF CONTENTS

CONTRIBUTOR

Yasser M. El-Wazir, M.D., Ph.D.
Associate Professor of Physiology
Department of Physiology
Faculty of Medicine
Suez Canal University
Ismalia, Egypt

PREFACE

Given that the understanding of physiology is conceptual in nature, this text carefully and methodically develops the most important concepts underlying the functions of the heart, lungs, and circulation (i.e., the cardiopulmonary system). In taking this approach, it is the authors' intention that students will find the text helpful not only in understanding the most important elements of cardiopulmonary physiology but also in providing a useful review of the heart, lungs, and circulation in preparation for Step 1 of the USMLE.

It will be helpful at the outset of the student's preparation for a career in medicine to bear in mind two fundamental questions in the study of the function of living systems: how does the system use energy to overcome the tendency to become disordered, and how does the organism control the rate of utilization of energy? The first issue is the cornerstone of biochemistry. The second of these grand thematic questions is the "focus concept" around which this text is organized. Historically, this concept has been presented and discussed in terms of *homeostasis*: the maintenance of a stable "internal environment." The body maintains its physiologic integrity—homeostasis—using what are called biofeedback systems, feed-forward systems, and a few other related mechanisms. Of these, biofeedback is undoubtedly the most important. The concept is familiar to almost everyone: the thermostat in a building controls the rate of utilization of natural gas or electricity (i.e., energy) to maintain a comfortable room temperature (i.e., a stable internal environment) despite rising or falling environmental temperature (the perturbation). The concept of homeostasis is so important that the authors have adopted several tools to facilitate its presentation. One of these, the *cycle diagram*, appears in almost every chapter. One of the major messages of any cycle diagram is that no single organ or organ system functions autonomously within an organism (Chapter 7). Instead, the organs of the cardiopulmonary system function as an integrated whole, just as they also interact with other organ systems to maintain total body function despite changes in the environment or of the organism's behavior. Once mastered, the cycle diagram becomes an effective mechanism to summarize the way almost any system functions.

The first chapters of this text develop concepts that are generally applicable across the cardiopulmonary system, such as an explanation of homeostasis itself (Chapter 1). The function of the lungs and circulation, like virtually every other organ system, is governed by the laws of physics; Chapter 3, accordingly, reviews some of the physical principles that are most relevant to the flow of fluids and actions of applied forces. Chapter 4 explains the principles of muscle function that are applied in later chapters to explain the ability of the heart to move blood or the respiratory muscles to cause air to flow. The middle chapters of the text describe features specific to each of the three components of the cardiopulmonary system: the heart, the vasculature, and the lungs. The student should take care to discern those portions of these chapters that deal with the *control* of cardiopulmonary function. Finally, the last chapter reunites the three elements of the cardiopulmonary *system* to show how they function together during exercise.

Case studies, a liberal use of margin notes, and review questions with explanations are found throughout this text to help the reader appreciate how an understanding of cardiopulmonary physiology ultimately leads to a more effective clinical practice. Finally, references at the end of the chapter are intended to assist the student in augmenting the concepts presented with additional detailed information.

Daniel R. Richardson, David C. Randall, and Dexter F. Speck

ACKNOWLEDGMENTS

The authors gratefully acknowledge the assistance of the faculty of the Department of Physiology, College of Medicine at the University of Kentucky, for their help and forbearance during the preparation of this manuscript. We are especially grateful to our students who have ultimately made this effort possible. We also express our sincere appreciation to Fence Creek Publishing whose support has been invaluable. Finally, we acknowledge the inestimable help of our editor, Ms. Jane Edwards: we owe her tuition!

INTRODUCTION

Cardiopulmonary System is one of ten titles in the *Integrated Medical Sciences (IMS) Series* from Fence Creek Publishing. These books have been designed as course supplements and aids for board review for first- and second-year medical students. Rather than focusing on the individual basic science disciplines, the books in the *IMS Series* have been designed to highlight the points of integration between the sciences, including clinical correlations where appropriate. Each chapter begins with a clinical case, the resolution of which requires the application of basic science concepts to clinical problems. Extensive use of margin notes, figures, tables, and board-review questions illuminates core biomedical concepts with which medical students often have difficulty.

Each book in the *IMS Series* shares common features and formats. Attempts have been made to present difficult concepts in a brief and focused format and to provide a pedagogical aid that facilitates both knowledge acquisition and review.

Given the long gestation period necessary to publish a book, it is often impossible for publishers to keep pace with the changes and advances that occur so rapidly. However, the authors and the publisher recognize the need to have access to the most current information and are committed to keeping *Cardiopulmonary System* as up to date as possible between editions. As the field of cardiopulmonary physiology evolves, updates to this text may be posted on our web site periodically at http://www.fencecreek.com.

We hope that the student finds the format and the text material relevant, interesting, and challenging. The authors, as well as the Fence Creek staff, welcome your comments and suggestions for use in future editions.

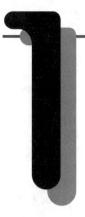

HOMEOSTASIS AS A FRAMEWORK OF CARDIOPULMONARY FUNCTION

CHAPTER OUTLINE

INTRODUCTION OF CLINICAL CASE

A 5′6″, 210-lb, 64-year-old male business executive had a physical examination prior to his retirement from corporate work [1]. His blood pressure on 3 separate days was more than 180 mm Hg systolic and 115 mm Hg diastolic. Additional relevant findings included an elevated total peripheral resistance (TPR) with cardiac output (CO) within the normal range.

HOMEOSTASIS: THE FOCUS CONCEPT OF PHYSIOLOGY

Focus Concepts. An understanding of both a focus concept and homeostasis is fundamental to the integrative approach taken in this text. Most disciplines have a core around which, or toward which, the various components of the discipline are related and can be understood as a whole. For example, the central concept of physics is energy balance. From an instructional point of view, central (or focus) concepts can be quite helpful in serving as landmarks to help students navigate their way through the maze of factual information.

Homeostasis. The *focus concept of physiology is homeostasis.* In classic terms, homeostasis is the maintenance of internal stability. The French physician Claude Bernard (1813–1878) was the first person to formalize this concept. In his words, "All vital mechanisms, however varied they may be, have only one object, that of preserving constant the conditions of life in the internal environment" [2]. The term homeostasis, from the Greek words *homis*, meaning "like," and *stasis*, meaning "standing still," was coined by Walter Cannon, the chairman of the Department of Physiology at Harvard University in the 1920s and 1930s.

*The political process is an example of **social homeostasis**.*

Chronobiology is a subdiscipline of the biologic sciences that investigates the mechanisms of body rhythms.

This change in blood flow occurs because by-products of tissue metabolism have a general vasodilatory effect.

Bernard applied the concept of internal consistency to the fluid environment in which cells live, now referred to as the interstitial fluid. However, through the work of Cannon, the concept of homeostasis has been expanded to include stability of any physiologic variable, such as blood pressure, as well as stability of a whole organism and societies of organisms. Therefore, within the life sciences, homeostasis includes both physiologic and behavioral facets.

Stability. Bernard was conceptually, but not factually, correct in his use of the term *constant.* As it is now understood, the internal environment is not constant, but it is stable. The difference between consistency and stability can be illustrated through the example of body temperature regulation. Body temperature has a circadian rhythm: it tends to be low in the early morning (about 36°C) and high in the early afternoon (about 37°C). Body temperature is regulated around each of these two *set points* at the appropriate time of day (e.g., 36°C in the morning and 37°C in the afternoon). Thus, at any particular time of the day, body temperature is stable, but it is not constant, since the regulatory set points are subject to change. Furthermore, considering that temperature is a measurement of heat concentration, the internal heat of the body is anything but constant, since the body is continually producing and eliminating heat. However, as long as heat production equals heat dissipation to the environment, body temperature will be stable.

Dynamic Equilibrium and Steady State. The stability of most physiologic variables occurs through the process of *dynamic equilibrium*, or *steady state*. The distribution of ions between the inside and outside of cells is a very important example of variables that remain stable through the process of dynamic equilibrium. For example, potassium ions (K^+) are constantly entering and exiting cells by way of carrier mechanisms and ion channels in the plasma membrane. However, under steady-state conditions, the rate of K^+ efflux from cells equals the rate of K^+ influx into cells; that is, in the steady state, K^+ exchange is occurring, but there is no *net* flux in or out of a cell. Therefore, the cell is in a state of dynamic equilibrium with respect to the exchange of K^+.

Using the example of temperature regulation, it can be stated that each set-point temperature is in a steady-state condition. For the total body to remain homeostatic, it is often necessary for some physiologic variables to change values from one steady-state condition to another in accordance with changing regulatory demands. Consider blood flow to a tissue, such as skeletal muscle. As the metabolic demands of the tissue change from one level to another, blood flow keeps pace, changing from one steady state to another in accordance with the ongoing level of metabolism. Such changes require the integration and interaction of a variety of physiologic mechanisms. For example, maintaining a stable oxygen supply to muscle tissue during exercise involves the interaction of mechanisms that control lung ventilation, lung perfusion, cardiac output, muscle blood flow, and oxygen uptake into muscle fibers.

Homeostasis Defined. For the purposes of this text, "homeostasis" is defined as *the maintenance of internal stability by action and interaction of physiologic mechanisms*. Adopting the notion that physiologic mechanisms, no matter how complex they may be, are focused toward maintaining stability within the internal environment (i.e., total body homeostasis) provides an organizing framework within which physiologic functions and their mechanisms can be understood. This is why homeostasis is considered to be *the* focus concept of physiology and why this text emphasizes the integrative aspects of the cardiopulmonary system.

MECHANISMS OF HOMEOSTASIS

Negative Feedback. The classic mechanism of homeostasis is negative feedback, as illustrated in Figure 1-1. In this system, any change in the variable being regulated (e.g., blood pressure) is detected by a sensor. The sensor transmits information about the variable in the form of an afferent signal to a transfer component. The transfer component integrates all incoming sensory information; then it makes, in essence, an "executive decision," resulting in a series of instructions in the form of efferent signals to one or more effector mechanisms. The net effect of these instructions is to *drive* the variable in the opposite direction from its original change. The *dashed line* between the sensor and the transfer component (i.e., the afferent signal) indicates that there is an inverse relationship between these two components; that is, a decrease in sensory information that would occur with a decrease in the variable causes the transfer component to increase efferent signals to the effector mechanisms and vice versa. In this manner, the efferent mechanisms serve to correct a change in the variable. It is important to note that inverse relationships in a negative feedback loop do not always occur between the sensor and the transfer component. They may exist anywhere in the loop. The key to a negative feedback regulatory system is that there must be an *odd number of inverse relationships* within the regulatory loop. If there is an even number of inverse relationships, or no inverse relationships, then a positive feedback loop results.

> Medication that either enhances or inhibits effector mechanisms in essence modifies the effectiveness of feedback regulatory systems.

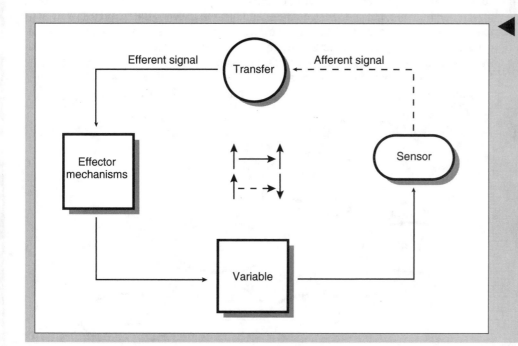

◄ **FIGURE 1-1**
Components of a Negative Feedback System. *As indicated at the bottom of the figure,* solid lines *indicate direct relationships between components;* dashed lines *indicate inverse relationships. In direct relationships when one component increases, the connected component also increases and vice versa. In inverse relationships, an increase in one component elicits a decrease in the connected component and vice versa. Negative feedback systems have one or an odd number of inverse relationships between components. (*Source: *Reprinted with permission from Richardson DR:* Basic Circulatory Physiology. *Boston, MA: Little, Brown, 1976, p. 140.)*

Positive Feedback. An example of positive feedback is given in Figure 1-2, which shows how an increase in blood viscosity can contribute to a reduction in tissue blood flow [3]. Chapter 6 shows that under certain conditions blood viscosity increases as blood flow decreases. This is indicated in the figure by the *dashed line* (C) between tissue blood flow and blood viscosity. An increase in viscosity contributes to an increase in resistance to the flow of blood, as indicated by *line A*. As resistance increases, tissue blood flow further decreases, indicated in the figure by *dashed line B*. Thus, in situations, such as hemorrhagic shock, which are characterized by low tissue blood flow, a positive feedback cycle is generated in the relationship between blood flow, blood viscosity, and resistance to flow. This positive feedback cycle contributes to the progressive degeneration associated with hemorrhagic shock. Many pathophysiologic conditions are characterized by positive feedback relationships of this nature. However, positive feedback cycles are not always pathologic in nature. Many serve a useful purpose in total body homeostasis. The foremost example of these cycles is the blood clotting mechanism, which serves an obvious protective function in maintaining blood volume.

> The voltage-dependent sodium (Na+) current at the onset of an action potential is another example of physiologic, as opposed to pathologic, positive feedback.

Labeling, or not Labeling, Components of a Feedback Diagram. This text often uses negative feedback diagrams to represent regulatory interactions. In constructing these loops, *solid lines* are used to indicate direct relationships between components and *dashed lines* to represent inverse relationships. However, the various components of the system (i.e., variable, sensor) are not always labeled, since these may not be apparent. For example, consider Figure 1-3. Figure 1-3A shows the regulation of blood pressure by

FIGURE 1-2 ▶

Example of a Positive Feedback Relationship Between Physiologic Variables. *Positive feedback cycles are characterized by no inverse relationships or an even number of inverse relationships, as depicted here.*

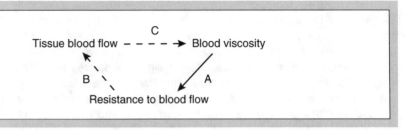

Most of this CNS transfer occurs in the medullary region of the brainstem.

what is known as the carotid sinus reflex. Here the components of the system, as illustrated in Figure 1-1, are easily identified. Arterial pressure is obviously the variable of interest, the carotid sinus is the sensor, the central nervous system (CNS) contains the transfer component, and the effector mechanisms are TPR and CO. Figure 1-3B depicts a negative feedback relationship between plasma water, plasma colloid osmotic pressure, and the absorption of interstitial fluid. Note that in this example, there is one inverse relationship: between plasma water and plasma colloid osmotic pressure. Therefore, this is a negative feedback system; however, it is not clear if plasma water or plasma colloid osmotic pressure should be designated as the regulated variable. *Both* plasma water and colloid osmotic pressure are being regulated. This example emphasizes the fact that the classic components of a feedback loop (i.e., variable, sensor) are terms borrowed from engineering, which may or may not apply in biologic regulation.

FIGURE 1-3 ▶

(A) This is a negative feedback system in which the components of the system, as depicted in Figure 1-2, can easily be identified. (B) This is an example of a negative feedback system in which the interacting variables cannot be labeled clearly as variable, sensor, and so on. In this example, and in most negative feedback systems in physiology, all interacting variables are regulated. CNS = central nervous system; TPR = total peripheral resistance; CO = cardiac output.

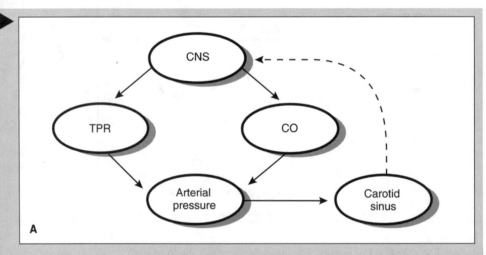

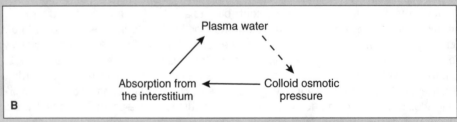

Figure 1-3 illustrates the point that in considering physiologic regulation it is best to depict feedback loops as interactions of regulated variables without attempting to label exactly what is being regulated. Furthermore, rarely, if ever, is the maintenance of a physiologic variable controlled by a *single* feedback system. Usually multiple feedback systems interact around a particular variable. This interaction is illustrated in Figure 1-4, an expansion of Figure 1-3B, which shows that plasma water is also determined by the amount of water retained by the kidneys under the influence of antidiuretic hormone (ADH). Most of the physiologic variables encountered in this text are governed by multiple regulatory systems.

Feed-forward. In addition to multiple feedback systems, a process known as *feed-forward regulation* may also be involved in orchestrating homeostasis. An example of feed-forward

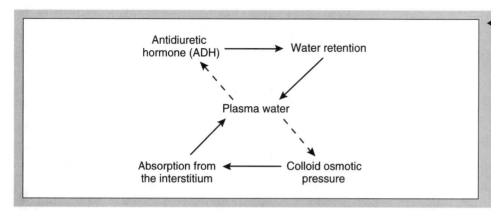

FIGURE 1-4
This is an extension of Figure 1-3B, illustrating the fact that physiologic variables (i.e., plasma water) are regulated by the interaction of several negative feedback systems.

is given in Figure 1-5, which illustrates what happens when a region of skin, such as that of a hand and arm, is exposed to cold (e.g., submersion of the arms in cold water). In this situation, cold receptors in the skin send sensory information to the CNS, resulting in an increase in heat conservation mechanisms (e.g., generalized cutaneous vasoconstriction), thereby buffering heat loss from the exposed skin. This process minimizes, or can even prevent, a change in body temperature; however, it is not a feedback system, since the cutaneous region being exposed to cold is not warmed by this process. Rather, information (i.e., cold skin) is fed forward into a feedback regulatory system (for body temperature), resulting in an increase in efficacy of the system. Another example of feed-forward is the increase in insulin secretion elicited during the digestion of a meal. In this case, the feedback system for regulating glucose is being primed *before* significant postprandial absorption of glucose can occur.

This system also works in reverse; that is, exposure of a region of skin to heat elicits a general cutaneous vasodilation and may initiate sweating.

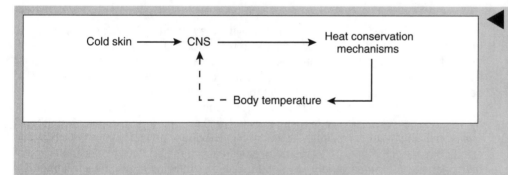

FIGURE 1-5
An Example of Feed-forward. In this case, cooling of the skin sends sensory information into the central nervous system (CNS), resulting in an increase in heat conservation mechanisms, which maintain body temperature. This system prevents or minimizes a fall in body temperature during cold exposure. However, if body temperature rises, the feed-forward effects are reduced, as indicated by the inverse relationship (dashed line) between body temperature and the CNS.

Regulation as a Hierarchial Tree. While this text uses negative feedback and feed-forward mechanisms to describe most regulatory interactions, in some cases, it is beneficial to describe a regulatory system in terms of a hierarchial tree of interacting variables with the variable of interest being placed at the top of the tree. Figure 1-6 is an example of a hierarchial tree that depicts the regulation of blood pressure. (At this point in the text, the reader does not need to be familiar with the different variables to understand the process, which is explained in later chapters.) At the apex of the tree is mean arterial blood pressure (MAP), the variable of primary interest. The first level of regulation illustrates that MAP is directly dependent upon each of two variables, CO and TPR. The second level of regulation shows that CO is dependent upon heart rate (HR) and stroke volume (SV), and that TPR is governed by the degree of blood vessel constriction and the viscosity of flowing blood.

TPR is the collective effect of all forces that oppose the movement of blood from the aorta to the right atrium.

Beyond the third level of regulation, the number of variables at each level becomes extensive. Therefore, at this level, and beyond, it is simpler to pick a particular path of interest and follow it. Figure 1-6 shows the path related to HR. In this context, the third level of blood pressure regulation illustrates that HR is determined by a balance between the positive effects of sympathetic activity and the negative effects of parasympathetic activity. The fourth level shows that both the sympathetic and parasympathetic systems

After reading Chapter 9, "The Heart as a Pump," come back to Figure 1-6 and construct a similar path of events leading to SV.

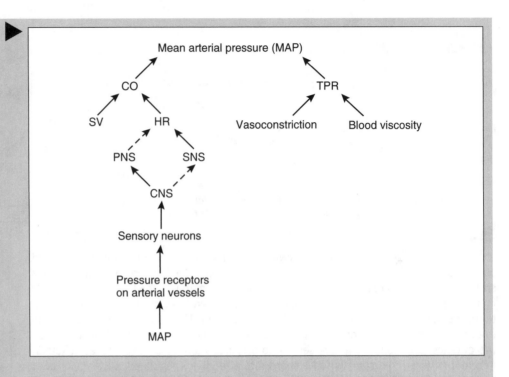

FIGURE 1-6

Example of a Hierarchial Tree Diagram of the Regulation of a Physiologic Variable. *The regulation of mean arterial pressure (MAP) is shown to occur at several levels. The first level simply indicates that blood pressure is determined by cardiac output (CO) and total peripheral vascular resistance (TPR). The second level shows the determinants of CO and TPR. Beyond this level, the number of variables can become extensive. To simplify, the pathway of heart rate (HR) is used. Here, HR is shown to be decreased by the parasympathetic branch of the autonomic nervous system (PNS) and increased by the sympathetic branch (SNS). Beyond this point, a single pathway is shown, leading from the central nervous system (CNS) to MAP. The solid and dashed line conventions show that an increase in MAP elicits an increase in PNS and a decrease in SNS activity. Collectively, these changes reduce HR. A reduction in HR decreases CO, which, in turn, lowers arterial pressure. Thus, the pathway from MAP to CO to HR and beyond to MAP again can be represented as a negative feedback loop. This approach to analyzing physiologic regulation illustrates that negative feedback loops are nested in arrays of broader interrelationships among physiologic variables.*

are controlled by the CNS. For the sake of brevity, the remaining levels are arranged in a linear path that actually ends in arterial blood pressure. Thus, it can be seen that one of the controlling factors of a variable (i.e., MAP) is the variable itself (i.e., arterial pressure is, in part, self-controlling). A negative feedback loop can be constructed using the pathway of MAP to CO to HR and beyond (or, rather, back) to MAP.

Figure 1-6 shows that an increase in MAP results in sensory information processed by the CNS, decreasing in sympathetic (*dashed line*) and increasing in parasympathetic (*solid line*) activity. This results in a reduction in HR due to an increase in the inhibitory effects of parasympathetic activity and to a decrease in the excitatory effects of sympathetic activity. Altering a variable by simultaneously changing excitatory and inhibitory regulators in opposite directions is quite common in physiology. The process is analogous to an accelerator and brake system in an automobile. A driver can slow down a car much faster by releasing the accelerator and pushing on the brake than by releasing the accelerator alone. Other examples of physiologic accelerator–brake systems include: vasodilation by simultaneous withdrawal of vasoconstrictor and increase of vasodilator influences; and increase in the rate of glucose clearance from the blood by simultaneous withdrawal of the hormone glucagon and increase of the hormone insulin.

On the surface, using the hierarchial tree approach to portray the interaction of physiologic variables in maintaining homeostasis may seem unnecessarily complex. However, the advantage of this approach is that it illustrates that negative feedback loops are nested in arrays of much broader interrelationships among physiologic variables, facilitating an understanding of how individual feedback loops fit within the context of more broad-based regulatory systems.

Hierarchial Regulation as an Example of Fractal Organization. The term *fractal* was coined to refer to the geometric patterns formed when objects are *fragmented* into smaller and smaller generations with each offspring generation representing the original parent form [4]. Figure 1-7 presents an example from *Fractal Physiology* (1994) by Bassingthwaighte et al., which shows the fractal patterns formed by successive dichotomous branching of a single line [5]. As their text points out, patterns such as this are remarkably similar to many branching patterns seen in nature (e.g., the successive

Fractal mathematics is a component of a more broad-based regulatory theory called chaos.

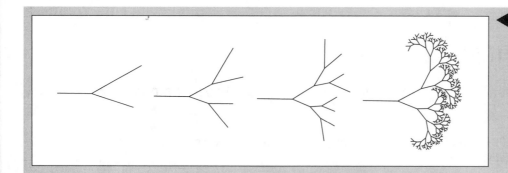

FIGURE 1-7
Example of a Fractal Pattern Formed by Dichotomous Branchings of a Single Line. *Many anatomic structures, such as the circulatory pattern in a tissue, are thought to be fractal in nature. (Source: Reprinted with permission from Bassingthwaighte JB, Liebovitch LS, West JB: Fractal Physiology. New York, NY: Oxford University Press, 1994, p. 364.)*

branchings of a natural tree and of the pulmonary *tree*, as shown in Chapter 5). These investigators, and others in the physical and natural sciences, have shown that the formation of many natural structures, such as the microcirculation of a tissue, can be explained by fractal geometry.

In addition to natural structures being fractal, it is presently thought that temporal variations in natural variables also follow fractal rules. In this regard, what appear to be random fluctuations of a variable over time—say, mean arterial pressure—may not be random but rather determined by the moment-to-moment interactions of the many variables that control arterial pressure. In this context, the hierarchial tree approach to physiologic regulation, as exemplified in Figure 1-6, can be considered as a structural representation of the fractal organization of factors that influence a particular physiologic variable. In this text, both feedback loops and hierarchial tree (i.e., fractal) organizations are used to describe how homeostasis is achieved.

RESOLUTION OF CLINICAL CASE

The patient in the case presented at the beginning of this chapter had primary hypertension (i.e., essential hypertension). Although the causes of essential hypertension are not entirely known, it is possible to propose a hypothesis based on disruption of blood pressure homeostasis. First, the patient's elevated TPR in the presence of normal CO indicates that the hypertension is due to widespread vasoconstriction in the circulatory system. A variety of factors, such as job-related stress, could have caused the initial insult to the system in the form of a rise in blood pressure due to sympathetic induced vasoconstriction or increase in CO. Normally, feedback regulatory systems, outlined in Figure 1-3A, counter these insults and maintain a normal blood pressure. However, if the elevation in blood pressure is frequent enough or persistent enough, then a mechanism known as *myogenic vasoconstriction* can take over and sustain the hypertension. Myogenic vasoconstriction is a local regulatory mechanism in which the small arterioles vasoconstrict in response to an increase in blood pressure. As discussed in Chapters 11 and 12, this mechanism serves to maintain a near normal capillary pressure, thereby preventing edema. Under normal conditions, severe myogenic vasoconstriction occurs only in the lower extremities when a person stands up and intravascular pressure in the legs rises due to the force of gravity. However, under conditions of hypertension, a systemic increase in myogenic vasoconstriction can occur that contributes to an elevated TPR. Because TPR is a determinant of arterial blood pressure, this sets up a *positive feedback cycle* in which an increase in arterial pressure causes myogenic vasoconstriction, which causes an increase in TPR, which causes a further rise in arterial blood pressure.

As indicated previously, the exact cause of essential hypertension is not known. This chapter explores a hypothesis based on a context in which a normal physiologic mechanism, myogenic vasoconstriction, becomes pathologic and disrupts normal homeostasis.

Essential hypertension is defined as hypertension of unknown origin.

REVIEW QUESTIONS

Directions: For each of the following questions, choose the **one best** answer.

1. Which of the following situations involving the cardiopulmonary system is an example of a negative feedback system?

   (A) An increase in blood pressure elicits vasoconstriction, which contributes to an increase in blood pressure

   (B) Cholesterol contributes to atherosclerosis, which reduces blood flow; a reduction in blood flow promotes the uptake of cholesterol into blood vessels

   (C) An increase in colloid osmotic pressure in the blood elicits the absorption of fluid from the interstitium into the blood; an increase in absorption of fluid from the interstitium reduces colloid osmotic pressure in the blood

   (D) A decrease in blood flow to the intestines increases the level of cardiotoxins in the circulating blood, which reduces cardiac output (CO); a reduction in CO reduces arterial blood pressure, which reduces blood flow to the intestines

2. Consider the following statement. An increase in tissue metabolic activity increases the concentration of metabolites in the interstitium. An increase in metabolites in the interstitium elicits dilation of arterioles. Dilation of arterioles increases tissue blood flow. An increase in tissue blood flow removes metabolites from the interstitium. This statement describes

   (A) positive feedback of tissue metabolism

   (B) negative feedback of tissue blood flow

   (C) negative feedback of interstitial concentration of metabolites

   (D) positive feedback of arteriole diameter

3. In accordance with the information in Figure 1-6, an increase in mean arterial blood pressure could be elicited by a decrease in

   (A) blood viscosity

   (B) vasoconstriction

   (C) sympathetic nervous system (SNS) activity

   (D) parasympathetic nervous system (PNS) activity

   (E) stroke volume

4. Consider the following sequence of events. Anticipation of exercise elicits an increase in epinephrine secretion. Epinephrine elicits an increase in plasma glucose. Plasma glucose is used to provide energy for muscle contractions. This series of events depicts

   (A) feed-forward control of muscle metabolism

   (B) negative feedback control of epinephrine secretion

   (C) positive feedback of plasma glucose

ANSWERS AND EXPLANATIONS

1. **The answer is C.** An increase in colloid osmotic pressure in the blood elicits the absorption of fluid from the interstitium into the blood. An increase in absorption of fluid from the interstitium reduces colloid osmotic pressure in the blood. This is the only choice in which a change in a variable, colloid osmotic pressure, elicits mechanisms that oppose the change in a negative feedback manner. The other choices describe positive feedback situations.

2. **The answer is C.** The statement in the question describes negative feedback of the interstitial concentration of metabolites. This is a negative feedback situation that maintains homeostasis of the interstitial concentration of metabolites. Tissue blood flow is not maintained, but rather it is increased as a mechanism to maintain homeostasis of tissue metabolites.

3. **The answer is D.** Of the choices given, a decrease in PNS activity is the only one that elicits an increase in blood pressure. This is achieved by the withdrawal of an inhibitory effect, that of PNS, on heart rate (i.e., a letting up of the break).

4. **The answer is A.** The sequence of events described in the question depicts feedforward control of muscle metabolism. Glucose is a major substrate for muscle metabolism during exercise. By this mechanism, the anticipation of exercise feeds forward to increase plasma glucose in readiness for an increase in metabolism.

REFERENCES

1. Van Wynsberghe D, Cooley GM: *Case Histories in Human Physiology*. Dubuque, IA: Wm. C. Brown, 1990.
2. Bernard C: *Les Phénomènes de la Vie, Paris, 1878*. Cited in: Cannon WB: Organization for physiological homeostasis. *Physiol Rev* 9:339–341, 1929.
3. Richardson DR: *Basic Circulatory Physiology*. Boston, MA: Little, Brown, 1976.
4. Mandelbrot BB: *The Fractal Geometry of Nature*. San Francisco, CA: Freeman, 1983.
5. Bassingthwaighte JB, Liebovitch LS, West BJ: *Fractal Physiology*. New York, NY: Oxford University Press, 1994, p 364.

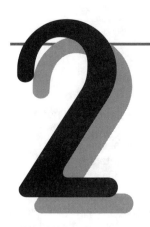

FOCUS CONCEPTS OF THE CARDIOPULMONARY SYSTEM

FOCUS CONCEPTS EXPANDED

Chapter 1 defined the focus concept of a discipline as the core around which the various components of the discipline are oriented. In this context, it was stated that homeostasis is *the* focus concept of physiology. This chapter describes what we consider to be the focus concepts of the cardiopulmonary system, a subdiscipline of physiology. An understanding of these concepts will help the reader to remain oriented while processing the factual information presented in subsequent chapters.

FOCUS CONCEPTS OF THE CARDIOPULMONARY SYSTEM

To a certain degree, focus concepts are subjective in nature and depend upon how the author of a text or the instructor of a lecture intends to approach the material. This text centers on two major focus concepts of the cardiopulmonary system: (1) *maintenance of the interstitial environment,* and (2) *maintenance of arterial blood pressure*; that is, the various actions of the cardiopulmonary system are focused toward one or both of these functions. In terms of a hierarchy, focus concept 2 is subservient to 1 in that the maintenance of arterial blood pressure is necessary to perfuse tissues with blood and, thereby, maintain homeostasis of the interstitial environment. However, many facets of arterial blood pressure regulation operate independently of tissue environment considerations. Therefore, it is treated as a separate focus concept.

Maintenance of the Interstitial Environment

Relation to Homeostasis. As discussed in Chapter 1, stability of the internal environment is the hallmark of homeostasis. The interstitial fluid that bathes all cells is foremost among the internal compartments that must remain stable for homeostasis to occur. In this context, homeostasis is centered around the maintenance of interstitial fluid volume, composition, and temperature. The cardiopulmonary system plays a major role in this maintenance.

Role of the Cardiopulmonary System. The role of the cardiopulmonary system in temperature regulation was touched on in Chapter 1. The interaction of factors associated with the composition and volume of the interstitial environment are presented as a concept map in Figure 2-1. Concept maps differ from feedback control diagrams in that they simply indicate linkages without necessarily specifying the nature (e.g., direct or inverse) of those linkages.[1]

As indicated in Figure 2-1, the interstitial environment serves as an intermediary between tissue metabolism and the composition and volume of blood. Nutrients from the blood pass through the interstitium on their way to the tissue cells, and products of tissue metabolism (e.g., carbon dioxide [CO_2]) pass through the interstitium into the blood. In the steady state (i.e., under homeostatic conditions), there is a balance between tissue metabolism and the composition and volume of blood. The cardiovascular system plays a key role in this balance by providing adequate blood flow and blood pressure so that the delivery of nutrients and the removal of by-products meet the ongoing metabolic needs of the tissues served by the blood. Details of this interaction are given in Chapters 11 and 12.

FIGURE 2-1

Linkages and Interactions of Factors Associated with the Composition and Volume of the Interstitial Environment.

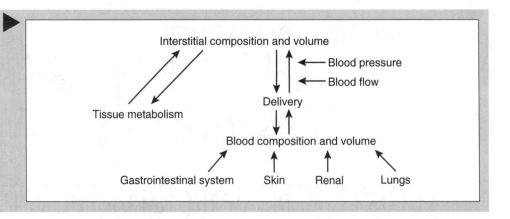

The gastrointestinal (GI) system, skin, kidneys, and lungs are collectively the major organ systems responsible for maintaining the composition and volume of blood. The digestive and absorptive processes of the GI system provide nutrients as well as water to the blood. The sweating mechanism of the skin is a major determinant of plasma and interstitial volume; to a large extent, evaporative loss of water through this mechanism is governed by the regulation of skin blood flow. This subject is discussed in Chapters 11 and 20. The renal system is to a very large degree responsible for both the volume and composition of plasma and, hence, interstitial fluid. (While many of the mechanisms of renal function are beyond the scope of this text, certain key features are described in Chapters 13 and 20.) In addition to their obvious role of maintaining proper levels of blood oxygen and carbon dioxide, the lungs metabolize certain hormones (e.g., catecholamines) and maintain acid–base balance. In terms of volume regulation, the lungs are a source of variable water loss because exhaled air is saturated with water vapor. These aspects of pulmonary function are discussed in detail within several chapters of this text.

[1] For further information on concept maps see Stewart J, Vankirk J, Rowell R: Concept maps: a tool for use in biology teaching. *Am Biol Teach* 41:171–175, 1979.

Maintenance of Systemic Arterial Blood Pressure

A stable systemic arterial blood pressure is necessary so that individual organs and tissues can be perfused with blood to meet their blood supply needs. Figure 2-2 provides a *forest* overview of linkages of key factors responsible for the maintenance of systemic arterial blood pressure.

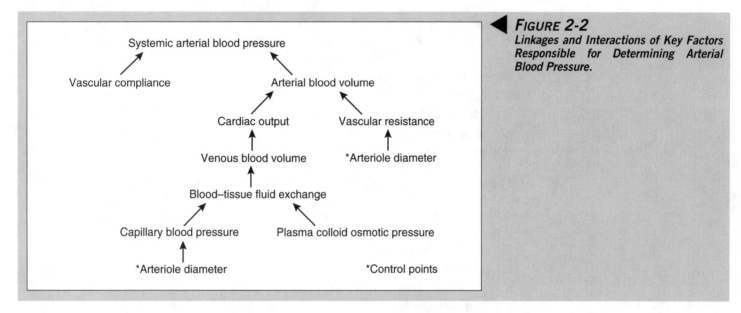

FIGURE 2-2
Linkages and Interactions of Key Factors Responsible for Determining Arterial Blood Pressure.

First, as described in Chapter 3, arterial pressure is determined by an interaction of the compliance of the arterial vessels and the arterial blood volume. Specifically, pressure is proportional to volume divided by compliance. Although arterial compliance definitely changes on a long-term basis (e.g., vessels tend to become stiff with age), arterial compliance remains within a relatively narrow range on a moment-to-moment, or even daily, basis.

In contrast to arterial compliance, arterial blood volume, and hence blood pressure, are subject to moment-to-moment variations within a homeostatic range. These variations are determined by the interactions of cardiac output (CO) and vascular resistance. An increase in CO *places* extra blood in the arterial system; an increase in vascular resistance *reduces the exit of blood* from the arterial system. The result of both of these interactions is that arterial blood volume and, therefore, blood pressure increase. Chapter 10 details how CO and vascular resistance interact to determine acute and steady-state changes in arterial blood pressure.

Chapter 9 describes the importance of venous blood volume in determining CO, and Chapter 12 outlines the mechanisms by which interstitial fluid serves as a reservoir to buffer changes in plasma volume. Fundamentally, these mechanisms involve an interaction of capillary blood pressure and the colloid osmotic pressure of the circulating plasma. As noted in Chapters 11 and 12, arteriole diameter is an important control point for both vascular resistance (hence, arterial blood pressure) and capillary hydrostatic pressure (hence, blood–tissue fluid exchange).

Figure 2-2 outlines interactions of some, not all, of the key elements in the determination of arterial blood pressure. As indicated in Chapter 1, the hierarchical tree approach to blood pressure regulation (see Figure 1-6) depicts numerous levels of regulatory variables, which collectively can be considered as a *fractal* organization. In this context, seemingly random variations in a variable are actually determined by specific moment-to-moment interactions of the many factors that determine that variable. The major homeostatic benefit of a multidimensional regulatory organization is that the variable being regulated tends to be quite stable. This text touches on only a few of the many factors that regulate arterial blood pressure.

REVIEW QUESTIONS

Directions: For each of the following questions, choose the **one best** answer.

1. Dehydration refers to the net loss of water from plasma and interstitial fluid. This being the case, to maintain homeostasis of plasma osmolality, urine osmolality must be

   (A) isotonic

   (B) hypotonic

   (C) hypertonic

   (D) iso-osmotic

   (E) hypo-osmotic

2. As indicated in Figure 2-2, a decrease in arteriole diameter (i.e., vasoconstriction) increases resistance, which increases systemic arterial blood pressure, while vasoconstriction of arterioles reduces capillary blood pressure. The net effect of these actions is to maintain homeostasis of

   (A) interstitial fluid volume

   (B) cardiac output

   (C) tissue blood flow

   (D) capillary blood flow

ANSWERS AND EXPLANATIONS

1. The answer is C. To maintain homeostasis of plasma osmolality, urine osmolality must be hypertonic because the net loss of water from plasma makes plasma hypertonic. To restore plasma to an isotonic state, the kidneys must retain water. To do this, they must excrete a hypertonic urine. The terms iso-osmotic and hypo-osmotic are the same as isotonic and hypotonic.

2. The answer is A. There is a tendency for arterial pressure to increase capillary blood pressure, which is countered by the tendency for vasoconstriction to reduce capillary blood pressure. Since capillary blood pressure is a main determinant of the amount of fluid filtered from the capillaries into the interstitial fluid, maintenance of capillary blood pressure maintains homeostasis of interstitial fluid volume.

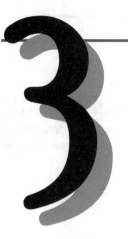

PHYSICAL PRINCIPLES UNDERLYING CARDIOPULMONARY FUNCTION

CHAPTER OUTLINE

INTRODUCTION OF CLINICAL CASE

A 65-year-old man was brought to the clinic by his daughter. She was worried about a sore on her father's foot that would not heal. On interview, the father stated, "My leg feels 'tight' when I walk a short distance." He acknowledged that he had had these symptoms for the past 2 years and that they had become progressively worse. Physical examination revealed a 1 × 1.5 cm ulcer on the dorsum of the left second toe with some edema (swelling) on the foot and ankle. His physician palpated the pulsations in some of his major vessels. On a scale of 0 to 4 (0 = no pulse; 4 = very strong pulse), the arterial pulses were as follows:

Left and right radial and brachial arteries = 3+   Right dorsalis pedis = 0+
Left and right femorals = 1+   Left dorsalis pedis = 0
Right popliteal = 0+   Right posterior tibialis = 0+
Left popliteal = 0   Left posterior tibialis = 0

FUNDAMENTAL PHYSICAL MEASUREMENTS

One of the themes of this text is that *fundamental principles of physics underlie many aspects of cardiopulmonary function*. It will be productive, therefore, to review some elementary principles of physics.

Measurements of Length, Mass, and Time. Physiology and medicine both require accurate measurements of physical phenomena. The sciences in general have adopted the meter (m), or centimeter (cm), kilogram (kg) or gram (g), and second (sec) as the fundamental units of length, mass, and time, respectively.

Higher-Order Measurements. Reliable determinations of area and volume are particularly important in cardiopulmonary physiology. *Area* is measured in square meters (m^2) or square centimeters (cm^2). *Volume* is commonly expressed in cubic meters (m^3) or cubic centimeters (cm^3, or simply "cc"). Another common volumetric unit is the liter (L), the volume occupied by one kg of water. One milliliter (mL; 1/1000 L) equals one cc. Therefore, syringes calibrated in cc's can be used to administer drugs whose *concentrations* (mass per volume) are given in milligrams (mg) per mL.

The measurement of time involves two more concepts. Moving a given length in a certain time yields a *velocity*, given in either m/sec or cm/sec. Neurologists, for example, measure how rapidly action potentials are conducted along nerves in m/sec. The dimensional units of area/time are not widely used in medicine, but volume/time is very important. The volume of blood ejected by the heart per minute is *cardiac output (CO)*. The CO of a 70-kg man is about 5 L/min. CO increases with body size, so this important variable is often *normalized* by dividing by the individual's body surface area. The resulting value, the *cardiac index (CI)*, is measured in units of $L/min/m^2$ (dimensionally equivalent to $L/min/m^2$). Cardiologists use the CI to compare the pumping capability of a patient's heart to that of a healthy person, irrespective of the person's body size. Likewise, the pulmonary physician normalizes the maximum amount of air a person can exhale in 1 second (the forced expiratory volume, or FEV_1) by dividing by body surface area. The results of this computation allow the physician to detect the presence of airway obstruction, regardless of the patient's body size.

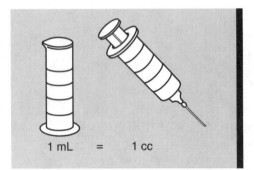

1 mL = 1 cc

FORCE, TENSION, AND STRESS

The words "force," "tension," and "stress" have very specific meanings in physiology and in medicine. Remembering Newton's classic statement that F = ma, the abbreviation a in this equation refers to acceleration: a progressive change in the velocity of the mass, m. Therefore, acceleration is the first time derivative of velocity (dv/dt) or the second time derivative of length (d^2l/dt^2). For example, the blood inside the heart is essentially at rest just before the beginning of the heartbeat. The ventricles must physically accelerate this blood to *eject* it from the heart into the pulmonary artery or aorta. Therefore, according to Newton's law, the heart muscle must develop force in order to produce CO. The unit of force, the Newton, is expressed in $kg \cdot m/sec^2$. The dyne, also a unit of force, is expressed in $g \cdot cm/sec^2$. In cardiopulmonary physiology, the words "force" and "tension" both refer to this phenomenon.

The physician can compare the force-generating capabilities in muscles of different size by dividing (normalizing) the contractile force by the cross-sectional area of the muscle. The result is the force/area, or *stress*. Stress measurements allow the physician to compare the force-generating capability of muscles of different size, just as the CI allows the physician to make CO comparisons between patients of different weight and body surface.

Stress = force/area.

ENERGY AND WORK

The *energy* that a system possesses allows it to perform *work*. Most physics texts include an illustration that shows how applied force can move a block horizontally along a surface. Another common figure shows how force applied to a piston compresses gas in a cylinder. The physicist would say that the energy expended and the work performed are equal to the force applied times the distance moved or the "pressure" applied times the change in volume. Energy can manifest in two forms: kinetic and potential.

Kinetic Energy. An object, or mass, possesses *kinetic energy* as a result of its physical movement; in equation form, $E = \frac{1}{2}mv^2$. This chapter considers kinetic energy from two perspectives. First, an amount of energy, E, must be expended to accelerate a mass to a given velocity, v. For example, the heart uses energy to impart a velocity to the blood and, thereby, to eject it from the ventricle. Second, if a moving mass were to hit another object, it could do work on that object; in the process, it would give up its motion. Therefore, a moving hammer hitting a nail into a block of wood trades its energy of motion to drive the nail forward. In short, kinetic energy is the ability of a moving mass to do work.

Potential Energy. A substance possesses *potential energy* when the ability to do work is stored within it. Later, this energy may be released, and under proper conditions, work is performed. Energy is expended and then stored, for example, when a mass is lifted and held above the surface of the earth. If this mass is allowed to fall back to earth, its potential energy may be converted into work. The energy stored in a column of fluid, or *hydrostatic pressure*, equals its density (g/mL, given as the Greek letter "rho," or ρ) times the acceleration of gravity (g, 980 cm/sec/sec) times the height, h, above the surface. This ρgh energy is important to the discussion of pressure, which follows.

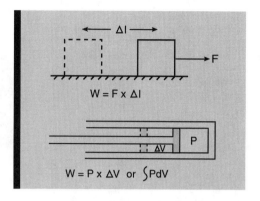

$$W = F \times \Delta l$$

$$W = P \times \Delta V \text{ or } \int PdV$$

PRESSURE

Pressure is among the most important forms of potential energy in the study of the cardiopulmonary system. *Pressure gradients*, or differences in pressure from one location to another, account for the movement of blood from the heart to the smallest vessels of the microcirculation and back to the heart again. Likewise, gases move into and out of the lungs because of pressure gradients. In addition, gases enter and leave the blood to and from tissues as a result of differences in their "partial pressures."

Formal Definition of Pressure. Pressure is defined as the force per unit area exerted by air or other fluid against the walls of its container. For example, car tires typically hold 28 to 30 pounds per square inch (psi) of air. The physicist usually measures pressure in dynes/cm² instead of psi. Consider the results of the following simple dimensional analysis.

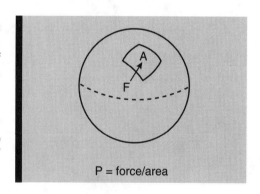

P = force/area

$$\text{Pressure} = \text{dyne/cm}^2 \times \text{cm/cm} = \text{dyne-cm/cm}^3$$

The formal units of pressure are multiplied by unity (i.e., by 1:cm/cm) to show that *pressure actually measures the energy (dyne-cm) inherent within a volume (cm³) of fluid.* Thus, pressure is a measure of potential energy.

Physiologic Definition of Pressure. In physiology and medicine, pressures are usually given in millimeters of mercury (mm Hg) or perhaps centimeters of water (cm H_2O). What does this mean, and what can it teach us about the nature of pressure? To help answer these questions, imagine a water tower 10 m (1000 cm) tall, which has been filled by a man carrying water from a pump up a ladder to the top of the tower and dumping it (*top,* Figure 3-1A). The man has performed work, and the energy that he expended has been stored as water pressure. The water would rise 1000 cm in an upright tube connected to the base of the tower. This water gauge would indicate not only the volume of water available for use but also, as a very practical definition, that the water pressure at the base of the tower was 1000 cm H_2O.

FIGURE 3-1 ▶

Dissipation of Pressure Energy in a Simple Water System. (A) Energy expended by the man carrying water from a pump to a water tower appears as potential energy of pressure. If the water is 10 m deep in the tower, the pressure at the bottom of the tower is equal to 10 m water. Water in the gauge on the side of the tower rises 10 m and is a direct measurement of water pressure. (B) Water pressure from the tower dissipates along the local water system. Consequently, the height of the water shooting out of the garden hose, which gives an approximate measure of the local pressure, decreases for hoses farther from the tower. Pressure energy is further dissipated by an obstruction. Water pressure for the last homeowner, with this simple water distribution system, is almost zero.

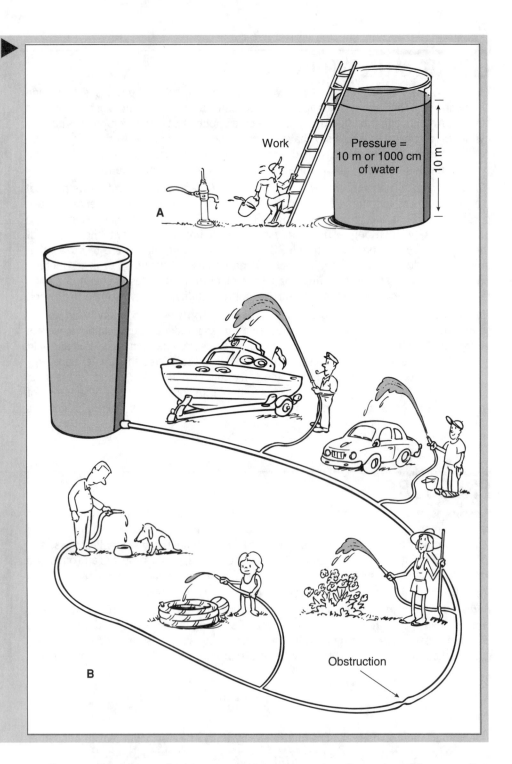

Because it is inconvenient to measure long column lengths such as 10 m, we often ask how high the pressure would lift a column of mercury. Since mercury is ≈13.6 times more dense than water, if the gauge were filled with mercury, the level would rise to only 1000/13.6, or ≈74 cm (or 740 mm). This is the basis for measuring pressures in *millimeters of mercury* (mm Hg). Thus, using the ρgh definition of pressure, mm Hg can be converted to dynes/cm²:

$$1 \text{ mm Hg} = 13.6 \text{ g/cm}^3 \times 980 \text{ cm/sec}^2 \times 0.1 \text{ cm} = 1333 \text{ dynes/cm}^2$$

To extend the water tower analogy, imagine that the tower supplies water to several houses at progressively greater distances along a pipeline (Figure 3-1B). Homeowners near the tower would find that when using their garden hoses, the water would rise almost 10 m into the air. However, individuals living at progressively greater distances along the pipeline would find that the water from their hoses would rise less and less as they live farther and farther from the source. There is also obstruction at one point in the system (see Figure 3-1B). Beyond this point, the water in the hoses is under much less pressure. Gardeners living near the end of this simple system would find the pressure within their water hoses to be very low indeed. Clearly, the pressure energy is consumed in transporting water away from the source and especially in overcoming the hydraulic resistance of the obstruction. In physiologic terms, by the time the blood in the *circulation* returns to the right atrium, most of its pressure has been *dissipated*, much as would happen were the last homeowner simply to allow the water from his hose to dribble into his dog's bowl.

Transmural Pressure. The volume of a tire or balloon clearly depends upon the pressure of the gas inside and vice versa. If a helium-filled balloon were released, however, its volume would increase as it rose in the atmosphere, even though the total number of gas molecules inside is unchanged. Conversely, were the balloon somehow forced below the surface of a lake, its volume would decrease. This phenomenon is best understood in terms of *transmural pressure*: the pressure difference between the inside and outside (i.e., "across the wall") of the balloon. Like the water in the tower example, the atmosphere exerts a pressure at the earth's surface. On a typical day, atmospheric pressure will lift a column of mercury 760 mm (or ≈30 in), almost as high as in the water tower example. Like the helium balloon, the volume of a pilot's chest would increase measurably were he or she to fly at high altitude in an unpressurized aircraft. Typically, atmospheric pressure is assigned a value of zero, and only the pressure inside a vessel is considered. This simplistic approach is often inadequate to the study of cardiopulmonary physiology, however. Chapter 5, for example, shows how changes in the transmural pressure of the thoracic vessels and heart as a result of respiration help move blood from the periphery back to the heart.

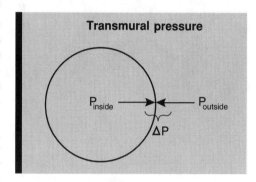

Partial Pressures of Gases. According to Dalton's law of *partial pressures*, each gas in a mixture of gases exerts pressure proportional to its presence in that mixture. The atmosphere is composed of approximately 79% nitrogen and 21% oxygen. Therefore, the pressure exerted by O_2 in inspired air is about 0.21×760 mm Hg = 160 mm Hg. Nitrogen exerts ≈600 mm Hg. Inspired air is quite dry when the humidity is low. This air rapidly becomes saturated with gaseous water as it traverses the upper airways. At body temperature (37°C–38°C), water vapor in humidified air exerts a pressure of 47 mm Hg. This vapor pressure must be included in computations of the partial pressures of the gases in the mixture. These considerations are important because differences in the partial pressure of a gas from one place to another determine the movement of the gas (e.g., between the air sacs in the lungs and blood in the *pulmonary capillaries*).

RESISTANCE

It is not possible to insert a catheter or probe into the body and measure resistance directly. Instead, resistance must be computed by dividing the pressure gradient by the flow produced by that gradient. For example, *total peripheral resistance (TPR)* is a measurement of the resistance to blood flow offered by the entire systemic circulation; likewise for *pulmonary vascular resistance (PVR)*. The formula for computing TPR is

$$TPR = \frac{P_{Ao} - P_{RA}}{CO},$$

where P_{Ao} is the mean (average) arterial blood pressure, P_{RA} is the pressure inside the right atrium, and CO is cardiac output. This is the hydraulic equivalent of the well-known Ohm's law in electricity ($I = E/R$). TPR is often computed by simply dividing mean aortic pressure by CO, since right atrial pressure is almost 0 mm Hg.

Resistors in Series. The resistance to the flow of fluids, or *hydraulic resistance*, is similar in many ways to electrical resistance. In both cases, resistances connected in series— one after another—are cumulative; the total resistance (R_T) equals the sum of the first resistance (R_1) and the second (R_2) through the nth (or last) resistor:

$$R_T = R_1 + R_2 + \cdots + R_n.$$

In portal systems, hydraulic resistances are connected in series. If three resistors of equal value were connected in series, the total resistance would be three times as great as the resistance of each individual resistor.

Resistors in Parallel. Most vascular beds are connected in parallel in the systemic circulation, and computation of their total hydraulic resistance differs from that for resistors in series. The total resistance for a parallel circuit is computed as:

$$\frac{1}{R_T} = \frac{1}{R_1} + \frac{1}{R_2} + \cdots + \frac{1}{R_n}$$

Sometimes it is easier to understand this relationship when it is rewritten as:

$$R_T = \frac{1}{\frac{1}{R_1} + \frac{1}{R_2} + \cdots + \frac{1}{R_n}}$$

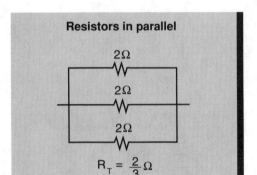

Resistors in parallel

2Ω

2Ω

2Ω

$R_T = \frac{2}{3}\Omega$

If three resistors of equal value were connected in parallel, the total resistance would be less than the value of any individual resistor. In fact, the total resistance is always less than the resistance of any individual component. In Chapters 10 and 11, these properties of resistors connected in parallel are shown to be especially important in two ways. First, arterial blood pressure can be controlled by appropriate changes in the resistances of many individual vascular beds. Second, it is possible to control the flow of blood through a given vascular bed by controlling the resistance of that vascular bed.

Poiseuille's Law. The factors that determine hydraulic resistance were first described by the French physician Jean Poiseuille. The general principles determined by Poiseuille hold for the conditions of flow found in most healthy vessels. *Poiseuille's law* is usually given in a form that relates the flow through a vessel ($\dot{Q}$) as a function of the pressure at its "input" side (P_1), its "output" side (P_2), its radius (r) and length (l), plus the viscosity of the blood (η) flowing through the vessel:

$$\dot{Q} = (P_1 - P_2)\frac{\pi r^4}{8\eta l}$$

The term, $P_1 - P_2$, is simply the pressure gradient driving flow through the vessel. The most significant feature of this relationship is that the radius is raised to the fourth power; therefore, very small changes in a vessel's radius result in very large changes in flow through that vessel.

Many people conclude *erroneously* that resistance to fluid flow is due to friction with the vessel wall. This is not what the radius (r) term in Poiseuille's law means. In fact, the resistance to flow is due to dissipation of energy within the fluid itself. Suffice it to say, Poiseuille's law explains why very small changes in the radius of arterioles or bronchioles due to contraction or relaxation of smooth muscle in their walls yield large changes in resistance to the flow of blood or air, respectively.

COMPLIANCE

Unstressed Vascular Volume. Imagine for a moment that you have a child's balloon in your hand. The balloon initially has little or no air inside it. If you were to puff gently on the stem, you could pop open the balloon with very little effort. It would probably look like a miniature version of itself when inflated. Likewise, a certain volume of blood is required to fill the circulation. Like the balloon, with this small volume of blood, there would be very little pressure inside the vessels. The volume of blood required to fill the heart and vessels in this way is called the *unstressed vascular volume.* Under normal physiologic conditions, the volume of blood in the veins approximates this unstressed situation while the arteries are filled (stressed) above this volume.

Pressure–Volume Relationship. Imagine now that you begin to blow up the balloon and stop at intervals to record both the pressure and volume of the gas inside. (For the moment, assume the pressure is zero outside the balloon.) You could then use this series of observations to plot a *pressure–volume relationship* such as that shown in Figure 3-2A. Initially the volume of the balloon increases quickly, even though you did not blow into the balloon with much pressure. This is because the *compliance* of the balloon is initially relatively high. In fact, this experiment allows you to measure the compliance by dividing the change in volume (Δ volume, or ΔV) by the corresponding change in pressure (Δ pressure, or ΔP). Figure 3-2B shows slopes at two positions along the pressure–volume relationship. *The ΔV is identical in both cases.* However, *the increase in pressure for the first observation, ΔP_1, is much smaller than for the second, ΔP_2.* The slopes shown in the figure are $\Delta P_1/\Delta V$ and $\Delta P_2/\Delta V$; therefore, the compliances, C_1 and C_2, are equal to the "inverse slope," or $\Delta V/\Delta P_1$ and $\Delta V/\Delta P_2$, respectively. The inverse slope is easily computed by dividing 1 by the actual slope (1/slope = inverse slope). *In this example, the compliance is large initially and decreases as the balloon is filled.*

Physiologic Examples. The pressure–volume relationship and the compliance of the ventricles during diastole determine how much blood fills the heart in preparation for the next beat; this volume of blood is called the *preload*. Cardiologists are very concerned about the preload in their patients' hearts. Likewise, the compliance of the lung and chest wall determines how much air is drawn into the alveoli with each breath. However, one often needs to know the transmural pressure rather than only the pressure inside the heart or inside the air sacs.

FIRST AND SECOND LAWS OF THERMODYNAMICS

Definitions. The principles inherent within the first and second laws of thermodynamics apply to virtually every function carried out by all living creatures. The first law can be recognized from the previous discussion: *energy may be changed from one form to another, but it can be neither created nor destroyed.* The second law asserts *that a system will inevitably fall into disarray with time if no work is performed upon it; that is, its entropy will increase.* Physicists usually discuss the second law using a variable called "entropy," which is abbreviated by the letter "S." Entropy measures how "disorganized" a specific collection of interacting objects is. The entropy of a *system* increases as the relationship between its component elements becomes more random, or less organized. For our purposes, the second law means that any natural system, including a biologic system, must expend energy to maintain orderly, coherent function (i.e., homeostasis).

Order of a System. The concept of "order" occurs throughout physiology and medicine. For example, assume there is initially a high concentration of molecules of a given substance at one location within a beaker of water and that none of these molecules is to be found outside this region. This would be the case for molecules of sucrose immediately after suspending a sugar cube in a beaker of water. This steep concentration difference in sucrose molecules from one location in the beaker to another is an example of a highly ordered system. The probability of finding such a nonuniform distribution of sucrose molecules in a passive (nonenergy expending) system is extremely low. Within seconds, the sugar cube's order starts to break down as individual sucrose molecules in the cube dissolve in the water and move into the surrounding liquid because of their molecular motion. This *Brownian motion* is due to the thermal energy of the molecules. The process is called *diffusion*. Within a short time, the concentration of sugar becomes uniform throughout the beaker. Figure 3-3 shows the concentration of sugar in a cross section of the beaker immediately after inserting the cube (t_0) and at two later times. The graph labeled t_∞ shows no differences in the concentration of sugar molecules at any point in the cross section after sufficient time has elapsed. The diffusion process is spontaneous and represents the second law in action. Diffusion explains, for example, the net movement (or *flux*) of oxygen from the air sacs (or *alveoli*), where it is relatively concentrated, into the pulmonary blood, where it is relatively depleted.

FIGURE 3-2 ▶

Derivation of the Pressure–Volume Relationship and Compliance. (A) Filling a balloon in successive stages provides data for a pressure–volume relationship. Each data point represents a single set of measurements during the course of inflating the balloon. Cardiovascular physiologists tend to plot pressure on the ordinate; pulmonary physiologists tend to plot lung volume on the ordinate. (B) Data from part A may be used to construct a pressure–volume curve. The inverse slope of this curve yields compliance. The balloon's compliance at low volumes is relatively high with respect to higher volumes. P = pressure; V = volume; ΔV = change in volume; ΔP = change in pressure; C = compliance.

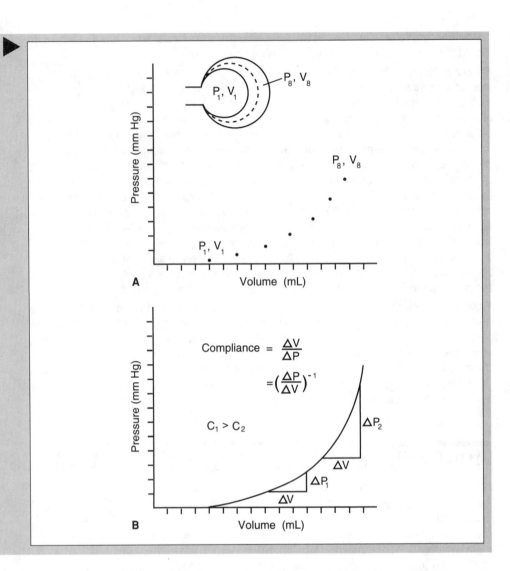

FIGURE 3-3 ▶

Demonstration of the Action of the Second Law of Thermodynamics. The second law of thermodynamics mandates that a highly ordered system, represented by a sugar cube, becomes progressively more disordered. Graphs show the concentration of sugar for a cross section of the beaker and sugar cube immediately after immersing the cube ($t = 0$), at two intermediate times (t_1 and t_2), and after many minutes have elapsed (t_∞). Uniform distribution of sugar across the beaker at t_∞ represents a disordered state. This process is called diffusion.

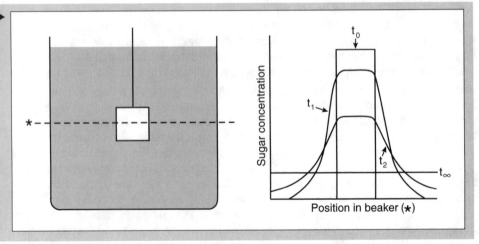

FLOW IN A CLOSED (CIRCULATORY) SYSTEM

The principles learned in the last section can now be applied to understanding the *circulation*. The simple model in Figure 3-4 will help. It includes a pump, which can be thought of as a simple heart with an input side at the atrium and an output at the aorta. When the pump is activated, "blood" flows from the heart, through some relatively stiff (i.e., low-compliance) elastic tubes to a hydraulic resistance, and then back to the heart through some fairly compliant tubes.

The input and output pressures are measured with glass tubes at the atrium and aorta, respectively. If the pump were initially turned off, the pressures inside the arteries and veins would be very low, and they would be equal. With the pump off, no energy is expended on the circulatory system. This uniform (low-order) pressure distribution is a static state, which the second law of thermodynamics demands when no energy is being expended. The value of the pressure, however low, is not zero. The actual value is determined in large part by the unstressed volume of the tubes and the heart and by their overall compliance; this topic is discussed in Chapter 10 where the concept of mean circulatory pressure is discussed.

The graphs of atrial and aortic pressure show that when the pump is turned on, the pressure in the aorta *increases* remarkably while the pressure inside the veins *decreases* somewhat. Once the pump has been working for a few moments, CO will equal the difference between the pressure in the aorta and the atrium divided by the value of the resistance. Several important applications of the physical principles follow. First, the pump must perform work to produce the increase in arterial pressure. Second, *fluid flows "down" the pressure gradient from aorta to atrium*. Finally, the pressure energy is dissipated as the blood moves around the circulation (especially when it moves through the hydraulic resistance), so that very little energy is left when it finally returns to the heart. The analogy to the community water system is now clear.

Although it is obvious that turning on the pump increases arterial pressure, perhaps it is not so obvious why atrial pressure decreases or why the size of these two pressure changes differs. The first problem can be solved by referring to the graph in Figure 3-4, which shows the changes in the volume of blood contained within the arterial and venous sides of the circulation. Obviously, the pump must obtain the blood it pumps into the aorta from the veins. Therefore, *the heart decreases the volume of blood on the venous side and transfers an equal volume into the arterial side of the circulation*. The pressure–volume relationship in Figure 3-3 shows that reducing the volume of blood inside the venous side of the circulation must *decrease* venous pressure. Finally, since the compliance of the venous system (C_v, represented by the thin-walled tube) exceeds the compliance of the arterial side (C_a, represented by the thick-walled tube), the pressure decrease in the veins is smaller than the pressure rise in the arteries. This is true even though the change in volume is identical in the arterial versus venous portions of the circulation.

FIGURE 3-4 ▶
Simple Hydraulic Pump and "Circulatory System" with Low-Compliance Arteries (Thick-Walled Tubes) and High-Compliance Veins (Thin-Walled Tubes). Fluid flows through the restriction representing peripheral resistance. Activating the pump results in increased pressure in the artery and decreased pressure in the vein because the pump is transferring blood from the venous to the arterial "side" of the circulation. (Source: Reprinted with permission from Richardson DR: Basic Circulatory Physiology. Boston, MA: Little, Brown, 1976, p 80.)

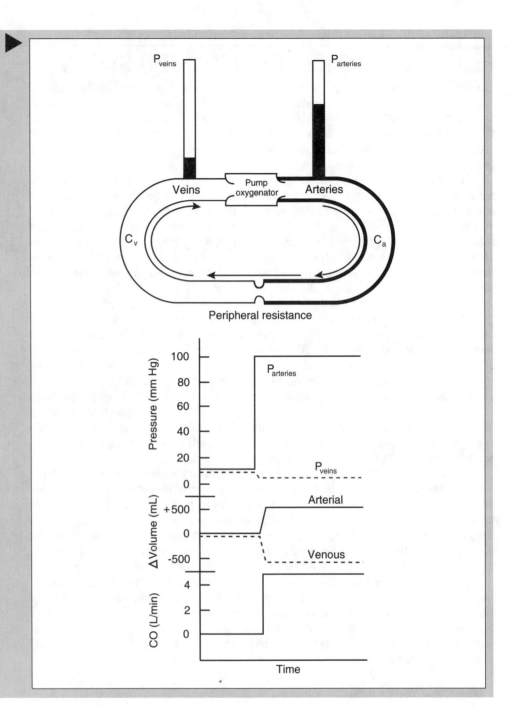

SUMMARY

Understanding the fundamental implications of the first and second laws of thermodynamics should clarify important concepts in Chapters 1 and 2. Homeostasis, the maintenance of an ordered state, can be attained only through the expenditure of energy to offset the tendency of all systems to become disordered. We can use fundamental physical concepts to understand how force generated by muscle contraction produces pressure gradients to cause air or blood to move, carrying the oxygen necessary to produce the high-energy compounds that are the "energy currency" of the body.

RESOLUTION OF CLINICAL CASE

The patient in this case has *peripheral vascular disease*. The lumens (inside diameters) of his arteries, especially in his left leg, have narrowed, probably as a result of tobacco smoking or eating a fat-rich diet. The pulse taken at the various arteries indicates the fluctuation of pressure inside the vessel: pressure is high during systole as the heart ejects blood into the aorta, and then drops during diastole as blood drains into the venous system. The strength of the pulse decreases in progressively more distal vessels. This is because the narrowing lumen creates a high resistance to flow, which dissipates a large proportion of the pressure energy inside the artery. (This is analogous to the drop in pressure that results from the obstruction in the homeowners' water system.) As a result, the circulation to the toe, far from the heart, is so poor that tissue oxygen demands cannot be met. Tissue necrosis (death) resulted because of the prolonged hypoxia. If the venous outflow from the vascular bed is also constricted, a balance of pressures can be created to increase the filtration of water from the capillaries into the interstitium. This may create *edema*, water collected within the tissue space. A vascular surgeon might attempt to revascularize the compromised areas by bridging a graft around localized, severe obstructions.

REVIEW QUESTIONS

Directions: For each of the following questions, choose the **one best** answer.

1. A pressure of 1 cm H_2O is equivalent to
    (A) 10 mm H_2O
    (B) 10 mm Hg
    (C) 10 dynes/cm^2
    (D) 9.8 m/sec^2
    (E) 10 Newton/cm^2

2. When are pressures measured in cm H_2O rather than mm Hg?
    (A) When the blood flow velocity at the measurement point is very rapid
    (B) When the pressure to be measured is above the level of the heart
    (C) When the person is exercising
    (D) When the pressure is relatively low, such as in the veins rather than the arteries
    (E) When mercury toxicity is a concern

3. During inspiration, the pressure inside the chest decreases. This tends to cause
    (A) a decrease in the transmural pressure for the atria and ventricles
    (B) an increase in the volume of blood inside the chambers of the heart
    (C) a decrease in the rate of flow of blood into the heart
    (D) a flow of air out of the lungs
    (E) a decrease in the rate of return of blood to the heart

4. The pressure gradient moving blood through the pulmonary circulation is
    (A) left atrial pressure minus aortic pressure
    (B) right atrial pressure minus pulmonary arterial pressure
    (C) aortic pressure minus right atrial pressure
    (D) pulmonary arterial pressure minus left atrial pressure
    (E) aortic pressure minus left atrial pressure

ANSWERS AND EXPLANATIONS

1. The answer is A. Because 1 cm equals 10 mm, 1 cm in height of water is the same as 10 mm height. Also, 1 cm H_2O equals 0.74 mm Hg or 987 dynes/cm^2.

2. The answer is D. Low values of pressure, such as venous pressure or airway pressure, are often measured in cm H_2O. This allows the physician to read and describe the pressure more accurately.

3. The answer is B. A decrease in intrathoracic pressure increases the transmural pressure across the atria and ventricles. This tends to increase the volume of blood inside the heart and the rate at which blood returns to the heart from the periphery (see Chapter 9).

4. The answer is D. Just as in the systemic circulation, blood moves through the pulmonary circulation because of a pressure gradient.

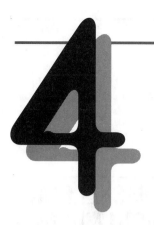

PHYSIOLOGY OF MUSCLES INVOLVED IN THE CARDIOPULMONARY SYSTEM

CHAPTER OUTLINE

INTRODUCTION OF CLINICAL CASE

A 12-year-old boy was brought to the emergency room by his parents one spring afternoon. He was in obvious respiratory distress. His parents explained that he had been mowing the lawn when he suddenly complained of difficulty breathing (*dyspnea*). The child's breathing was obviously labored with wheezing and unsuccessful attempts to inspire deeply. The muscles of his chest wall were contracting in a rigorous, grossly exaggerated manner. His skin had an unnatural paleness (*pallor*) with a cold sweat. His heart rate was 120 beats per minute (normal $\approx$ 90 bpm). The partial pressure of oxygen in his arterial blood (Pao_2) was 80 mm Hg (normal $\approx$ 100 mm Hg). Arterial carbon dioxide partial pressure ($Paco_2$) was 58 mm Hg (normal $\approx$ 40 mm Hg).

MUSCLE PHYSIOLOGY AND CARDIOPULMONARY FUNCTION

The ability of the cardiopulmonary system to move air and blood depends upon muscle contraction and relaxation that is of appropriate strength and timing. The theme of this chapter is that *a solid foundation in the fundamental nature of the development of force and shortening is essential to understand the normal function of the heart, blood vessels, and respiratory system.* An important corollary is that the adaptive powers of the cardiopulmonary system may allow adequate supply of oxygen and nutrients to the peripheral tissues despite advanced states of cardiopulmonary diseases such as congestive heart failure, atherosclerosis, and emphy-

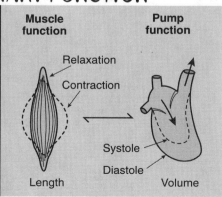

sema, at least when the patient is at rest. In such cases, the physician must consider the basic properties of muscle function when diagnosing and treating the disease.

COMPARATIVE PHYSIOLOGY OF SKELETAL, CARDIAC, AND SMOOTH MUSCLE

The cardiopulmonary system uses all three types of muscle: skeletal, cardiac, and smooth. These three classes of muscle share many features, since they are all excitable tissues containing cellular elements designed to generate force. This force produces pressure gradients within the cardiopulmonary system that result in flow of air or blood. The pulmonary pump depends upon several distinct types of striated muscle, while the cardiac pump uses exclusively cardiac muscle. The distribution systems of both the airways and blood vessels contain smooth muscle, which is important for regulating the bronchial and vessel diameters and, therefore, resistance to the flow of air and blood.

A comprehensive treatment of the basic physiology of excitable tissues and muscle is beyond the scope of this text. Fortunately, the details can be gleaned from other sources [1–3]. It is necessary to examine only select features of muscle structure and physiology that directly influence the function of the cardiopulmonary system. Table 4-1 summarizes the similarities and differences among the three types of muscle.

TABLE 4-1 ▶

Similarities and Differences among Skeletal, Cardiac, and Smooth Muscles

	Skeletal	Cardiac	Smooth
Similarities			
Contain actin and myosin			
Depend on Ca^{2+} release for contraction			
Are influenced by neural input			
Differences			
Location in cardiopulmonary system	Diaphragm Accessory muscles Upper airway muscles Intercostal muscles Abdominal muscles	Heart	Trachea Bronchioles Arteries Veins
Innervation	Somatic nervous system	Autonomic	Autonomic
Nerve terminals	Neuromuscular junction	Varicosities	Varicosities
Neurotransmitters			
Excitatory	Acetylcholine	Norepinephrine	Norepinephrine
Inhibitory	None	Acetylcholine	Acetylcholine
Major source of Ca^{2+}	Sarcoplasmic reticulum	Sarcoplasmic reticulum	Extracellular
Sarcoplasmic reticulum	Triad	Diad	Poorly developed
Inherent automaticity	None	Yes	Yes/maybe
Actin–myosin relationship	Sarcomere	Sarcomere	Diffuse
Length–tension curve	Limited range	Limited range	Wide range
Velocity of contraction	Fastest	Fast	Slow

ELECTROPHYSIOLOGIC PROPERTIES OF MUSCLE

Membrane Potentials

The similarities among skeletal, cardiac, and smooth muscles begin with the fact that the cells of all three muscle types maintain a negative intracellular potential. This potential ranges from about −85 millivolts (mV) in some cardiac fibers to around −50 mV in some smooth muscle. Like neurons, these potentials are maintained largely by the selective permeability of the cell membrane for different ion species and the electrochemical gradients that are thereby established; the *equilibrium potentials* for the relevant ions are described by the Nernst equation. Action potentials also show considerable variability between and among the various muscles, depending upon their specific permeabilities and activities. The important variations in action potential configuration within the heart are examined in detail in Chapter 8.

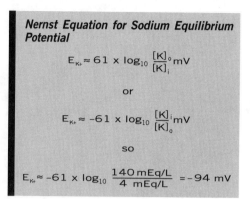

Nernst Equation for Sodium Equilibrium Potential

$$E_{K+} \approx 61 \times \log_{10} \frac{[K]_o}{[K]_i} \, mV$$

or

$$E_{K+} \approx -61 \times \log_{10} \frac{[K]_i}{[K]_o} \, mV$$

so

$$E_{K+} \approx -61 \times \log_{10} \frac{140 \, mEq/L}{4 \, mEq/L} = -94 \, mV$$

Initiation of Contraction in Skeletal Muscle

The mechanisms that initiate contraction differ in important ways among the three classes of muscle. Onset of force generation in skeletal muscle is directly triggered by depolarization of the α-motor neuron in the ventral horn of the spinal cord. The neuronal action potential is propagated to the end plate region of the motor axon and, via a chemical synapse, leads to an *end plate potential* (EPP) in the postsynaptic membrane of the skeletal muscle. The EPP triggers a muscle action potential, which, in turn, elicits a process known as *excitation–contraction coupling*; this culminates in muscle contraction. An α-motor neuron typically innervates more than a single skeletal muscle cell. The α-motor neuron and the muscle cells it innervates are collectively called a *motor unit*. Three major attributes of motor unit function are:

1. A single presynaptic action potential elicits an EPP of sufficient magnitude to depolarize the skeletal muscle to threshold. This means that no "decision" is made at this synapse; that is, *once the α-motor neuron has been brought to threshold, the muscle fibers of the motor unit will always contract.*

2. *The EPP is always excitatory.* There is no equivalent to an inhibitory postsynaptic potential (IPSP) in the end plate region. Inhibition of motor unit contraction always occurs within the central nervous system (CNS)—ultimately at the α-motor neuron itself.

3. *Recruiting additional motor units or increasing their frequency of contraction by processes within the CNS increases the force generated by the overall skeletal muscle.* In effect, the brain increases or decreases the work performed by skeletal muscle by controlling the number and frequency of action potentials of motor units active at any given moment.

Syncytial Nature of Cardiac Muscle

Cardiac muscle cells are electrically coupled to one another by *gap junctions*, which allow movement of small ions between cells. As a result, *once a single myocyte reaches threshold, a wave of depolarization sweeps over the entire "sheet" of cardiac muscle.* (Chapter 8 explains that pacemaker cells within the sinoatrial [SA] node trigger each heartbeat by spontaneously depolarizing to threshold.) From an electrophysiologic perspective, therefore, the atria and ventricles function as though they were a single organic entity. This property is denoted by characterizing the myocardium as a *functional syncytium*. This syncytial property of the myocardium has two important consequences:

1. *The ventricles (and atria) function in an integrated, coordinated fashion.* Once the heartbeat has been triggered by the pacemaker, all the muscle cells depolarize and contract in a coordinated manner.

Key Question
Since additional motor units cannot be recruited, how does the myocardium increase or decrease the amount of work it performs?

2. *The heart cannot recruit more muscle fibers to increase or decrease the amount of work it performs, since all cells contract during each heartbeat.* Therefore, the mechanisms whereby the body increases and decreases cardiac output differ in kind from those used to increase or decrease force generation in a skeletal muscle, such as the biceps.

Electrophysiologic Characteristics of Smooth Muscle

The transmembrane potential in smooth muscle ranges from about -50 to -70 mV. As in other muscle, this intracellular electronegativity results in part from the relative permeabilities of sodium (Na^+) and potassium (K^+). In addition, however, the electrogenic Na^+/K^+ exchange pump, which extrudes 3 Na^+ for every 2 K^+ returned to the cell, may render the cell $\approx 6-8$ mV more electronegative than would be explained by the electrochemical equilibrium alone. Since the rate of the exchange pump may vary over time, the cell's transmembrane potential may also be labile. This and other factors contribute to slow oscillations in the resting membrane potential that occur in many smooth muscle cells. These oscillations may induce changes in contractile tension even without the generation of action potentials. Furthermore, these slow oscillations may propagate from cell to cell, since many smooth muscle fibers are electrically coupled through gap junctions. Finally, smooth muscle has *voltage-dependent calcium (Ca^{2+}) channels* that often conduct current even in the "relaxed" state; this inward flow of Ca^{2+} can result in modest levels of active tension in the basal state—the so-called *basal tone*. This basal tone is particularly important in vascular smooth muscle in small vessels (arterioles) that help determine the resistance to blood flow.

Action potentials in smooth muscle, when they occur, generally are due to currents carried primarily by Ca^{2+} rather than Na^+. Understanding the role of Ca^{2+} fluxes across the cell membrane and to and from intracellular stores is key to understanding contractile function in smooth muscle. The process by which cell depolarization triggers contraction is called *electromechanical coupling*. The predominant membrane channel in this case is an "L-type" (long-opening) voltage-dependent Ca^{2+} channel; opening of these channels allows Ca^{2+} to enter the cell under its electrochemical gradient. (As discussed in the section on ligand-gated channels below, there is another mechanism by which Ca^{2+} may enter the cell without the membrane depolarizing.) If Ca^{2+} enters the cell, it must be removed in equimolar amounts. Long-term Ca^{2+} balance is achieved by adenosine triphosphate (ATP)–driven pumps and Na^+/Ca^{2+} exchange mechanism.

Ligand-gated Channels

The membranes of skeletal, cardiac, and smooth muscle cells contain not only voltage-gated channels but also *ligand-gated channels* or *receptor-operated channels* (ROC). The membrane proteins that form these channels influence the instantaneous permeability of the membrane to small ions and can ultimately give rise to action potentials. Skeletal muscle cells have the simplest design with only one ligand-gated channel: an acetylcholine-activated, nonselective cation channel (mostly Na^+). The receptors coupled to these channels can be activated pharmacologically by nicotine and are consequently referred to as *nicotinic receptors*; they are blocked by neuromuscular blocking agents such as curare. As previously noted, the flow of positive ions into the cell through this channel is exclusively excitatory because it always depolarizes the myocyte. The receptors that activate the Na^+ channel are clustered within the synaptic cleft of the neuromuscular junction.

In contrast to the limited variety of ligand-gated channels in skeletal muscle, the membranes of cardiac and smooth muscle cells contain muscarinic acetylcholine (ACh) receptors, several types of catecholaminergic receptors, and numerous other receptors activated by "putative" (i.e., supposed) neurotransmitters. These receptors are linked to a variety of channels or second messenger systems that endow their cells with unique functional properties. For example, binding of a norepinephrine molecule to an adrenergic receptor in some smooth muscle cells activates an intracellular cascade to increase the conductance of a Ca^{2+} channel; this produces contractile tension with no

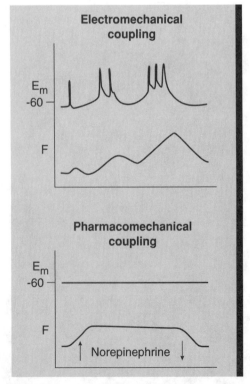

Electromechanical coupling

E_m
-60

F

Pharmacomechanical coupling

E_m
-60

F

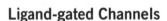

Norepinephrine

detectable change in membrane potential (and certainly without an action potential). The basis of this *pharmacomechanical coupling* is rather complicated. It depends not only upon the ROC but also upon a membrane-bound "G protein" linked to the receptor. The G protein activates an enzyme (phospholipase C), which, in turn, catalyzes the conversion of phosphatidylinositol 4,5-bisphosphate (PIP_2) to an intracellular second messenger, inositol 1,4,5-triphosphate (IP_3). The latter acts on the sarcoplasmic reticulum to release Ca^{2+}. Note that the ROC allows extracellular Ca^{2+} into the cell, while the G-protein chain ultimately releases Ca^{2+} from intracellular stores. Therefore, the smooth muscle contraction depends upon both intra- and extracellular sources of Ca^{2+}. (See Chapter 11, Figure 11-18 for further clarification.)

Cardiac muscle also increases force generation in response to increased sympathetic nervous activity or increased levels of circulating catecholamines. The *adrenergic receptors* responsible for this *positive inotropism* (or increased *contractility*) are distributed fairly uniformly over the cell membrane, since there is no structure equivalent to the neuromuscular junction. The neurotransmitters are released by postganglionic neurons of the autonomic nervous system from *varicosities* that arise along the course of the axon; they then diffuse to the myocyte's cellular membrane, where they bind to a *beta (β)-receptor*. (There are actually several varieties of β-receptors; this is a β_1 subtype.) In general, activation of adrenergic receptors *modulates*, rather than triggers, cardiac or smooth muscle contraction. This contrasts markedly with the role of ACh released at the neuromuscular junction of skeletal muscle, where the ACh directly triggers contraction via the EPP. Note that different ROCs may exist for the same neurotransmitter. For example, catecholamines can interact with alpha$_1$ (α_1)-receptors in smooth muscle to promote contraction or with β_2-receptors to promote relaxation.

The membranes of some cardiac and smooth muscle cells also contain channels that produce a spontaneous or *pacemaker* depolarization. This inherent *automaticity* of cardiac and smooth muscle leads to the important principle that *the depolarization and resultant contraction is usually generated within the muscle itself and is only modulated by the neural control mechanisms.*

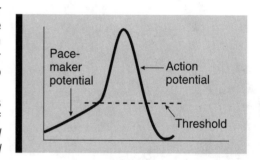

STRUCTURAL AND MECHANICAL PROPERTIES OF MUSCLE

Ultrastructure of Muscle

All three muscle types contain "thin" actin and "thick" myosin filaments that interact in the presence of Ca^{2+} to form cross bridges. These filaments are organized in both skeletal and cardiac muscle into small, subcellular functional units known as *sarcomeres*. These structures are easily seen in appropriately stained preparations under the microscope (Figure 4-1). In *striated* (i.e., skeletal and cardiac) muscle, the thin filaments appear to originate from the "Z lines"; the Z lines, in turn, demarcate the individual sarcomeres. Literally thousands of sarcomeres may be connected end-to-end to form an individual muscle fiber.

Sarcomeres, as such, cannot be discerned in smooth muscle. The thick and thin filaments of smooth muscle are not organized in a parallel manner, as in skeletal and cardiac muscle, but rather in a more random-appearing, crisscross pattern. Even here, actin fibers coupled to *dense bodies* within the cytoplasm (or dense bands on the inner surface of the membrane) interact with myosin to generate force. The dense areas also form linkages between adjacent cells and between smooth muscle cells and the interstitial matrix. The remainder of this discussion develops concepts that may be explained on the basis of the sarcomere in striated muscle, though analogous mechanisms may exist for smooth muscle.

Under appropriate conditions, the formation of the cross bridges between actin and myosin "slides" the filaments together, thereby shortening the cell [4]. This biochemical process produces force or tension within the muscle. As part of this process, the Z lines move closer together as the individual sarcomeres shorten. This interaction has been well

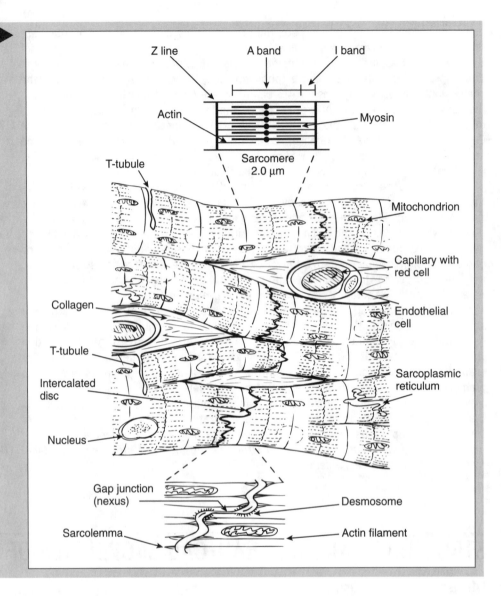

FIGURE 4-1 ▶

Section of Myocardium Cut Parallel to Fiber Axis Based upon Electron Microscopic Studies. *The myocyte is composed of many individual sarcomeres. The interaction of actin and myosin results in force development. Intercalated discs are the sites of low intercellular electrical resistance as a result of gap junctions.* (Source: *Adapted with permission from Levick JR:* An Introduction to Cardiovascular Physiology, *2nd ed. Oxford, UK: Butterworth-Heinemann, 1995, p 26.*)

First Answer to Key Question
Increasing the initial length of the muscle increases the amount of work the myocardium can perform.

---

described at the biochemical and structural levels and is known as the *sliding filament hypothesis*.

Length–Tension Relationships

One of the major predictions of the sliding filament hypothesis is that the force-generating capacity of the sarcomere depends upon its length. This effect of muscle length upon active development of force by the sarcomere results in *length–tension relationships* in the whole muscle. A thorough understanding of these relationships is critically important, especially with respect to skeletal and cardiac muscle function.

The *left* portion of Figure 4-2 demonstrates these relationships. It shows a skeletal muscle attached to a force transducer. The active element in the transducer changes its electrical properties (e.g., resistance) as the force exerted by the muscle increases or decreases. The lever is very stiff, however, so that when the motor nerve innervating the muscle is stimulated, the muscle develops tension but does not shorten appreciably. This is called an *isometric contraction*. The resulting electrical signal is fed to an amplifier whose output causes a writing pen to deflect in proportion to the force applied to the transducer.

The tracing at the *right* of Figure 4-2 shows a single isometric muscle *twitch* that results from stimulating the motor nerve. When this recording was made, the paper was pulled under the writing pen at a rapid speed (100 mm/sec), so the actual shape of the force recording is visible. Before the muscle contracts, the transducer detects a *passive tension* (or resting tension) of ≈ 10 g.[1] This force is due to the elastic properties of the muscle, much as a rubber band exerts a force when stretched. When the muscle contracts, it produces an *active tension* as a result of the interaction of the thick and thin filaments within the individual muscle fibers. The *total tension*, therefore, equals the sum of the passive and active tensions.

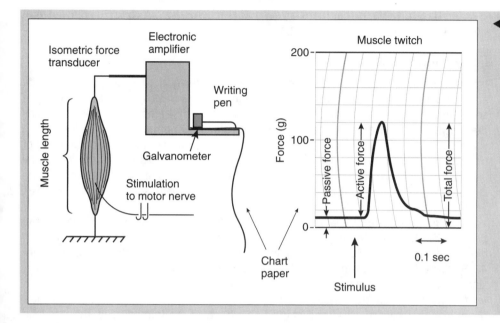

◀ *FIGURE 4-2*
Experimental Apparatus (left) to Measure Isometric Muscle Twitch (right). *The muscle motor nerve is stimulated to induce contraction. The force transducer changes contractile tension into an electrical signal, which is amplified electronically and converted to an ink tracing on the chart paper by a galvanometer. When the paper moves rapidly under the ink pen, the form of the twitch may be seen. Passive (resting) force, active (developed) force, and total force may be determined for the twitch.*

Although the length of the muscle does not change during the contraction, it is possible to change its length for any given contraction by raising or lowering the force transducer. This initial length is called the *preload*. By changing the initial length of the muscle, the effects of different preloads upon all three tensions—passive, active, and total—can be tested. Figure 4-3A shows sets of three muscle twitches, each set at four increasingly longer muscle lengths or preloads. When these recordings were made, the paper moved very slowly (1 mm/sec), so each twitch appears simply as a vertical line. The point at which the length is changed is designated as Δl. Note that *all three components of the twitch tensions increased as the length of the muscle increased.*

Figure 4-3B depicts the effects of muscle length upon passive, active, and total tensions. Recall that Figure 4-2 defines each of these three components. Each line was formulated using the data for the four series of contractions described above plus several others at shorter and longer lengths. The *passive length–tension relationship* shows that the muscle exerts relatively little tension at short lengths but bears progressively more as it is stretched to longer lengths. Notice especially the shape of the *active length–tension relationship*: the contraction of the muscle produces only modest force at shorter lengths, but force increases as the muscle is stretched more. *There is a point, however, at which further stretch upon the muscle decreases active tension.* This length is usually termed L_{max} or L_o (for "optimal").

As mentioned earlier, the shape of the active length–tension relationship can be explained by the sliding filament hypothesis: at optimal overlap between thick and thin filaments, the maximum number of active sites are available for mutual interaction. In striated muscle, the attachments to the bone generally keep the muscle stretched to near optimal lengths, or the *in situ* length of skeletal muscle is approximately equal to L_{max}. This explains why the ability of the respiratory pump to generate force can be decreased by compression of the chest wall and abdomen or by breathing at near maximal lung volumes. In marked contrast to skeletal muscle, the healthy myocardium functions on

---

[1] Notice that the force recording is calibrated simply in grams, rather than g/cm/sec[2] (see Chapter 3). This is because the acceleration (a) resulting from the force of gravity at the earth's surface is a constant (9.8 m/sec[2]) and, by tradition, is simply ignored in the equation F = ma. All that remains in the equation defining force, therefore, is the mass, in grams.

the *ascending limb* of its active length–tension relationship. This means that the stretch on the individual muscle fibers at the end of the filling phase is still less than L_{max}. Therefore, *a mechanism is built into the way heart muscle functions, which enables the myocardium to perform more work by increasing preload*. Chapter 10 demonstrates that this mechanism is the basis of Starling's law of the heart, which explains how cardiac output can be altered in accordance with the volume of blood delivered to the heart. Chapter 10 also explains that there is yet another mechanism for controlling myocardial work that does not require increasing preload.

Force–Velocity Relationship

Isometric contractions do not allow the muscle to shorten and, therefore, do not provide any information on two key parameters of muscle function: shortening (Δl) and velocity of shortening ($\Delta l / \Delta t$). These two factors are closely related to the amount of blood ejected by the ventricles with each heartbeat—the *stroke volume*—and the *rate of ejection* of this volume of blood (i.e., power). It is hard to imagine two more important parameters of cardiac pump function! We can study muscle shortening and velocity of shortening by using a different type of muscle contraction as illustrated in Figure 4-4. The process that is described below yields *the most fundamental descriptor of muscle function: the force–velocity relationship*.

In Figure 4-4A, the *initial length* of the muscle is established by a light weight, the *preload* (P). As shown in Chapters 9 and 10, this preload corresponds to the volume of blood in the left or right ventricle at the very end of diastole: *end diastolic volume*. Figure 4-4B shows that the maximum length of the muscle can never exceed this initial value, since a stop is placed that prevents additional lengthening. In Figure 4-4C, a heavier *afterload* is suspended on the muscle; the muscle is "unaware" of the presence of this additional load, however, until *after* it starts to contract. In the human body, the afterload corresponds roughly to the *arterial blood pressure* in the heart or the weight being lifted for skeletal muscle. In general terms, afterload establishes the work the muscle must perform. In Figure 4-4D, the muscle is excited and starts to generate tension. Note, however, that *the muscle cannot shorten until it generates force equal to the sum of the preload and afterload*. The *isometric contraction* in Figure 4-4D is analogous to *isovolumic contraction* in the ventricles discussed in Chapter 9. Finally, the muscle is able to shorten (Figure 4-4E). There are several critical features of this shortening phase of the contraction.

1. The tension generated by the muscle is constant and equal to the sum of the preload and afterload throughout this *isotonic* phase of contraction.
2. The amount of shortening, Δl_a, is equal to the difference between the initial length, l_1, and the final length, l_2.
3. The velocity of shortening may be calculated by knowing Δl and the time course of the contraction.
4. This phase of contraction corresponds to the *ejection* of blood from the ventricles in an intact heart.

The "payoff" for our efforts comes when we express these relationships using the principles outlined in Chapter 3. Surprisingly, the task is not difficult, and the results are key to our understanding of the ability of the heart to pump blood around the circulatory system. Figures 4-5A and B plot the length and force of the muscle, respectively. The *solid lines* show the contraction given in Figures 4-4A through E. (The *broken lines* and Figure 4-4F will be discussed in a moment.) The preload that determines this initial length can be read at P on the force recording in Figure 4-5B. The stimulus is delivered at S, and the muscle starts to contract. Although force increases, there is *no change in length until the muscle generates a force equal to the sum of the weight of the preload and afterload (P + A)*. This is the *isometric contraction* that occurred in Figure 4-4D. Once the muscle develops a force equal to P + A, the tension remains constant at this value—the muscle is contracting *isotonically*. Figure 4-5A shows that *the muscle shortens only during the isotonic phase of contraction*. The rate of shortening—or the velocity of shortening—can be estimated by taking the slope of this curve. *For this*

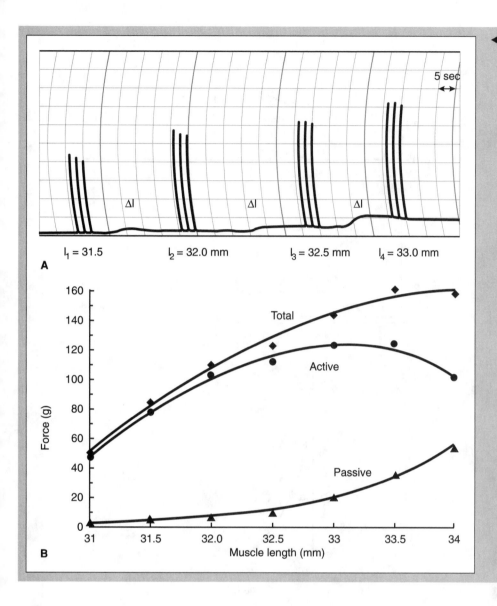

A

$l_1 = 31.5$ $l_2 = 32.0$ mm $l_3 = 32.5$ mm $l_4 = 33.0$ mm

B

FIGURE 4-3

Use of Series of Isometric Contractions at Different Lengths to Derive the Length–Tension Relationships. (A) Force recordings show three individual isometric twitches for four different initial lengths (preloads) of muscle. The chart paper moved slowly in this record, so the form of twitch cannot be seen. Increases in length (Δl) of muscle augment passive, active, and total tensions for the twitches. (B) Data are plotted to show length–tension relationships. As preload increased, passive tension increased. Active tension also increased until ≈33 mm (L_{max}), beyond which it decreased. The active length–tension relationship shows that the muscle progressively increases its force development as it is stretched to L_{max}.

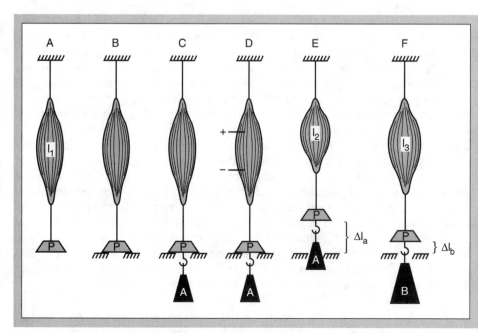

FIGURE 4-4

Experimental Arrangement to Derive Force–Velocity Relationship. Preload (P) determines initial length (A); the addition of "stop" (B) fixes muscle length at a value determined by preload. Heavier afterload (A) is added to muscle (C), which is then stimulated to contract (D). Muscle cannot shorten (Δl) until it develops a tension equivalent to the sum of preload and afterload (E). Adding a heavier afterload (F) results in a decrease in muscle shortening ($\Delta l_a > \Delta l_b$). (Source: Adapted with permission from Pollack GH: Maximum velocity as an index of contractility in cardiac muscle. A critical evaluation. Circ Res 16:113, 1970.)

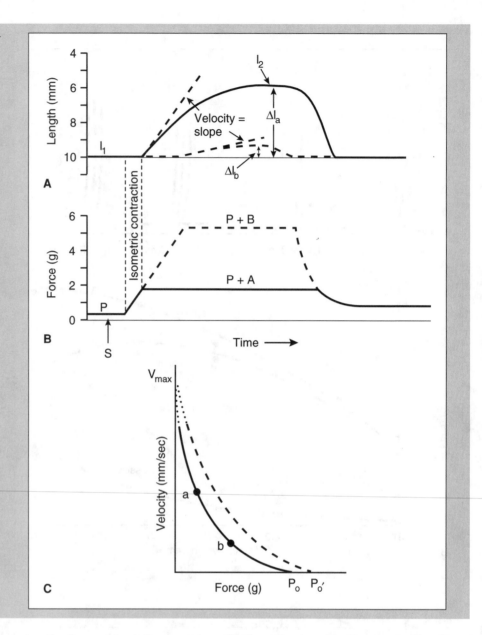

FIGURE 4-5 ▶

Length (A) and Force (B) Data for Contraction with Light Afterload (solid line) and Heavy Afterload (broken line), as in Figure 4-4. The actual values shown on the ordinate were chosen arbitrarily, and shortening is shown as an upward deflection in panel A. The initial length seen in panel A equals l_1 from Figure 4-4; l_1 has been assigned a value of 10 mm. The muscle is stimulated to contract at S. Force increases, but length is unchanged during the isometric phase of contraction (vertical lines). Once active tension equals the sum of preload (P) and afterload (A), the muscle shortens isotonically by the amount Δl_a (panel A), which equals Δl_a in Figure 4-4. This total force is plotted against the velocity of shortening ($\Delta l/\Delta t$, panel A) as point a in panel C for light afterload. Increasing afterload to B results in greater force development (P + B) and smaller shortening (Δl_b). These data are plotted as point b in panel C. The solid line in panel C shows the force–velocity relationship for contractions from constant preload. V_{max} represents the theoretical maximum velocity of contraction; P_o is the maximum load muscle can lift. If preload is increased (broken line, panel C), maximum load increases to $P_{o'}$, though V_{max} is not changed markedly. (Source: Adapted from Braunwald E, Ross J Jr, Sonnemblick EH: Mechanism of Contraction of the Normal and Failing Heart, 2nd ed. Boston, MA: Little, Brown, 1976, p 45.)

contraction from preload, P, we now have the force developed by the muscle (P + A) and the velocity of shortening; these two values are plotted as point a in Figure 4-5C.

In Figure 4-4F, suppose we replace the original afterload, A, with a much heavier weight, **B**. Note, however, that *the preload remains the same, so that the initial length is still l_1.* If we stimulate the muscle to contract as before, it will not begin to shorten until the developed tension equals the larger value, P + **B**. In Figure 4-4F, the final length is l_3, and the total shortening equals Δl_b. The muscle shortens less in Figure 4-4F than it did in Figure 4-4E ($\Delta l_a > \Delta l_b$). *This difference in shortening cannot be explained by the length–tension relationships because the preload is identical in both contractions!*

This second contraction is shown in the *broken line* in Figure 4-5. The total load in this contraction (P + **B**) exceeds that of contraction a (P + A). The shortening and velocity of shortening are much less in this second contraction. Once again, the total force and velocity are plotted as point b in Figure 4-5C. If we were to test the effects of many additional values of afterload on the muscle force and velocity of shortening and add them to the graph in Figure 4-5C, we would construct the *solid line* shown there. This is called the *force–velocity relationship*. Some of the most important principles inherent within this relationship, or the experiments used to derive it, are as follows:

1. The length that the muscle shortens decreases as the load that the muscle must lift increases. In other words, as the load decreases, the shortening increases.

2. The velocity of shortening decreases as the load the muscle must lift increases, and vice versa.

3. There is a certain maximal load that the muscle can just barely lift, designated P_o in Figure 4-5C.

4. The curve may be extrapolated to a maximum velocity of shortening, V_{max}, which would theoretically be observed if the afterload were zero and the muscle did not even have to lift the preload and its own weight.

These principles are applied in Chapter 9 to understand how the heart functions as a pump.

Effects of Changes in Preload on Force–Velocity Relationship. Each of the contractions used to construct the *solid line* in Figure 4-5A and B was obtained with the same preload. However, active tension increases, at least up to a point, as the preload increases. How would an increase in preload alter the force–velocity relationship? The *broken line* in Figure 4-5C shows a force–velocity relationship for a greater value of preload. Once again, however, each point on this new curve was taken from the new value of (increased) preload. The salient point is that increasing the preload shifts the force–velocity relationship to the right such that P_o (now designated $P_{o'}$) increases. This is simply another way to show that the myocardium can increase the work it performs with increased preloads (if, of course, its length does not exceed L_{max}).

Effects of Changes in Inotropic State on Force–Velocity Relationship. One of the most critical differences between cardiac and skeletal muscle is that *cardiac muscle, but not skeletal muscle, is quickly able to increase active tension development without increasing its initial length (or preload).* Suppose we were to record an isometric twitch from a cardiac papillary muscle, much as we did earlier for the skeletal muscle. The *solid line* in Figure 4-6 shows such a twitch for a given preload. *Without changing this preload*, we now add some epinephrine to the bathing medium in which the muscle is suspended and repeat the contraction. (Epinephrine activates the myocardium's β_1-receptors.) The *broken line* shows this second contraction. These data demonstrate the following important characteristics of an *increase in contractility*:

1. The active tension is significantly increased *without* an increase in preload.

2. The rates of tension rise ($+\Delta F/\Delta t$) and fall ($-\Delta F/\Delta t$) are both markedly increased.

3. The duration of the twitch decreases.

An increase in myocardial contractility is also called a *positive inotropism*.

> ***Second Answer to Key Question***
> *Increasing the inotropic state allows the myocardium to increase the amount of work it performs (and the rate at which it performs that work).*

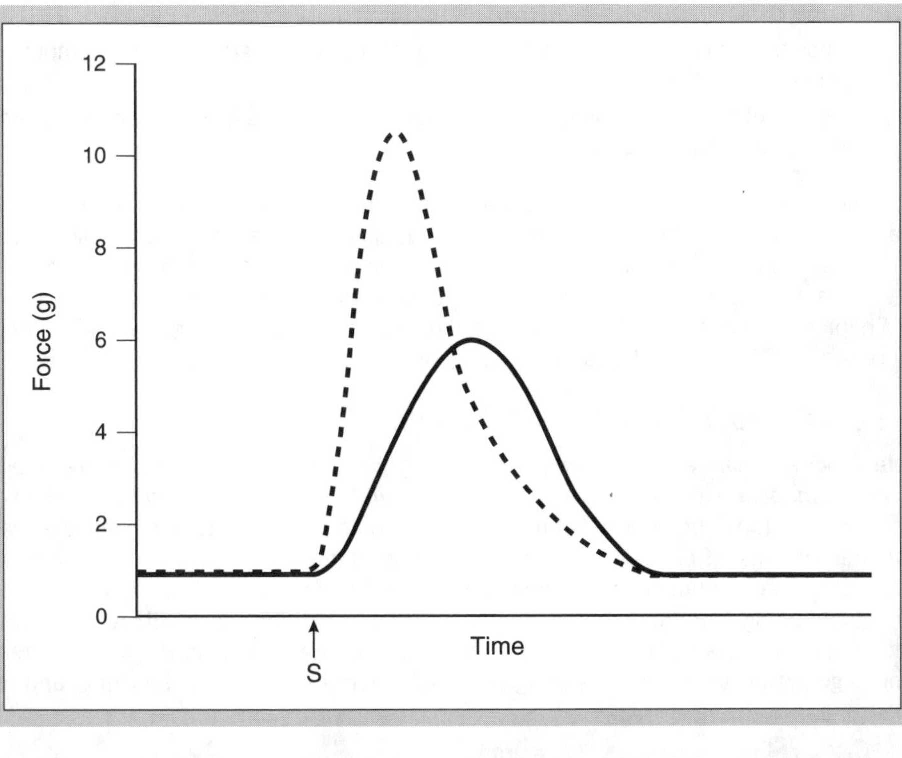

◀ ***FIGURE 4-6***
Isometric Cardiac Muscle Twitches for Control (solid line) ***Contraction and after Stimulation with Epinephrine*** (broken line, ***Positive Inotropism***). *Preload is identical for two twitches, but an increase in contractility yields an increase in active tension, the rate of tension rise and fall, and a shortening of duration of twitch relative to control.*

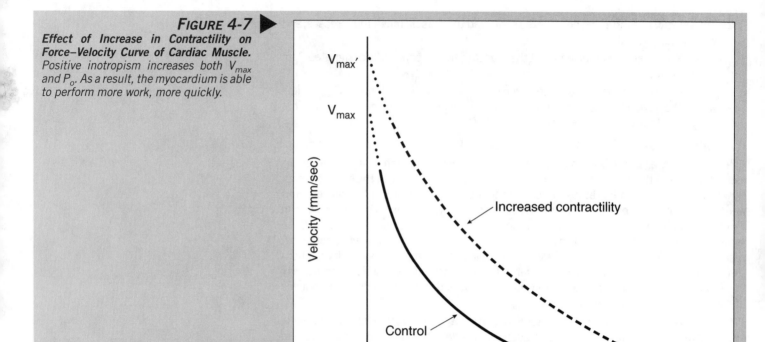

FIGURE 4-7 ▶

Effect of Increase in Contractility on Force–Velocity Curve of Cardiac Muscle. *Positive inotropism increases both V_{max} and P_o. As a result, the myocardium is able to perform more work, more quickly.*

Since a simple isometric contraction does not teach anything about muscle shortening, it is important to examine the effects of a positive inotropism on the force–velocity relationship as compared to the control relationship. Figure 4-7 shows a force–velocity relationship for the control state (*solid line*) and for an increase in contractility (*broken line*). Since there is no change in the initial length of the papillary muscle, *both curves are from the same preload.* Two of the important principles from the comparison of these two relationships are:

1. A positive inotropism causes the muscle to develop a greater force without an increase in preload.
2. The rate of force development and the maximum theoretical velocity of shortening are significantly increased.

Increased sympathetic nervous activity increases the contractility of cardiac muscle via activation of β_1-adrenergic receptors. Conversely, withdrawal of sympathetic tone decreases the contractile state: a negative inotropism. In short, *increased sympathetic nervous activity enables the myocardium to generate more force, more quickly.* As shown in Chapter 9, a positive inotropism allows the ventricles to eject a larger stroke volume more rapidly. The cellular basis for a positive inotropism is explained in Chapter 8.

Contractile Function in Smooth Muscle

One important feature of vascular and pulmonary smooth muscle is that they are able to maintain moderate levels of force for long periods with low energy expenditure. Although Ca^{2+} controls the interaction of actin and myosin in both striated and smooth muscles, the two mechanisms differ in important ways. In striated muscle, release of Ca^{2+} from the sarcoplasmic reticulum increases intracellular "free" Ca^{2+}. This Ca^{2+} binds to troponin, thereby inducing conformational changes in the position of tropomyosin with respect to the actin filaments. As a result, cross bridges are formed between actin and myosin, and tension is generated as these cross bridges "cycle"—forming, "flexing," breaking, and re-

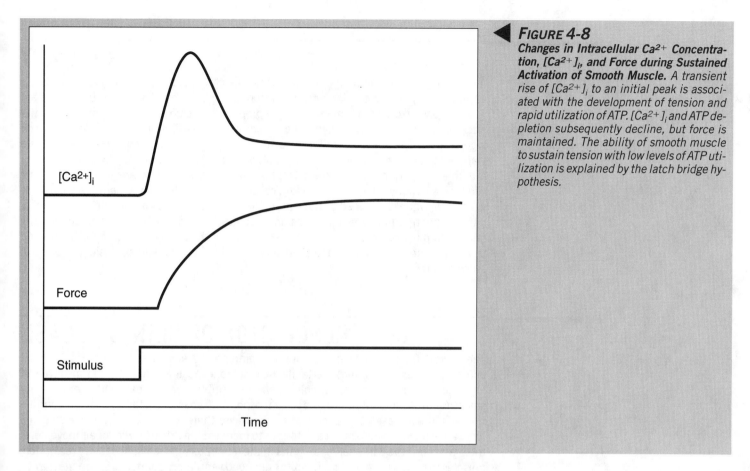

FIGURE 4-8
Changes in Intracellular Ca²⁺ Concentration, [Ca²⁺]ᵢ, and Force during Sustained Activation of Smooth Muscle. *A transient rise of [Ca²⁺]ᵢ to an initial peak is associated with the development of tension and rapid utilization of ATP. [Ca²⁺]ᵢ and ATP depletion subsequently decline, but force is maintained. The ability of smooth muscle to sustain tension with low levels of ATP utilization is explained by the latch bridge hypothesis.*

forming. Smooth muscle, however, lacks troponin; instead, interaction of actin and myosin depends upon a *covalent phosphorylation of the cross bridge.*

The relationships shown in Figure 4-8 establish a basis for understanding this covalent mechanism for control of contraction in smooth muscle. When a sustained contraction is triggered in smooth muscle, there is an initial peak in intracellular Ca^{2+} concentration. This initial peak is associated with a rather rapid rate of cross bridge phosphorylation and rather rapid utilization of ATP. Force increases as the actin and myosin interact. These high levels are not sustained, however, and the initially rapid rate of phosphorylation—and ATP expenditure—slows. Nonetheless, contractile tension remains high!

The explanation for the varying rate of ATP utilization involves the changing levels of intracellular Ca^{2+}. *The interaction of actin and myosin occurs only when the cross bridges are phosphorylated by the enzyme, myosin light chain kinase.* Another key player is a protein in the cytoplasm, *calmodulin,* which binds with Ca^{2+} that is released from intracellular stores or that enters the cell through a plasma membrane channel. Myosin kinase is activated when it binds to the calcium–calmodulin complex. With the initial, higher levels of Ca^{2+}, the cross bridges are allowed to *cycle* in a manner somewhat analogous to skeletal muscle. Although slow by skeletal muscle standards, this cycle allows tension to increase at a modest rate and consumes ATP at a fairly rapid rate (though, again, slow by skeletal muscle standards). As intracellular Ca^{2+} falls, a very slow cycle begins to dominate control of contraction. Another enzyme, myosin phosphatase, is thought to dephosphorylate the cross bridge, leaving it *bound* to the actin. The actin and myosin dissociate very slowly from this rigor-like complex when another molecule of ATP is used. This very slow cycle is referred to as the *latch bridge mechanism* and offers a satisfying explanation for the ability of smooth muscle to maintain tension without fatiguing and with relatively low utilization of ATP.

SUMMARY

A knowledge of the physiology of cardiac and skeletal muscle is essential to understanding the ability of the cardiac and respiratory pumps to cause a flow of blood and air, respectively. Likewise, a firm grasp of the properties of smooth muscle clarifies how the arterial, venous, and respiratory "trees" control the distribution of blood and air. Each type of muscle is able to alter force development in response to changes in length and load. Some of these responses are due to the "intrinsic" properties of the sarcomere; for example, the critically important length–tension relationships are explained by the sliding filament hypothesis. Conversely, cardiac and smooth muscles can alter their force generation when stimulated by the autonomic nervous system. This "extrinsic" control of muscle function produces increases and decreases in contractility. The force–velocity relationship is the most fundamental description of the ability of muscle to shorten and develop tension; it is sensitive to changes in both the intrinsic and extrinsic properties of muscle function.

RESOLUTION OF CLINICAL CASE

The child in the case presentation at the beginning of the chapter was suffering from an acute bout of *asthma*, almost certainly the result of exposure to high springtime levels of airborne pollens. Exposure to pollens in susceptible persons can cause bronchiolar smooth muscle to contract, perhaps to the point of *spasm* (sustained, severe contraction). This decreases the lumen of the airways, thereby dramatically increasing the resistance to air movement. In an attempt to increase the driving force for air movement, the brain recruits additional motor units in the respiratory muscles. Accessory respiratory muscles may also be recruited. Despite enhanced ventilatory effort, gas exchange may be diminished, leading to hypoxia and hypercapnia. (See blood gas values at the beginning of the chapter.) The stress also increases sympathetic nervous activity, which explains the elevated heart rate and cold sweat. Skin pallor results from the low oxygen content in the arterial blood vis-à-vis cutaneous vasoconstriction. A *β-agonist* (i.e., a drug that stimulates β-receptors such as isoproterenol or albuterol) was administered to the child via an inhalant. Within a breath or two, the child's respiratory distress resolved because of the relaxation of the bronchiolar smooth muscle caused by the β-agonist. Arterial blood gases quickly returned to normal, and, after advising the child and the child's parents to minimize pollen exposure, the child was dismissed with a prescription for a small device that administers puffs of inhalant when needed. The child, his color returned to normal, explained to his father as they left the physician's office that he would no longer be able to mow the grass.

REVIEW QUESTIONS

Directions: For each of the following questions, choose the **one best** answer.

1. Conduction of the electrical depolarization from one muscle cell to the next in the myocardium has which of the following characteristics?

   (A) It depends upon an elaborate system of nerve fibers within the heart

   (B) It depends upon low-resistance electrical connections between myocytes

   (C) It is controlled by the presence or absence of γ-receptors on the individual myocytes

   (D) It is possible because the resting membrane potential of the individual myocytes ≈ 0 mV

   (E) It occurs in Purkinje fibers but not in other cardiac muscle

2. The "active length–tension relationship" is most closely related to

   (A) the effect of changes in the amount of blood in the ventricle at the end of diastole upon force generation by the myocardium

   (B) the effect of changes in afterload upon the amount of blood ejected with each beat of the heart

   (C) the relationship between pressure and tension in the wall of the ventricle during diastole

   (D) changes in the pressure inside the ventricle as it is filling with blood during diastole

   (E) the tension generated by smooth or skeletal muscle when intracellular calmodulin is exhausted

3. Which of the following statements regarding an increase in contractility is correct?

   (A) An increase in cardiac parasympathetic nervous activity typically increases contractility

   (B) It occurs because of increased stretch on the muscle prior to onset of contraction

   (C) The primary result of an increase in contractility is that the muscle shortens more slowly

   (D) Activation of β-adrenergic receptors on cardiac muscle by circulating epinephrine increases the inotropic state

   (E) An increase in contractility is accompanied by a decrease in the rate of rise in muscle tension during isovolumic contraction

4. Which of the following statements about the force–velocity curve is correct?

   (A) An increase in cardiac contractility results in a decrease in V_{max}, indicating that the rate of muscle shortening is decreased

   (B) Elevating the preload on heart muscle in deriving a force–velocity relationship is analogous to decreasing the volume of blood inside the heart at the end of diastole

   (C) The increase in P_o (maximum load the muscle can lift) in the force–velocity relationship as a result of a positive inotropism is related to the intact heart's ability to perform more work when stimulated by the cardiac sympathetic nerves

   (D) The velocity of shortening of the papillary muscle is analogous to the rate of filling of the blood during diastole in the intact heart

   (E) A shift in the force–velocity curve upwards and to the right is an example of a positive dromotropism

ANSWERS AND EXPLANATIONS

1. **The answer is B.** The conduction system of the heart is composed of muscle fibers, not nerves, which are specialized for rapid cell-to-cell propagation of the depolarization, which originates at the sinoatrial node.

2. **The answer is A.** Changes in the preload on the heart can alter force generation by the myocardium, according to the principles of the active length–tension relationship. These concepts are developed in Chapters 9 and 10.

3. **The answer is D.** A positive inotropism results when either circulating epinephrine from the adrenal gland or norepinephrine from the sympathetic nerve varicosities interacts with a β_1-receptor on the myocyte.

4. **The answer is C.** A positive inotropism, such as occurs with sympathetic stimulation of the myocardium, allows the muscle to perform more work (e.g., increase in P_o), more rapidly (e.g., increase in V_{max}).

REFERENCES

1. Nicholls JG, Martin AR, Wallace BG: *From Neuron to Brain*, 3rd ed. Sunderland, MA: Sinauer Associates, 1992.
2. Kandel ER, Schwartz JH, Jessell TM: *Principles of Neural Science*, 3rd ed. New York, NY: Elsevier, 1991.
3. Hille B: *Ionic Channels of Excitable Membranes*, 2nd ed. Sunderland, MA: Sinauer Associates, 1992.
4. Irving M, Gabriella P: Motions of myosin heads that drive muscle contraction. *News Physiol Sci* 12:249–254, 1997.

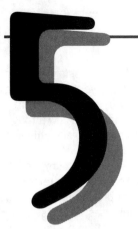

DESIGN OF THE CARDIOPULMONARY SYSTEM

INTRODUCTION

This chapter focuses on the common design principles of the cardiovascular, lymphatic, and respiratory systems. Additional specific features of each of these are elaborated in Chapters 9 and 14. Although there are many differences between these systems, there are also several compelling similarities. Muscle pumps generate pressure gradients necessary to move the blood, lymph, and air, respectively, through all three distribution systems. The cardiovascular and respiratory distribution "trees" involve bifurcating conduits that exhibit some degree of resistance, capacitance, compliance, and control of their diameter. The presence of strategically placed valves helps to maintain directed flow throughout many of the conduits. Ultimately, both systems use small-diameter, thin-walled structures with very high cumulative surface areas to accomplish the goal of the system: that is, an adequate exchange of nutrients, gases, waste products, and water to and from the body tissues.

PUMPS

The heart acts as a typical "push" type of pump, generating a positive driving pressure to initiate the flow of blood through the circulation. It is often useful to think of the heart as two separate pumps: the right heart producing flow through a low-pressure pulmonary circulation, and the left through the systemic circulation. The cardiac muscle described in Chapter 4 is responsible for developing this force with each beat of the heart. The periodic nature of the pump's contractions gives rise to pulsatile flow patterns with the

Pulmonary Circulation
Vessels or blood flow associated with "nutritive" gas exchange in the lungs.
Systemic Circulation
Vessels or blood flow associated with "metabolic" gas exchange in all tissues.

When a soldier stands motionless at attention for a long time, there may be significant blood volume lost to the leg. Muscle contractions are helpful in preventing this fluid shift that can contribute to fainting.

Clench your hand tightly for a few seconds and then open your hand. Your palm appears white because the blood has been forced out of the capillaries and veins by the high intramuscular pressure. Slowly a red flush develops from the reactive hyperemia that follows periods of ischemia. If you keep your hand clenched for a long time, the reduced blood flow may result in pain.

*Pressure = flow × resistance, R = P/V
For resistances in series:*
  $R_T = R_1 + R_2 + R_3 \cdots$

R_1 R_2 R_3

For resistances in parallel:
  $1/R_T = 1/R_1 + 1/R_2 \cdots$

R_1

R_2

R_3

highest pressure and highest flow velocity through the major arterial vessels occurring during systole. Two of the heart valves prevent backflow through the ventricles during their "off" cycle, while the elastic properties of the major arteries permit temporary storage of some of the pressure. This stored, or *diastolic*, pressure maintains flow through the systemic and pulmonary vessels, while the left and right ventricles are filling in preparation for the next heartbeat.

The respiratory system includes both an inspiratory and an expiratory pump, each dependent on striated muscle. Although these pumps are capable of generating relatively large pressures under extreme conditions, they routinely operate at pressures well below those of the cardiovascular system (see Chapter 3). For our purposes, it is useful to consider the inspiratory pump as a "vacuum" pump generating a negative pressure that "pulls" air into the lungs. In contrast, the expiratory pump develops a positive pressure in the lungs to "push" air from the lungs. During quiet breathing, the expiratory pump does not require active muscle contraction. Instead, air leaves the lungs as a result of the passive elastic recoil properties of the inspiratory pump and lung.

A third pump that is important to the function of both the venous system and the lymphatic system is the *muscle pump*. As skeletal muscle contracts, it generates pressure on the surrounding tissues, which is then transmitted to surrounding vessels. This pressure forces fluid from the contracted regions into adjacent areas with quiescent (or no) muscles that are subject to much lower pressures. The muscle pump moves fluid from regions of higher to lower pressure. Numerous unidirectional valves are found in both the venous and lymphatic vessels. These valves permit forward movement from the contracted segment and then prevent any backward flow when the muscles are relaxed. Thus, this mechanism contributes significantly to flow in the peripheral portions of the systemic and lymphatic vessels. This muscle pump is profoundly important in preventing blood from pooling in the lower extremities during prolonged standing. When periodic muscle contraction is prevented by prolonged inactivity, the resulting pooling of blood in the dependent structures decreases the useful blood volume, and fainting may ensue.

Although this muscle pump serves an important constructive function in the venous circulation, it can occasionally be counterproductive in many contractile tissues. During the period of contraction (the *duty cycle*), blood flow through a muscle may be temporarily impeded or even stopped by the high pressures developed outside the vascular walls. Such an action may decrease the total blood flow that a region receives. This "throttle effect" is especially significant in the coronary circulation. However, since most muscles do not remain contracted for long periods of time, the intermittent flow that occurs when the muscle is relaxed is usually sufficient to maintain adequate perfusion.

DISTRIBUTION SYSTEMS

The vessels that serve as pathways for blood, air, and lymph are often organized as a bifurcating structure similar to the branching of a tree (see Chapter 1, Figure 1-8). This fractal organization may be maintained throughout numerous subdivisions of the system. It is often described in terms of successive generations in which a parent structure gives rise to two or more "daughter" structures, which can, in turn, produce their own daughters. For the pulmonary system, most of the branching has been modeled as a *regular dichotomy* in which each parent vessel splits into two smaller vessels. Although the branching patterns in the cardiovascular tree are not as uniform, parent vessels still branch to form numerous smaller daughter vessels. At first glance, the reduced lumen in the daughter vessels suggests an increase in resistance since resistance is proportional to the fourth power of the radius (see Chapter 3). Although resistance increases rapidly as the radius decreases, it does not fully explain the resistances observed within the distribution systems, since at each bifurcation point the *total* cross-sectional area for fluid movement is usually increased despite a narrowing of each individual element.

At each successive branching generation, the total resistance for the entire generation may decrease, since an increasing number of conduits are added in parallel. An important physical principle from Chapter 3 is that $1/R_T = 1/R_1 + 1/R_2 + \cdots + 1/R_n$. The major resistance in the circulatory tree lies in the small arteries and arterioles; the major resistances for the respiratory tree lie in the trachea, bronchi, and upper bronchioles. At the level of the exchange vessels (capillaries and respiratory bronchioles), the resistance is actually quite low because: (1) the total cross-sectional area is very large; (2) there is little flow; and (3) there is an even smaller pressure gradient through each individual structure.

Although the branching patterns in vessels and airways are often symmetric, there can be differences in both the diameters and the angles of branching of the daughter vessels. These asymmetries produce the opportunity for turbulent flow or preferential flow through the larger and more direct pathways. As smaller vessels branch from the arterioles, the blood that enters the smaller vessels tends to be dilute in red blood cells (RBCs), leading to *plasma skimming*. In the airways, a major asymmetry of the bronchi leads to preferential distribution of inhaled particulates in the right middle lobes, resulting in a higher incidence of lung infection in this region.

Vasculature

Throughout the vasculature, all the different types of distribution vessels are lined by a single layer of endothelial cells. There are, however, considerable differences in the structure of the remaining components of the wall (Table 5-1). The walls of these vessels contain varying amounts of contractile smooth muscle tissue along with fibrous and elastic connective tissue. The larger vessels have walls thick enough to require their own circulation through small vessels known as the *vasa vasorum*.

Aorta. The aorta receives all the blood pumped with each contraction of the heart. It is usually described as an *elastic* artery because it has a relatively high elastin content and a modest amount of smooth muscle. The elastic properties of the aorta give it a relatively high compliance, which permits its expansion during systole and the subsequent reduction in volume during diastole. With a cross-sectional luminal area of about 4 cm^2, it sees an average flow velocity of about 20 cm/sec. During exercise, peak flow velocities exceed 150 cm/sec.

Arteries. At each successive branch point in the vascular tree, the total cross-sectional area increases by a factor of approximately 1.2–1.7. These distributing arteries contain a higher proportion of smooth muscle than the other vessels. Because of the extra layers of smooth muscle, the ratio of wall thickness to vessel diameter increases greatly. Extensive branching occurs from the main arteries, leading to a substantial increase in luminal cross-sectional area. Although there is a significant amount of vascular smooth muscle, the large arteries contribute little to the overall resistance to blood flow.

Arterioles. Within the tissue beds, the arteries lose much of their distensibility as they further branch and decrease in size to become arterioles. Arterioles have luminal diameters of about 5–100 μm with wall thicknesses of 2–6 μm. With their small lumens and their ability to change luminal diameter with smooth muscle contraction, these vessels produce the major resistance within the vascular tree. The smooth muscle is under neural and humoral influences, which play a major role in altering resistance and, therefore, modulating flow to the downstream tissues.

Capillaries. Capillaries are located distal to the arterioles. The capillary is the ultimate exchange vessel, and its thin wall is designed to optimize diffusion and transport. Like all the other components of the vasculature, it is lined by endothelial cells, but it lacks smooth muscle and any overlying adventitia. In fact, the endothelial cell itself provides the only structural element and the only barrier to exchange. Although the total volume of blood within the systemic capillaries is relatively small, the total surface area is huge, perhaps as large as 60 m^2 (Figure 5-1).

Venules and Veins. Blood leaving a capillary enters small vessels known as *venules*. Multiple venules converge to form *veins*. Although the gross structure of the venous tree resembles a mirror image of the arterial tree, the veins differ from their arterial counterparts in that the venous vessels have larger lumens, thinner walls, less smooth muscle, less elastin and collagen, and a greater distensibility. These characteristics help account for the fact that the veins are the major *compliance* vessels. In addition, since the veins

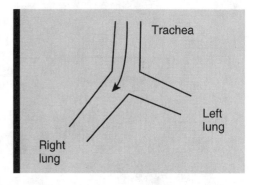

For resistance in the airways:

$$R_T = R_{trachea} + R_{main\ bronchi} + R_{bronchioles} + \cdots$$

$$1/R_{main\ bronchi} = 1/R_{left\ bronchi} + 1/R_{right\ bronchi}$$

$$1/R_{bronchioles} = 1/R_{bronchiole\ 1} + 1/R_{bronchiole\ 2} + \cdots + 1/R_{bronchiole\ n}$$

Trachea

Right lung

Left lung

Flow through the aorta = cross-sectional area × flow velocity.

$Q = 4\ cm^2 \times 20$ cm/sec = 80 cm^3/sec = (80 mL/sec)(60 sec/min) = 4800 mL/min.

(Remember that aortic flow ≈ cardiac output ≈ 5000 mL/min at rest.)

A previously stretched balloon requires very little pressure to inflate to the point at which it begins to stretch. From zero volume to this point, it behaves like a vein.

TABLE 5-1 ▶
Divisions of the Distribution Systems

	Pulmonary				
	Trachea	*Bronchi*	*Bronchioles*	*Respiratory Bronchioles/ Alveolar Ducts*	*Alveoli*
Generations	0	1–3	4–16	17–20	21–23
Diameter (cm)	1.8	1–0.5	0.5–0.06	.05–0.04	0.04
Length (cm)	12	1–5	0.2–1	0.1	0.05
Number	1	14	120,000	2,000,000	16,000,000
Total cross-sectional area (cm²)	2.5	2	3–180	10^3	10^5
Volume (mL)	30	20	120	300	1200
Cumulative no. of alveoli	0	0	0	10,000,000	300,000,000
Cumulative surface area (m²)	0.007	< 0.1	< 1	10	100
Wall thickness (mm)	5	1	0.05–1	0.0003	0.0003
Smooth muscle	Abundant	Abundant	Present	No	No
Cartilage	Yes	Yes	No	No	No
Goblet cells	Yes	Yes	Yes	No	No
Epithelium	Pseudostratified columnar		Cuboidal	Squamous	Squamous

	Cardiovascular						
	Aorta	*Artery*	*Arterioles*	*Capillary*	*Venule*	*Vein*	*Vena cava*
Diameter (mm)	25	8–0.6	0.1–0.01	0.01–0.003	0.1–0.01	1–15	30
Number of each	1	Increased	2×10^k	5×10^4	5×10^k	Decreased	2
Cross-sectional area (cm²)	4	20	500	3500	2700	100	18
Flow velocity at rest (cm/sec)	20	4	0.16	0.02	0.03	0.8	4
Wall thickness (mm)	2	1–0.1	0.01–0.002	0.0005–0.001	0.001–0.01	0.5	1–2
Smooth muscle	Modest	High	High	Absent	Very low	Low	Low
Elastin fibers	High	Moderate	Low	Absent	Very low	Low	Moderate
Collagen fibers	High	Medium	Low	Very low	Low	Low	Moderate

operate at low pressures, they normally function in an unstressed volume range, which contributes to their high compliance. Because of their high compliance, the large veins function as a major reservoir for blood.

Lymphatics

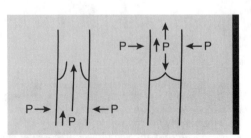

Branches of the lymphatic system are found in all tissues except bone, cartilage, epithelium, and the central nervous system (CNS). The lymphatic system is most similar to the venous side of the cardiovascular system in its structure and function. Flow originates in small, closed-end *lymphatic capillaries* that are highly permeable, since their endothelial lining lacks tight junctions between the individual cells. Fluid that enters the lymphatics is eventually returned to the circulation (from where it originally came) through a converging network of vessels. These vessels ultimately lead to the *main thoracic duct*, which empties into the subclavian veins. Like veins, the larger lymph vessels are relatively

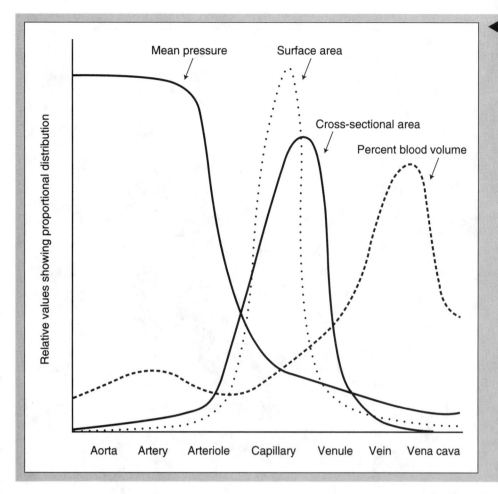

FIGURE 5-1
Alterations in Important Features of the Cardiovascular Tree. *Blood pressure, total surface area, total cross-sectional area, and the percent of total blood volume are plotted for each subdivision of the cardiovascular distribution system.*

compliant, contain unidirectional valves, and have a small amount of elastic tissue and smooth muscle. The smooth muscle in the lymphatic vessels contributes to the active pumping of lymph. Additional features that promote the return of lymph to the venous circulation include tissue pressures, the *muscle pumps* developed by skeletal muscle contraction, and the presence of unidirectional valves.

Airways

Upper Airways. The upper airways include the oral and nasal cavities, pharynx, larynx, and extrathoracic trachea (Figure 5-2). The musculature surrounding these regions consists exclusively of striated muscle innervated by the cranial nerves. Although the activity of some of these muscles can be controlled voluntarily, control is usually involuntary or "automatic." Many of these muscles exhibit a respiratory periodicity, which influences the diameter of the airway, usually producing a decreased resistance to airflow during inspiration. Bony or cartilaginous structures contribute to the stiffness of most of these airways. The region of the pharynx just orad to the larynx is the most collapsible region. The patency of this part of the upper airway can be compromised by the negative pressures developed during inspiration and may present a significant problem in some cases of obstructive sleep apnea. Collapse of this region contributes to turbulent airflow that can result in snoring. Although usually considered a social concern, snoring may have important clinical relevancy.

The structures associated with the nasal cavity perform the essential functions of warming, humidifying, and filtering the incoming air during normal nasal breathing. To increase the surface area and aid these functions, the air moves past the *turbinates*. The oral cavity and pharynx are important to both airflow and the ingestion of food and water, while the larynx acts as a crossroads for the digestive and respiratory systems. All of these structures are richly innervated and can participate in the reflex control of ventilation. Extensive neural reflex control is essential to prevent the swallowing of air and the aspiration of food.

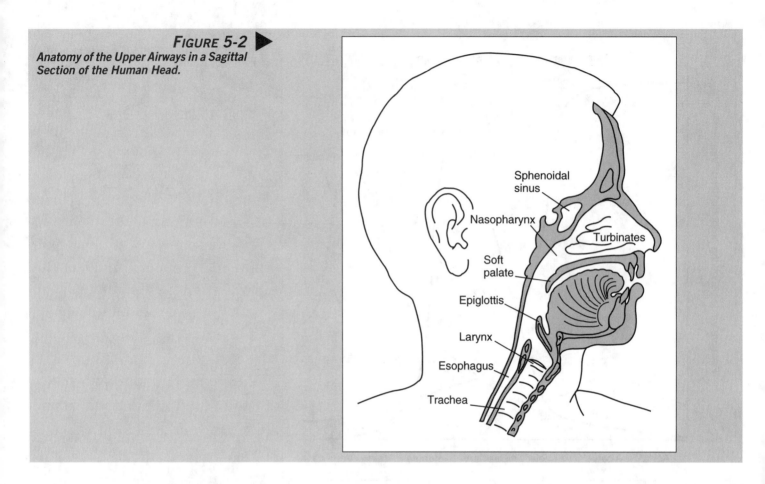

Sphenoidal sinus

Nasopharynx

Turbinates

Soft palate

Epiglottis

Larynx

Esophagus

Trachea

Larynx. The larynx contains several cartilaginous plates interconnected by striated muscles. In addition to speech and sound production, the larynx is very important in swallowing and preventing aspiration of ingested material into the airways. The epiglottis effectively prevents entry of food and liquid into the trachea.

Trachea. The trachea begins immediately below the larynx at about the level of the seventh cervical vertebra. It is composed of a series of horseshoe-shaped rings of cartilage connected by intercartilaginous ligaments. The smooth muscle of the trachea is located between the dorsal ends of the cartilaginous rings. Contraction of this muscle brings the ends of the horseshoe rings closer and decreases the internal diameter of the trachea. The smooth muscle is innervated by the recurrent laryngeal nerve. Sensory receptors are located primarily in the epithelium and smooth muscle; their afferent fibers project to the brain in the superior laryngeal nerve. A layer of ciliated columnar epithelial cells lines the trachea and promotes the active flow of the overlying mucous layer. This mucus plays an important role in trapping impacted particulate matter and transporting it toward the pharynx. In addition to the ciliated cells, some of the epithelial cells produce mucus.

The trachea extends into the chest cavity, where it is subject to a negative distending intrapleural pressure. The trachea bifurcates into the left and right main bronchi at the *carina*, a specialized area containing a high concentration of sensory receptors, which are thought to play an important role in the cough reflex (Figure 5-3).

Bronchi. The structure and function of the first several generations of bronchi are similar to those of the trachea. With each bifurcation, the airway diameter decreases substantially, leading to a very slight decrease in the total cross-sectional area (Figure 5-4; Table 5-2). The decreased area results in an increase in the flow velocity through this region. This contributes to the formation of turbulent flow (Figure 5-5) and the increased resistance to airflow often seen in this region (Figure 5-6). The main bronchi subdivide into *lobar bronchi* and then *segmental bronchi*.

TABLE 5-2
Changes in Radius and Area in the Upper Airways

	Diameter (cm)	Radius (cm)	Area (cm²)	Total Cross-sectional Area (cm²)
Trachea	1.8	0.9	2.54	2.54
Main bronchi	1.22	0.61	1.17	2.34
Lobar bronchi	0.83	0.42	0.55	2.21

Bronchioles. Further subdivisions of the bronchial tree become progressively smaller in their individual diameter and length. However, since they are increasing in number, the total cross-sectional area increases. Generations 4–16 are less than 1 mm in diameter and are usually considered to be *bronchioles*; the later generations are called the *terminal bronchioles*. Since minimal gas exchange occurs within the airways mentioned thus far, they are all classified as *conducting airways*, and their cumulative volume constitutes the majority of the *anatomic dead space*. The bronchioles are lined by ciliated cuboidal epithelial cells. The beating of these cilia moves debris-laden mucus back toward the pharynx, where it can be swallowed.

Since the terminal bronchioles lack any cartilaginous skeleton and have limited smooth muscle, their diameter is dependent on their interaction with adjacent lung tissue and the degree of subepithelial smooth muscle contraction. The physical coupling between the small airways and the lung parenchyma helps to maintain the patency of these structures. With larger lung volumes, this *tethering* effect causes an increased diameter and a decreased resistance.

Respiratory Bronchioles. As the bronchioles become even smaller, the epithelial lining begins to lose the mucus-secreting cells and eventually the cilia. The epithelial cells become flattened and form specialized gas exchange structures called *alveoli*. The alveoli appear in small numbers on the *respiratory bronchioles* (generations 17–19);

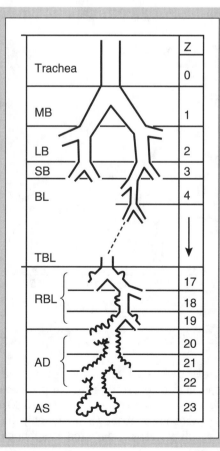

FIGURE 5-3
Diagram of the Regular Dichotomous Branching of the Human Airways. Each bifurcation provides another generation, as indicated on the right. The first 16 generations have relatively thick structural walls and do not contribute any significant gas exchange; hence, they are called the "conducting zone." Since generations 17–19 serve a conducting function and contribute some gas exchange, they are termed the "transitional zone." Generations 20–23 serve primarily for gas exchange and are therefore called the "respiratory zone." MB = main bronchi; LB = lobar bronchi; SB = segmental bronchi; BL = bronchioles; TBL = terminal bronchioles; RBL = respiratory bronchioles; AD = alveolar ducts; AS = alveolar sacs.

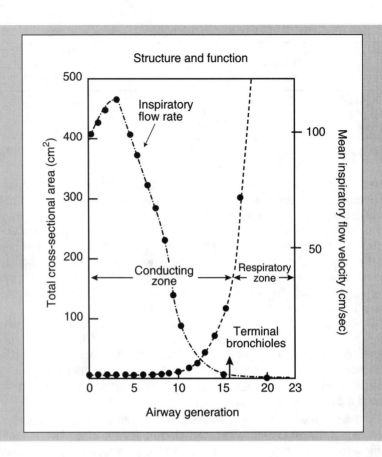

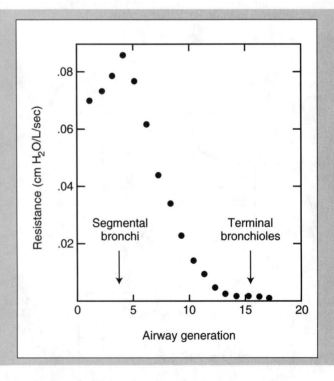

however, their density increases with each further branching. The last few generations of the airways are highly specialized to permit effective gas exchange and include the *alveolar ducts* and the *alveolar sacs.* In total, there are about 300 million alveoli, creating a total surface area for gas exchange of about 75 m² (roughly the size of a tennis court). Although the individual alveoli are usually depicted as spherical structures, their thin walls are subject to the surface tension and elastic properties of adjacent structures. Therefore, their shape is better depicted by a complex polyhedron typical of soap bubbles (Figure 5-7).

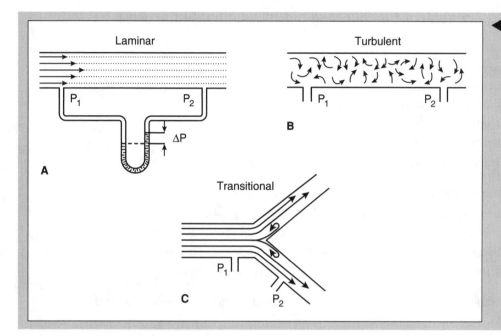

◀ **FIGURE 5-6**
Patterns of Fluid Flow Seen in the Cardiopulmonary System. *(A) In this figure, the flow is laminar. This flow pattern is usually observed in the larger vessels and facilitates movement of the fluid. (B) Turbulent flow decreases the amount of fluid effectively moved from one location to another. This pattern is often observed in response to rapid changes in conduit diameter or excessively high flow velocities. (C) Some turbulent flow occurs along with laminar flow. This pattern gives rise to "eddy" currents in a small stream. This flow pattern is often observed at the branch points or bifurcations.*

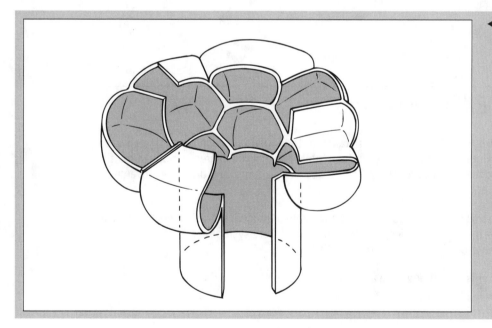

◀ **FIGURE 5-7**
Model of the Alveolar Shapes Surrounding the Alveolar Duct. *Note that the forces created by the adjacent structures give rise to a complex shape similar to stacked soap bubbles. (Source: Adapted with permission from Weibel ER: Morphology of the Human Lung. New York, NY: Academic Press, 1963, p 37.)*

REVIEW QUESTIONS

Directions: For each of the following questions, choose the **one best** answer.

1. The largest component of total resistance in the respiratory tree is generated by the resistance in the

    (A) trachea and bronchi

    (B) terminal bronchioles

    (C) respiratory bronchioles

    (D) alveolar ducts

2. Which distribution system is best matched with the muscle type of its primary pump?

    (A) Respiratory–skeletal; cardiovascular–smooth; lymphatic–smooth

    (B) Respiratory–smooth; cardiovascular–cardiac; lymphatic–smooth

    (C) Respiratory–skeletal; cardiovascular–cardiac; lymphatic–smooth

    (D) Respiratory–smooth; cardiovascular–skeletal; lymphatic–skeletal

3. Which circulatory vessel has the greatest ratio of smooth muscle to wall thickness?

    (A) Aorta

    (B) Arterioles

    (C) Capillaries

    (D) Veins

ANSWERS AND EXPLANATIONS

1. **The answer is A.** Although the resistance in the individual bronchioles is very great, these bronchioles are in parallel and the total cross-sectional area is much larger than in the trachea. There is very little flow in the alveolar ducts, and diffusive movement of oxygen predominates.

2. **The answer is C.** Both smooth muscle and skeletal muscle pumping mechanisms are important in the lymphatics; however, the respiratory system is strictly skeletal and the cardiovascular pump is strictly cardiac muscle.

3. **The answer is B.** Although the aortic wall contains significant muscle, the *proportion* of muscle is much larger in the arterioles.

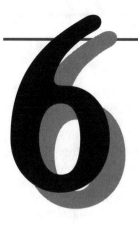

BLOOD AS A COMPONENT OF THE CARDIOPULMONARY SYSTEM

CHAPTER OUTLINE

INTRODUCTION OF CLINICAL CASE

A man in his mid-40s presented with abdominal "fullness," mild speech impairment, and episodes of extreme fatigue. He reported being bothered by frequent colds and related infections. Cold weather made his hands extremely painful, and there were ulcerated sores on his hands and fingers. Eye examination showed extreme dilation of retina arterioles, sluggish blood flow, clumping of red blood cells (RBCs), and hemorrhage of some vessels within the retinal circulation. A blood sample showed a low hematocrit, and an abdominal radiograph showed an enlarged spleen.

BLOOD COMPOSITION

The cardiopulmonary system serves to circulate blood at the flow rate and composition necessary to satisfy the metabolic demands of the body and to maintain homeostasis of the internal environment. With this in mind, it goes without saying that blood is the central element of the cardiopulmonary system.

This chapter describes some salient constituents and properties of blood that affect the cardiopulmonary system. A thorough description of all the elements of blood comes under the topic of hematology and is not necessary for an understanding of cardiopulmonary function.

Formed Elements

Blood is a nonhomogeneous fluid composed of formed elements suspended in a complex colloidal fluid called *plasma*. The formed elements are the erythrocytes (RBCs), leukocytes (white blood cells, WBCs), and thrombocytes (platelets). As shown in Figure 6-1, the formed elements are produced in the bone marrow and are all derived from the same stem cell. However, the myeloid cells arising from the first differentiation of the parent stem cell, in turn, give rise to the majority of the formed elements, the exception being the lymphocytes. The WBCs, which consist of the lymphocytes, neutrophils, monocytes, eosinophils, and basophils, are nucleated cells that function in the immune response. The platelets are not whole cells, but fragments of megakaryocytes. The platelets are named thrombocytes because of their role in the clotting process. In addition, the platelets contain a variety of vasoactive substances, some of which are discussed in conjunction with the regulation of blood flow in Chapter 11.

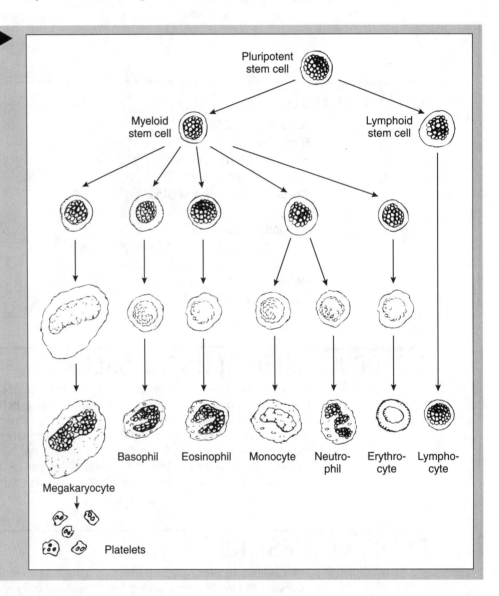

FIGURE 6-1 ▶
Flow Chart of the Formed Elements Produced in Bone Marrow. (Source: *Reprinted with permission from Vander AJ, et al.:* Human Physiology. *New York, NY: McGraw-Hill, 1994, p 401.)*

The RBCs, which function in blood-gas transport, are clearly the most important of the formed elements to consider in the study of cardiopulmonary function. In mammals, the RBCs lack a nucleus; therefore, they have a finite lifetime, averaging about 120 days. Consequently, RBC homeostasis, and hence homeostasis of blood-gas transport, requires a continuous balance between RBC death and production. Normally, RBC destruction occurs in the liver and spleen, which recycle the iron. The continuous destruction of

RBCs is balanced by a continuous production of the hormone erythropoietin from the capillary endothelial cells of the kidneys. Erythropoietin stimulates the production of RBCs by the bone marrow. The basal secretion of erythropoietin is normally adequate to maintain RBC homeostasis. However, under conditions in which the oxygen content of arterial blood decreases (e.g., at high altitudes), the decreased oxygen delivery to the kidneys increases erythropoietin synthesis and secretion.

The relative volumes of formed elements and plasma can be obtained by centrifuging a sample of anticoagulated blood at 1500 rpm for 30 minutes. As a result of their relative densities, the formed elements pack in the sample tube, as shown in Figure 6-2: the RBCs form the bottom layer, the WBCs and platelets form the next layer, and the plasma forms the top layer. This figure shows that in the normal state, plasma constitutes the largest portion of whole blood at about 55%, followed by the RBCs at 40%, with the WBCs and platelets constituting only about 5%.

About 50% of total body iron is found in the hemoglobin molecules within erythrocytes. Of the remaining iron, 25% is found in the liver ferritin and 25% occurs in heme-containing proteins in other body cells.

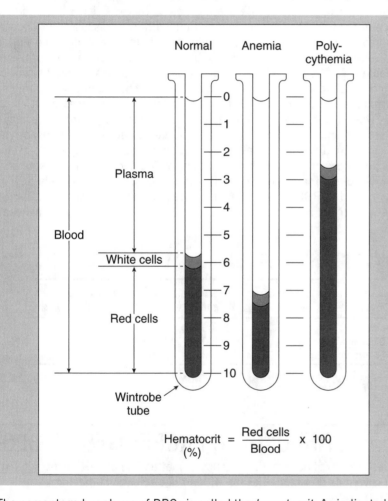

FIGURE 6-2
Distribution of Formed Elements in Normal, Anemic, and Polycythemic Human Blood. *(Source: Adapted with permission from Selkurt EE: Physiology 4th ed. Boston, MA: Little, Brown, 1976, p 243.)*

The percentage by volume of RBCs is called the *hematocrit*. As indicated in Figure 6-2, the hematocrit has clinical relevance, since RBC volume changes in a variety of disorders. For example, in polycythemia hematocrits as high as 70% can occur. Such high hematocrits significantly increase resistance to the flow of blood. At the other extreme, severe anemia can result in hematocrits too low to support adequate oxygen delivery.

As indicated in Figure 6-2, the number of RBCs in the circulation is far greater than the number of WBCs. However, the difference is even greater than indicated in this figure since, as shown in Figure 6-1, a RBC is much smaller than a WBC. A more accurate method of obtaining the relative numbers of the different formed elements is to place a drop of blood on a hemocytometer and count the number of cells in a cubic millimeter of blood. This procedure shows that normal blood contains about 5 million RBCs per cubic millimeter but only 5000–8000 WBCs in the same volume. Thus, RBCs

Anemia does not always result from a deficiency of total RBC volume. For example, in hypochromic anemia the number of RBCs per unit of blood may be normal, but the hemoglobin content of the RBCs is depressed. Iron deficiency anemia is a form of hypochromic anemia due to dietary lack of iron.

have a population density 600–1000 times that of WBCs. Despite their relatively small numbers, however, WBCs do affect circulatory dynamics. Because of their size and the fact that many WBCs can "cling" to endothelial cells, they have a tendency to "plug" capillaries. The stop–start flow pattern often seen in systemic capillaries frequently is due to intermittent WBC plugging.

Plasma Composition

Plasma is composed of about 90% water, 7% protein, and 3% inorganic and organic solutes. Of the constituents in plasma, the proteins are quite important in terms of circulatory function. For example, because capillary endothelial cells are in colloidal suspension and are relatively large, their permeability to the plasma proteins is small. Furthermore, protein concentration in plasma is much higher than it is within interstitial fluid. This protein separation creates a special type of osmotic force that tends to hold fluid in the circulatory system. The significance of this reaction with regard to the interchange of fluid between the plasma and interstitium is discussed in Chapter 12.

The three major types of plasma proteins are albumin, globulin, and fibrinogen. Their relative amounts, molecular weights, and percent concentrations in plasma are given in Table 6-1. The most abundant of the plasma proteins, albumins provide the major osmotic force tending to hold fluid in the circulation. In addition, albumins serve important roles as transport carriers for water-insoluble substances such as steroid hormones. This is one reason that children with protein-deficient diets may have compromised endocrine function. The globular proteins also serve as transport carriers (e.g., for sex steroid hormones) as well as functioning in the immune system as antibodies (immunoglobulins). Fibrinogen, the least numerous of the plasma proteins, plays a pivotal role in the blood-clotting process. Finally, globulin and fibrinogen have the ability to bind to RBCs, thereby altering the mechanical properties of circulating blood. The mechanical properties of blood as a fluid come under the general heading of *rheology*.

TABLE 6-1 ▶

The Plasma Proteins

Protein	Percent of Total	Molecular Weight	Concentration (g/100 mL plasma)
Albumin	55	69,000	4.0–6.0
Globulin	38	80,000–200,000	1.5–3.0
Fibrinogen	7	350,000–400,000	0.2–0.4

RHEOLOGIC PROPERTIES OF BLOOD

Rheology is the study of deformation and flow of matter. Therefore, the characteristics of blood that govern its flow properties fall within the discipline of rheology.

Basic Rheologic Principles

Under normal circumstances, whole blood moves through blood vessels, a process called *laminar flow*. Figure 6-3 illustrates the principle of laminar flow. *Part A* shows several rectangular blocks stacked and placed on a fixed plane. If the stack is struck evenly with a mallet such that the same force is applied to each block, then the stack will be displaced in the manner depicted in *part B* of the figure. When the same force is applied, each successive block from the fixed plane is displaced farther to the right in a given amount of time. If each block represents a unit *lamina*, then for a given applied force, each lamina moves with a velocity proportional to its distance from the fixed plane. In effect, each block, or lamina, has been sheared away from its neighbor in response to the applied force. The degree of shearing is determined by the magnitude of the applied force and the frictional resistance between the lamina that opposes their separation.

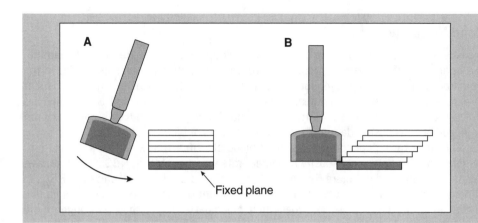

FIGURE 6-3
Laminar Displacement of Blocks as a Result of Being Struck by a Mallet. *Note that each succeeding block from the fixed plane is displaced farther than the one preceding it. (Source: Reprinted with permission from Richardson DR: Basic Circulatory Physiology. Boston, MA: Little, Brown, 1976, p 109.)*

In the flow of a liquid, such as blood through a vessel, the fluid appears to flow in discrete laminae or streamlines. This flow is illustrated in Figure 6-4, which shows an applied force, blood pressure, which represents the shear stress. In response to this stress, the respective laminae are sheared from each other, and the blood flows in such a manner that the velocity of the respective laminae increases from the wall to the center of the vessel in a streamline manner. The difference in velocity between adjacent laminae ($\Delta\dot{V}$) is the shear rate. In the circulatory system, shear rate is proportional to the velocity with which the blood is flowing through a vessel.

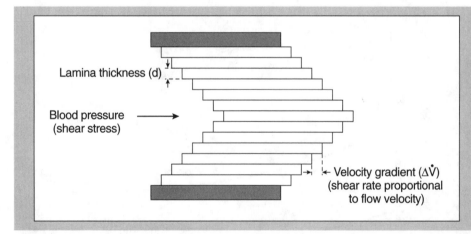

FIGURE 6-4
Illustration of Laminar, or Streamline, Flow in the Circulatory System. *The block analogy of Figure 6-3 is extended to represent the manner in which fluid flows through a vessel in discrete lamina. Blood pressure represents the shear stress, and in response to the shear stress, the laminae are separated from each other with the difference in velocity between two adjacent laminae, representing the velocity gradient.*

A characteristic feature of laminar flow is that the lamina next to the vessel wall remains stationary no matter how large the applied force. Thus, the velocity gradient of a laminar flowing fluid goes from zero at the wall to a maximum value at the center of the flow stream. Quantitatively, the velocity gradient, or shear rate, is defined as the velocity difference between two successive laminae ($\Delta\dot{V}$) divided by the thickness of the lamina (d). In equation form:

$$\text{Shear rate} = \frac{\Delta\dot{V}\ (\text{cm/sec})}{d(\text{cm})} = \frac{1}{(\text{sec})}$$

Therefore, shear rate is given in the unusual units of inverse seconds.

In a liquid, the frictional resistance opposing the separation of the laminae is termed the *viscosity* (η). In quantitative terms, viscosity is given as the ratio of shear stress to shear rate:

$$= \frac{\text{shear stress}}{\text{shear rate}} = \frac{\text{dynes/cm}}{1/\text{sec}} = \frac{\text{dynes sec}}{\text{cm}}$$

Blood Viscosity

Viscosity is a measurement of the internal friction opposing the separation of the lamina. This internal friction is largely responsible for the dissipation of pressure energy in the circulatory system. In a homogeneous fluid, such as water, the viscosity is independent of shear rate; that is, the ratio of shear stress to shear rate is a constant. Such fluids are termed *Newtonian fluids*. Blood, however, is not homogeneous but is a complex fluid composed of cells suspended in plasma. The viscosity of blood is dependent upon shear rate. The shear rate–dependent behavior of blood classifies it as a non-Newtonian fluid. The relationships between viscosity and shear rate for whole blood, RBCs in saline, and plasma are presented in Figure 6-5. Note that relative to whole blood, and even RBCs in saline, plasma has a low viscosity that is independent of shear rate. Thus, plasma is a Newtonian fluid. However, not only does whole blood have a high viscosity throughout the shear rate curve, but at shear rates below about 4 seconds^{-1}, blood viscosity increases sharply as shear rate decreases. Investigations into this relationship have shown that the high viscosity throughout the shear rate curve for whole blood is due to the absolute concentration of the RBCs (the hematocrit). This concentration is indicated in the *middle curve* in Figure 6-5, which shows a substantial viscosity for RBCs suspended in saline when compared to plasma alone.

> **Shear stress** represents an energy force, while **shear rate** represents motion due to the energy force. Therefore, viscosity is a resistance term (energy/motion). This is another example of the application of Ohm's law to nature.

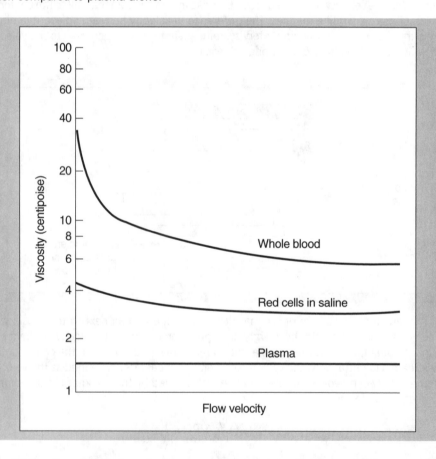

FIGURE 6-5
Relationship Between Fluid Viscosity and Flow Velocity for Whole Blood, RBCs in Saline, and Blood Plasma. *(Source: Reprinted with permission from Well RE: Rheology of the blood. The Microcirculation. Edited by Winter WL, Brest AN. Springfield, IL: Charles C Thomas, 1969, p 11.)*

RBCs affect blood viscosity because solid particles (RBCs) in a Newtonian fluid (plasma) cause a disturbance in the lamina or streamlines such that, in effect, the laminae become thicker, and separation of laminae becomes more difficult. Therefore, the viscous resistance is increased, and the overall viscosity of the fluid rises. As shear rate decreases, the RBCs tend to form aggregates, increasing their effective particle size, which, in turn, increases the viscosity of the blood. This tendency to form aggregates is minimal with RBCs suspended in saline. With whole blood, however, there is a marked increase in RBC aggregation and, consequently viscosity, at low shear rates.

Research into the phenomenon of RBC aggregation indicates that RBC aggregates are formed by cross-bonding of macromolecules on the surface of adjacent RBCs. The macromolecules that cross-bond in this manner are the plasma proteins, primarily globulin and fibrinogen. A percentage of these proteins is always bound to the surface of the RBCs in such a manner that their free ends are available for bonding with other RBCs. At high shear rates, the RBCs are oriented in a streamline manner that minimizes cross-bonding between proteins on separate RBCs; therefore, RBC aggregation is minimal. As shear rate decreases, however, RBC orientation becomes more favorable for cross-bonding of proteins. Thus, RBC aggregation increases, elevating the viscosity of the blood.

In brief, what we have learned thus far is that plasma is a Newtonian fluid in that its viscosity is independent of the rate at which the lamina are separated from one another (the shear rate). Whole blood, however, is non-Newtonian in that its viscosity is shear rate–dependent. This shear rate–dependent behavior of whole blood is due to the tendency of RBCs to form aggregations as a result of cross-bonding between plasma proteins that adhere to the surface of RBCs.

In all laminar flowing fluids, shear rate is proportional to shear stress. In the circulatory system, blood pressure serves as the shear stressing force. On the arterial side of the circulation where blood pressure is high, the shear rate of the blood is also high, and viscosity is relatively low. On the venous side, however, where blood pressure is quite low, shear rate is also low, and blood viscosity can be several times greater than that observed on the arterial side of the system.

Evidence indicates that in the circulatory system, shear rate is at its lowest point within the immediate postcapillary venules [1], probably because this region has the combination of a low blood pressure and a low mean cross-sectional flow velocity. In these vessels, blood viscosity is highest. This high viscosity may be a major source of the postcapillary contribution to vascular resistance.

Effect of Vessel Size on Blood Viscosity

The viscosity of whole blood is dependent upon the size of the tube or vessel through which the blood flows. The relationship between blood viscosity and tube size is presented in Figure 6-6. Note that with vessels of a radius greater than 1.0 mm, viscosity is independent of tube size; however, viscosity falls sharply as the tube radius decreases below this size. This direct relationship between blood viscosity and vessel size with vessels up to 1.0 mm in radius is known as the *Fahraeus-Lindqvist effect* (named after the investigators who discovered the phenomenon).

Since the range of vessel diameters in the microcirculation is approximately 0.004–

Observation of the retinal circulation by use of an ophthalmoscope allows the physician to view RBC aggregations directly in microvessels. An increase in RBC aggregations above normal is indicative of infectious disease. This is because with infection the concentration of circulating globular proteins is elevated.

An increase in RBC aggregation indicative of infection occurs mainly in postcapillary venules.

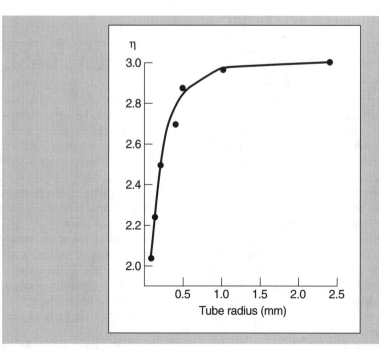

FIGURE 6-6
Relationship Between Viscosity (η) of Blood and Radius of the Tube Through Which the Blood Is Flowing: The Fahraeus-Lindqvist Effect. In this graph, viscosity is presented relative to that of water. (Source: *Reprinted with permission from Burton AC:* Physiology and Biophysics of the Circulation. *Chicago, IL: Year Book, 1965, p 53.)*

0.10 mm, the Fahraeus-Lindqvist effect is an important aspect of microcirculatory dynamics. As the vessels become smaller, that is, from arterioles to capillaries, blood viscosity decreases.

Rearranging the equation for Poiseuille's law, given in Chapter 3, and solving for vascular resistance, $(P_1 - P_2)/\dot{Q} = 8\,nl/\pi r^4$. This equation shows that a decrease in viscosity with smaller tube size tends to offset the effect of a decreasing radius on resistance to the flow of blood through a single vessel.

In terms of a mechanism, physiologists and biophysicists do not fully agree on an explanation for the cause of the Fahraeus-Lindqvist effect. One explanation, which seems at least theoretically sound, is the "plasma zone" hypothesis: near the wall of the vessel, a zone of blood exists that is relatively free of RBCs and, therefore, has a lower viscosity than that of plasma. As the vessel size decreases, the fraction of the blood that constitutes the cell free zone increases, and, therefore, the total effective viscosity decreases.

Nature of Blood Flow Through Capillaries

The consideration of blood as a laminar-flowing fluid is valid only for vessels of more than two or three RBCs in diameter (≈ 14–$20\,\mu$). At the level of the smallest blood vessels, the capillaries, RBCs tend to flow in single file and usually in a deformed shape. Flowing between the RBCs in a capillary is a bolus of plasma. According to Whitmore, within this bolus exist several eddy currents that make the plasma appear to traverse the capillary in a circular motion [2]. This mixing of the plasma as it flows through a capillary has the obvious physiologic significance of exposing all the plasma to the endothelial exchange surface area. This flow behavior adds a high degree of complexity to blood flow mechanics.

> The tendency for plasma to mix in eddy current fashion is thought to be a major reason why the circulatory time for plasma is lower than the circulatory time for RBCs.

In summary, the flow of blood in the circulation, particularly in microvessels, displays markedly non-Newtonian behavior. The characteristics of blood that make it non-Newtonian in the microvascular region are as follows:

1. At any particular vessel size, blood viscosity increases as shear rate decreases. This effect is significant in the venules where shear stress (pressure) is lowest.

2. In a microcirculatory network, blood viscosity is directly proportional to vessel diameter (the Fahraeus-Lindqvist effect).

3. At the capillary level, the laminar or streamline nature of blood flow is replaced by a flow pattern characterized by the single-file passage of RBCs, with a turbulent bolus of plasma flowing between the RBCs.

RESOLUTION OF CLINICAL CASE

The patient introduced at the beginning of the chapter has a bone marrow disorder known as *Waldenström's macroglobulinemia*. This disease is similar to multiple myeloma in that it is characterized by an abnormal production of the lymphocytes that secrete immunoglobulins. This disorder tends to "crowd out" the production of other formed elements, such as RBCs and the granulocytic leukocytes. The general disruption of formed element production is probably the cause of many of the symptoms and clinical findings in this case, such as a low hematocrit, frequent infections, and retinal hemorrhage.

The patient's speech impairment and tendency toward fatigue are part of a general symptom known as *paresis*, or incomplete paralysis. In this case, paresis probably is due to disruption of spinal nerves or the presence of ischemic areas of the brain.

Waldenström's macroglobulinemia is characterized by overproduction of an immunoglobulin known as IgM, a relatively large globular protein. The presence of abnormal amounts of a large globular protein markedly increases the incidence of RBC aggregation. The increased RBC aggregation gives rise to a *hyperviscosity syndrome*, which is interpreted as sluggish blood flow and RBC clumping in the patient's retinal vessels. The dilated arterioles in the patient's retinal circulation likely reflect an autoregulatory response to reduced blood flow.

Abnormal globulins, such as those produced in this disease, have a tendency to precipitate at low temperatures. This markedly increases blood viscosity, thereby reducing blood flow in extremities exposed to cold weather. Reduced blood flow to the extremities explains the patient's *Raynaud's* symptom of painful hands. Furthermore, reduced blood flow to the extremities vis-à-vis a compromised immune system explains the ulcers on the patient's hands and fingers.

Finally, in Waldenström's macroglobulinemia, the globular proteins infiltrate the lymph nodes and spleen. This infiltration probably accounts for the patient's sensation of abdominal fullness.

REVIEW QUESTIONS

Directions: For each of the following questions, choose the **one best** answer.

1. A deficiency in erythropoietin is associated with
   - **(A)** an increase in blood viscosity
   - **(B)** lymphocyte deficiency
   - **(C)** a reduction in hematocrit
   - **(D)** a decrease in platelet production

2. An increase in the synthesis of globular proteins, as occurs with an infection, elicits
   - **(A)** a reduction in hematocrit
   - **(B)** an increase in blood viscosity
   - **(C)** a decrease in clotting ability
   - **(D)** anemia
   - **(E)** a reduced capacity to transport steroid hormones

3. As blood moves from arterioles into capillaries, which of the following actions is likely to occur?
   - **(A)** Blood viscosity increases because flow velocity decreases
   - **(B)** Blood viscosity decreases because vessel diameter becomes smaller
   - **(C)** Resistance to the flow of blood decreases because vessel diameter becomes smaller
   - **(D)** Resistance to the flow of blood increases because proportionately more of the vessel surface area is exposed to plasma

4. As blood flow through a vessel decreases, resistance to the flow of blood
   - **(A)** increases because RBCs tend to aggregate
   - **(B)** increases because blood pressure increases
   - **(C)** increases because hematocrit increases
   - **(D)** decreases because blood viscosity decreases
   - **(E)** decreases because RBC aggregates tend to break apart

ANSWERS AND EXPLANATIONS

1. **The answer is C.** A deficiency in erythropoietin is associated with a reduction in hematocrit. Erythropoietin is the hormone that stimulates RBC synthesis. Without adequate production of RBCs, hematocrit is reduced. The lymphocytes and platelets are not as affected, and viscosity decreases rather than increases.

2. **The answer is B.** An increase in the synthesis of globular proteins, as occurs with an infection, elicits an increase in blood viscosity. An increase in globular proteins increases cross-bonding of RBCs, the mechanism of RBC aggregation. An increase in RBC aggregation results in an increase in blood viscosity. Hematocrit, hence anemia, is not affected. Clotting ability might increase, but it definitely does not decrease. Finally, since globular proteins, in part, transport steroids, the transport capacity for steroid hormones increases; it does not decrease.

3. **The answer is B.** As blood moves from arterioles into capillaries, blood viscosity decreases because vessel diameter becomes smaller. This is an expression of the Fahraeus-Lindqvist effect (see Figure 6-6). The flow velocity in capillaries is usually lower, but viscosity does not tend to increase, again as a result of the Fahraeus-Lindqvist effect. Resistance to flow does decrease in capillaries, but because the collective cross-sectional area of capillaries increases, not because vessel diameter of individual capillaries becomes smaller. Proportionately more of the vessel surface area is exposed to plasma in capillaries, but this causes resistance to decrease, not increase—the Fahraeus-Lindqvist effect.

4. **The answer is A.** As blood flow through a vessel decreases, resistance to the flow of blood increases because RBCs tend to aggregate. At any particular vessel diameter, as blood flow decreases, flow velocity and shear rate decrease. A decrease in shear rate elicits an increase in viscosity as a result of an increase in RBC aggregation. An increase in viscosity results in an increase in resistance to the flow of blood— Poiseuille's law. An increase in blood pressure elicits an increase in resistance, but this is due to myogenic vasoconstriction, not a decrease in blood flow. Hematocrit is the percentage of RBCs in whole blood. This variable is not affected by blood flow. A decrease in blood viscosity decreases, not increases, resistance. RBC aggregates tend to form, not break apart, as blood flow decreases.

REFERENCES

1. Chien S: Present state of blood rheology. In *Hemodilution: Theoretical Basis and Clinical Application*. Edited by Messmer K, Schmid–Schonbein H. Munich: Karger, 1972, pp 1–45.
2. Whitmore RL: A theory of blood flow in small vessels. *J Appl Physiol* 22:767–771, 1967.

7

FUNDAMENTALS OF CARDIOPULMONARY REGULATION

PRACTICAL AND CLINICAL IMPLICATIONS OF HOMEOSTASIS

The scientific and practical benefits of studying successively more discrete *components* of living systems have been repeatedly demonstrated. In fact, research at the cellular and subcellular levels is among the most aggressive in the medical sciences and has yielded qualitatively new insights into how biologic systems function. While science must break down living systems to analyze how the individual parts function, the clinician must assemble the insights gained from these reductionist studies to understand how the organism functions as a whole. This is why the wise physician takes a comprehensive medical history to evaluate his or her patient's physical condition from a broadly *integrative* viewpoint. Nonetheless, it is often difficult to view the results of highly focused studies within the context of the whole organism. The goal of this chapter is to explain some of the mechanisms the body uses to integrate and control the myriad parts of the human cardiopulmonary system.

HOMEOSTASIS AND INTEGRATIVE PHYSIOLOGY

Chapter 1 explains that homeostasis is the focus concept of this textbook: within a wide range of environmental conditions, biofeedback is able to maintain the constancy of a variety of physiologic variables despite harsh external challenges. Regulation of arterial blood pressure is an important example of homeostasis within the cardiovascular system. The body is normally capable of maintaining blood pressure within a relatively narrow range despite changing posture, going from a state of rest to one of rigorous physical activity, or gaining fluid through drinking or losing it by sweating. It is important to understand the mechanisms whereby this stability is achieved. However, there are some hidden consequences of how homeostatic systems are organized and function. It is vital that the physician understand these consequences as well as the fundamental regulatory mechanisms.

Three major systems are involved in maintaining blood pressure stability. First, changes in the function of the *heart and vasculature* directly alter arterial pressure. Heart rate (HR), stroke volume (SV), and peripheral vascular resistance are all influenced by the autonomic nervous system (ANS); a significant part of this neural regulation involves a

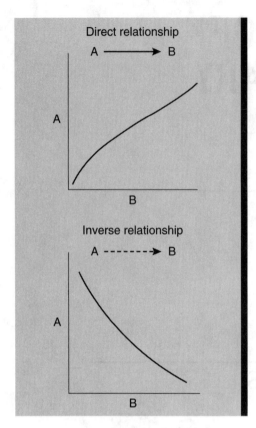

Direct relationship

A ——————➤ B

B

Inverse relationship

A - - - - - ➤ B

B

Despite the visual impression in Figure 7-1 that blood pressure is "the" regulated variable, in reality all variables within a closed "cycle of causation" are subject to tight regulation. In fact, sometimes physiologists find it convenient to regard CO as "the" regulated variable.

feedback cycle that regulates blood pressure known as the *baroreflex* (see Chapter 13). Second, changes in *renal function* also profoundly alter pressure by controlling the amount of salt and water retained within the body and, thereby, the total volume of blood within the circulation. Some components of the renal control of blood volume are also influenced by the baroreflex. In addition to direct renal control, fluid shifts into and out of the cellular and extracellular fluid compartments can play a significant role in stabilizing blood volume. Third, the *endocrine system* influences blood pressure in several ways, primarily by modulating the function of the other systems.

Figure 7-1 is a simplified presentation of some of the baroreflex pathways that operate upon cardiovascular and renal regulation of blood pressure. The cycle diagram portrays the qualitative nature of the relationships between variables within the cycle: a *solid arrow* linking two variables indicates a direct relationship such that an increase in the first variable acts to increase the second (or a decrease in the first leads to a decrease in the second); conversely, a *dashed arrow* indicates an inverse relationship between the two variables such that an increase in the first yields a decrease in the second (or vice versa). An odd number of *dashed arrows* within a cycle is required for negative feedback.

Although the cycles in panels A and B of Figure 7-1 look distinctly different—and deliberately convey two very different visual impressions—the physiologic relationships between the variables are identical in the two illustrations. Both depictions show that if blood pressure were to increase because of some external or internal challenge, the baroreflex would cause a decrease in cardiac and renal sympathetic nerve activity (SNA). One loop shows that the decrease in SNA would decrease myocardial contractility (see Chapter 3), which, in turn, would tend to decrease cardiac output (CO) [see Chapter 4]. The remaining loop shows that the decrease in SNA directed to the kidney would tend to reduce plasma volume because of a decrease in renal retention of salt and water. *Both the decrease in CO and the decrease in plasma volume offset the original increase in blood pressure, maintaining a stable blood pressure!* In addition, note that the different visual impact of the presentation of the cycles in panels A and B can be used to demonstrate two important hidden consequences of homeostatic feedback cycles.

The cycles in Figure 7-1A and B both focus upon arterial blood pressure, deliberately creating the impression that blood pressure is the central variable. Panel A, however, also emphasizes that the two pathways are "nested." Nesting refers to the existence of multiple parallel pathways focused around the regulated variable. This type of organization has two important consequences:

1. *Nesting multiple cycles increase the stability of the regulated variable.* As mentioned in Chapter 1, physiologic homeostatic systems have multiple levels of nesting that normally assure adequate maintenance of stability. This is loosely analogous to an engineer's design of multiple "backup" systems at critical points in important mechanical systems.

2. *Nesting may obscure disease processes that are occurring within one or more components of the overall system.* For example, blood pressure can be maintained even if myocardial function (inner cycle, Figure 7-1A) is seriously compromised, because renal function (outer cycle, Figure 7-1A) compensates via adjustments in plasma volume. Thus, a normal blood pressure can mislead physicians into believing that a patient is healthy unless they consider the wider implications of nested feedback control systems. This is a major consideration in Chapters 9 and 10.

Figure 7-1B emphasizes the coupling between the two cycles and de-emphasizes the nesting. The two cycles interact through their common element, arterial blood pressure. The function of the common element may be compared to the cogs on two coupled gears: a torquing force exerted on one gear is transmitted via the cogs to the other gear. The physiologic corollary is that *because feedback cycles interact through common elements, a pathologic disturbance in one physiologic system may adversely influence the function of the entire organism.* In Figure 7-1, for example, a degenerative process in the kidney (e.g., glomerulonephritis) can ultimately profoundly affect how the heart functions. Here is perhaps the most compelling rationale for an integrative approach to medical education and, eventually, to medical practice. *Because of the interaction between systems produced by coupled homeostatic systems, the physician must view that organ's function within the context of the whole body rather than focus myopically upon the function of a single organ.*

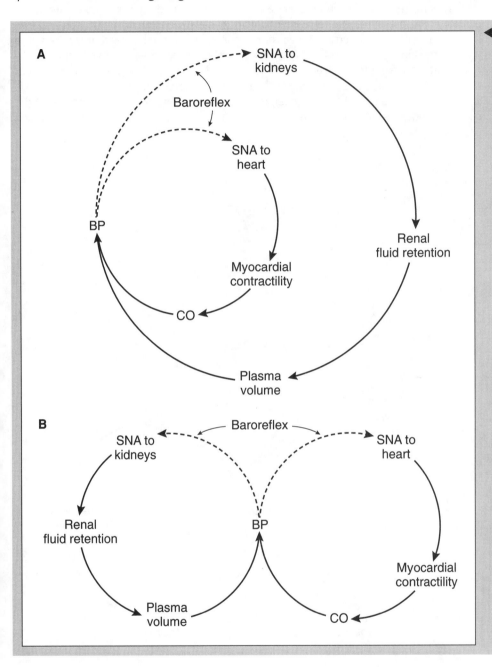

FIGURE 7-1
Biofeedback Cycles Focusing upon Control of Arterial Blood Pressure. *(A) This figure illustrates nesting of the two cycles. The outer loop portrays renal control of plasma volume; the inner loop focuses upon one aspect of the baroreflex control of cardiac output (CO). Nesting of cycles improves the stability of "the" regulated variable. (B) This figure illustrates the same physiologic relationships shown in panel A; however, this panel emphasizes the coupling of the "renal" pathway with the "cardiac" pathway via the common element, blood pressure. In reality, many systems are coupled by common elements throughout the body. As a result of this coupling, functional changes—or pathologic processes—in one system can influence many other systems throughout the organism. SNA = sympathetic nervous activity; BP = blood pressure.*

EXTRINSIC AND INTRINSIC HOMEOSTATIC SYSTEMS

Neuroendocrine homeostatic regulation of function depends upon a decision-making element, or transfer component (see Chapter 1), and upon efferent pathways that are located *outside* of the cardiopulmonary system; in particular, the transfer components of these "extrinsic" control systems are often within the central nervous system (CNS). *Extrinsic regulatory mechanisms generally are able to adjust respiratory or cardiovascular function within seconds to minutes of the onset of a challenge to homeostasis.* On the other hand, the cardiopulmonary system has a built-in, natural stability as a result of the inherent properties of the constituent tissues and organs. *Intrinsic control mechanisms*

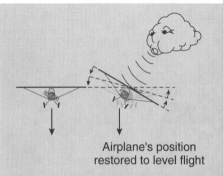

Airplane's position
restored to level flight

A small aircraft affords a good example of a system with both extrinsic and intrinsic stabilization. The pilot—who is ideally a good "transfer component"—may adjust the stick or rudder controls to minimize changes in the airplane's attitude in gusty flying conditions. Alternatively, aeronautic engineers design the distribution of the aircraft's center of gravity with respect to the wings in order to restore a level flight position naturally, even if the pilot elects simply to hold the "stick" steady when flight conditions are erratic.

sometimes respond more slowly to a perturbation than the reflexive cycles—perhaps even over days; however, they endow the organism with an inherent, long-term stability. Figure 7-2 illustrates how the combined actions of the kidney's ability to produce urine in proportion to renal perfusion pressure and the neurally mediated baroreflex interact to control blood pressure. The renal mechanism (cycle A), described by Guyton and colleagues [1, 2], does not require nerves or hormones to function; instead, it is inherent in the way the kidney works. This cycle appears to play a very important role in the day-to-day maintenance of blood pressure stability. Cycle B represents (only) one component of the arterial baroreflex. The "command center"—the transfer component—of this cycle is within the brainstem, and several other key components are anatomically not part of the circulation per se. The baroreflex is vital to maintaining moment-to-moment blood pressure stability.

FIGURE 7-2 ▶

Combined Action of Intrinsic and Extrinsic Feedback Cycles in Regulation of Blood Pressure. *(A) The left cycle is one example of an inherent stability attributable to physiologic mechanisms that do not require neurohumoral mediation. In this case, the ability of the kidney to increase urine excretion when blood pressure increases— pressure diuresis—provides long-term blood pressure stability. (B) The right cycle portrays one component of the arterial baroreflex. The baroreflex depends upon neural pathways that are external to the cardiovascular system. The baroreflex assures that blood pressure remains within a restricted range despite moment-to-moment external or internal challenges to the cardiopulmonary system. SNA = sympathetic nervous activity; BP = blood pressure.*

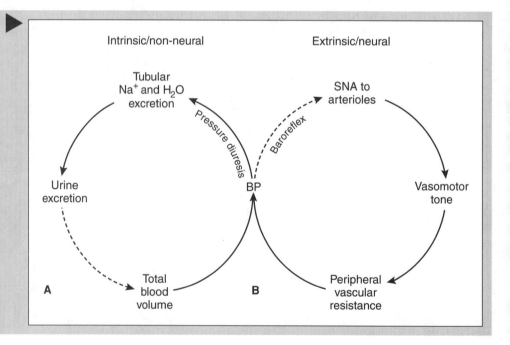

MULTIPLE LEVELS OF CARDIOPULMONARY CONTROL

Physiologic systems often have two (or more) levels of regulation. Many textbook descriptions of cardiopulmonary regulation are restricted to the brainstem's control of cardiopulmonary function. More recently, physiologists have begun to appreciate the potential importance of multiple "levels" of regulation (Figure 7-3). Although these may be arranged in a hierarchical manner, it is not at all clear that "higher" levels inevitably dominate "lower" levels in all cases. In fact, it may be more accurate to think of these different levels of control as "nested" systems that interact to achieve the appropriate regulation.

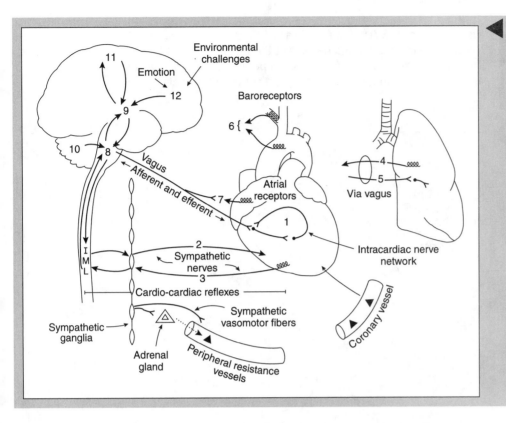

FIGURE 7-3
Multiple Levels of Extrinsic Regulation of Cardiopulmonary Function. Neural pathways include the intracardiac nerve network (1), efferent (2) and afferent (3) fibers carried in the sympathetic nerves, vagal afferent (4) and efferent (5) fibers innervating the lungs and bronchial tree, sensory fibers from the aorta and carotid sinus regions (6) and from the atria (7). The sympathetic ganglia, the intermediolateral (IML) column of the spinal cord, the brainstem (8), the diencephalon (9), the cerebellum (10), and "higher" centers (11) all participate in the regulation of the heart, lungs, and arteriolar resistance vessels of the circulation. Emotions or external challenges (12) can profoundly change cardiovascular and respiratory function. Circulating hormones (▲) transported from the adrenal gland (△) and other endocrine glands to the heart (via the coronary vessels) or to the vascular smooth muscle of the resistance vessels influence both the heart and vasculature.

At the "highest" level of control, the forebrain plays an important role in coordinating anticipatory responses for both the cardiovascular and respiratory systems. Hypothalamic regulation also participates in emotional and autonomic regulation for both systems. The fundamental neuro- and neurohumoral reflexes are integrated at the brainstem, using many common nuclei, even providing input to many of the same interneurons. Segmental control can occur through the autonomic ganglia and through the spinal cord somatic reflexes associated with the respiratory pump. At the "lower" levels of control, the "heart brain" [3], a network of neurons within the heart, appears to be capable of influencing cardiac function in cooperation with the CNS [4]. Axon reflexes may play an important role in regulating smooth muscle function in the airways and blood vessels. Additional control is exerted through the intrinsic properties of the cardiac and smooth muscle. It appears likely that these multiple control systems interact to assure a more effective and more efficient regulation than would otherwise be possible.

BIOFEEDBACK CYCLES AND DISEASE

Physicians are often called to deal with very ill patients whose cardiopulmonary systems are incapable of meeting any additional demands beyond those at rest. What accounts for the dramatic changes in function that occur in disease and at death? Figure 7-4 presents one view of this complex process. Panel A illustrates how a heart with a healthy myocardium responds to a change in the amount of blood delivered to it from the periphery (or pulmonary circulation): a change in preload (Chapter 4). The graph at the top of panel A shows an important relationship between the volume of blood in the ventricle at the end of diastole (EDV) and the resulting SV. This is known as "Starling's law of the heart" (see Chapter 10) and is explained in part by the myocardial active length–tension relationship presented in Chapter 4. A healthy ventricle would function within a normal operating range of preloads on the *ascending limb* of the relationship (*dark portion of curve*, panel A). The bottom portion of panel A expresses the relationships between EDV, SV, and end

SV equals the volume of blood inside the left ventricle at the end of diastole minus the volume at the end of systole: SV = EDV − ESV.

Note that the feedback cycle also "works" if the initial perturbation is a decrease in EDV; this tends to decrease SV, which increases ESV, which tends to increase EDV to a more normal value.

systolic volume (ESV) that prevail in a healthy heart: an increase in EDV tends to increase SV; an increase in SV would decrease ESV, which would, in turn, tend to decrease EDV. This cycle is stable because the original perturbation—an engorgement of the ventricle at the end of diastole—was offset by the action of the cycle.

FIGURE 7-4 ▶

Homeostatic Cycles in Health and Disease. (A) The top portion graphs Starling's law of the heart in the healthy person where end diastolic volume (EDV) remains within a normal range on the ascending limb (dark portion of curve). As a result, the feedback cycle representing Starling's law (bottom left) is homeostatic, as evidenced by an odd number of dashed arrows. (B) The top graph shows a depressed ventricular function curve with the heart operating at or near the plateau (dark portion of curve) of Starling's law. Since changes in EDV no longer produce changes in stroke volume (SV), the feedback cycle (bottom) is interrupted and can no longer effectively maintain homeostasis. (C) The top graph illustrates what would happen if a "descending limb" (dotted line) were to appear in Starling's law. The moment the heart started to operate on this portion of the curve, the relationship between changes in EDV and SV would be reversed from normal: an increase in EDV would decrease SV, and vice versa. The feedback relationships (bottom) would suddenly convert to a positive cycle, and death would quickly ensue. CHF = congestive heart failure.

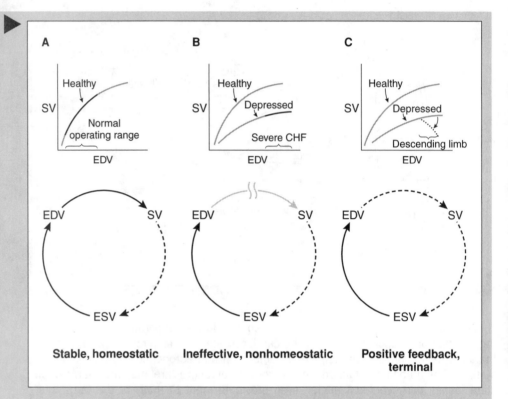

A feedback diagram with an even number (0, 2, 4, . . .) of dashed arrows is a positive cycle; the cycle amplifies disturbances rather than reducing them. In the cycle shown in the bottom portion of Figure 7-4C, an increase in EDV would decrease SV; since the heart ejects less blood, this would increase ESV and further increase EDV. This explosive cycle could last only a few heartbeats before the heart arrests in asystole.

Figure 7-4B shows what occurs in a patient with severe congestive heart failure (CHF). The Starling curve is depressed; consequently, SV is unacceptably low at normal preloads. Therefore, to maintain adequate output, EDV becomes so high that the ventricle functions on the plateau of the curve (*dark portion of curve*, panel B). *The fact that the curve is "flat" in this region means that the relationship between EDV and SV is effectively interrupted: increases (or decreases) in EDV no longer produce increases (or decreases) in SV.* This decoupling between two major elements in the feedback cycle (*dashed arrow*, bottom portion, panel B) means that the cycle is no longer functional: this important adaptive mechanism for regulating SV has failed. As a result, the stability of the overall cardiopulmonary system decreases. Although other nested elements may be able to maintain some degree of homeostasis, untreated patients with this condition typically are unable to walk across a room or sleep comfortably at night. Moreover, this means that heart size, instead of being maintained within a mechanically advantageous range (see the section entitled "Implications of Laplace's Law for Cardiac Pump Function" in Chapter 10), remains within high ranges of EDV at which even greater myocardial fiber damage can occur [5]. Such is the inevitable result when physiologic regulatory mechanisms fail to the extent that they can no longer maintain function when external or internal challenges occur.

Figure 7-4C illustrates one possible series of events that can cause immediate death in patients with end-stage CHF. As mentioned in Chapter 10, the existence of a "descending limb" (upper portion, panel C) in Starling's law of the heart has been hotly debated. Suppose for a moment that it does exist and that a patient's heart suddenly converts from operating on the plateau (panel B) to a descending limb (*dotted line*, top portion, panel C). This would change the normal *direct* relationship between EDV and SV (i.e., $\uparrow$EDV $\rightarrow$ $\uparrow$SV or $\downarrow$EDV $\rightarrow$ $\downarrow$SV) to an *inverse* relationship (i.e., $\uparrow$EDV $\rightarrow$ $\downarrow$SV or $\downarrow$EDV $\rightarrow$ $\uparrow$SV). As a result, the relationship between EDV and SV would now be represented by a *dashed arrow* (bottom portion, panel C) rather than the normal *solid arrow* (bottom portion, panel A). The normal homeostatic cycle becomes an "explosive" positive cycle, and death ensues within a very few heartbeats. It is a common clinical axiom that death occurs (only) when a major system fails. This failure may take the form of a regulatory cycle that can no longer maintain stability [6].

SUMMARY

The integrative control of cardiopulmonary function at multiple levels and within multiple nested cycles has three practical consequences for the physician. First, circulatory and respiratory function is amazingly resilient even when serious external and internal challenges occur. Second, the consequences of even serious failure of one or more components of the cardiopulmonary system may not be immediately obvious to the patient or the physician because compensatory changes in other components of mutually linked cycles maintain overall function. Third, the consequences of pathologic changes in one component of the cardiopulmonary system eventually have an impact on how other components function. Accordingly, the physician dare not consider any element of the cardiopulmonary system out of the context of the whole.

REFERENCES

1. Guyton AC, Jones CE, Coleman TG: *Circulatory Physiology: Cardiac Output and Its Regulation*, 2nd ed. Philadelphia, PA: W. B. Saunders, 1973.
2. Guyton AC, Coleman TG, Cowley AW: A system analysis approach to understand long-range arterial blood pressure control and hypertension. *Circ Res* 35:159–176, 1974.
3. Randall WC, Wurster RD, Randall DC, et al: From cardioacceleratory and inhibitory nerves to a "heart brain": an evolution of concepts. In *Nervous Control of the Heart*. Edited by Shepherd JT, Vatner SF. Amsterdam, B.V.: Harwood Academic Publishers, 1996, pp 173–199.
4. Ardell JL: Structure and function of mammalian intrinsic cardiac neurons. In *Neuro-cardiology*. Edited by Armour JA, Ardell JL. New York, NY: Oxford University Press, 1994, pp. 95–114.
5. Komamura K, Shannon RP, Ihara T, et al: Exhaustion of Frank–Starling mechanism in conscious dogs with heart failure. *Am J Physiol* 265:H1119–H1131, 1993.
6. Engelberg JE: On the dynamics of dying. *Integr Physiol Behav Sci* 32:143–148, 1997.

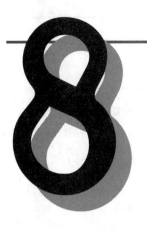

CARDIAC ELECTROPHYSIOLOGY AND THE ELECTROCARDIOGRAM

INTRODUCTION OF CLINICAL CASE

A 31-year-old woman experienced a brief loss of consciousness while driving. She regained control of her automobile upon reviving and immediately reported to the emergency room of a local hospital. She denied chest pain but reported that she had experienced periodic episodes of "skipped beats" in the past. She said it felt as though her heart was going to "jump out of my chest" for the beat following the skipped beat. On a few occasions in the past, her pulse had "disappeared" for up to 5 seconds, but she had never lost consciousness before. She had no history of *orthopnea* (i.e., difficulty in breathing except when sitting upright, which is characteristic of congestive heart failure [CHF]) or of dyspnea on exertion.

The woman was hospitalized, and her electrocardiogram (ECG) was monitored continuously on a telemetry ward. The ECG showed no evidence of acute myocardial infarction, nor did blood tests show changes in enzyme levels indicative of a heart attack. Her physician observed multiple incidents of premature ventricular contractions (PVCs) and episodes of nonsustained ventricular tachycardia. The QT interval ranged from 480–520 msec when her heart was beating in a sinus rhythm. During the hospitalization, the physician placed her on a β-adrenergic blocking agent. She was released from the hospital when the β-blocker had been titrated to a dose at which the ventricular tachycardia no longer occurred, although there were a few persisting PVCs. Her physician instructed her to call him immediately if her pulse disappeared again or if she experienced episodes of lightheadedness.

INTRODUCTION TO CARDIAC ELECTROPHYSIOLOGY

The cardiac action potential can be explained by the concentration gradients of ions across the cell membrane, by changes in the electrical characteristics of the cell membrane, and by the resulting flow of ionic currents into and out of the cell. *As knowledge of the individual components of the cell membrane continues to increase, it seems inevitable that a thorough understanding of cellular electrophysiology will become essential to the competent practice of medicine* (see Resolution of Clinical Case). Action potentials recorded from dissimilar parts of the heart, such as the sinoatrial (SA) node versus ventricular muscle, differ significantly. These differences also can be explained in terms of electrophysiologic properties of the membrane. Depolarization of the heart is highly coordinated because cardiac myocytes are electrically intercoupled via gap junctions. This integrated change in the polarization of countless myocytes results in an electrical signal that can be recorded on the body surface known as the ECG. The timing of the spread of the depolarization and repolarization of myocytes across the heart determines the various "waves" of the ECG.

General Characteristics of the Ventricular Muscle Action Potential

Figure 8-1 shows a transmembrane voltage recording from a ventricular myocyte that is initially at rest (*electrical diastole*) and then sustains an action potential (*electrical systole*). Notice the following general characteristics of this recording:

- The membrane potential (E_m) is *electronegative* (i.e., the inside of the cell is negatively charged relative to the outside of the cell) and *stable* during electrical diastole. Electrical diastole constitutes the resting phase, or *phase 4*, of the ventricular muscle action potential.
- The rate of change of voltage, dV/dt, is *extremely rapid* during the rising phase of the action potential. This rapid depolarization is called *phase 0*.
- E_m peaks briefly, and then starts to repolarize. This short-lived, partial repolarization constitutes *phase 1*.

- The limited repolarization of phase 1 is followed by a sustained *plateau* or *phase 2*, during which E_m remains near 0 mV for longer than 200 msec. This long plateau phase is one of the major differences between ventricular muscle action potentials and those of skeletal muscle or of typical neurons.

- The cell repolarizes during *phase 3*. The *effective refractory period*, during which no new action potential can be generated, does not end until the cell has largely repolarized.

> Proper function of the heart requires sequential periods of muscle relaxation and ventricular filling followed by muscle contraction and ejection. The tension developed by the muscle peaks prior to the end of the long effective refractory period. Therefore, **cardiac muscle cannot tetanize**. The inability of the myocardium to tetanize protects the heart from sustained contracture in an unremitting systole.

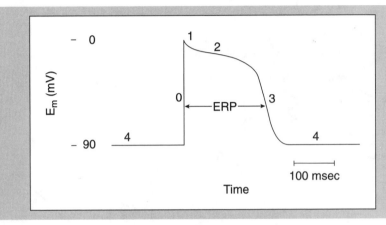

◀ **FIGURE 8-1**
A transmembrane potential (E_m) from a ventricular myocyte showing a typical action potential that consists of four phases. Another action potential cannot be elicited until the end of the effective refractory period (ERP).

Current–Voltage (I/V) Relationship

It is helpful when studying cardiac electrophysiology to review some fundamental laws governing the flow of currents around a circuit. The goal is to derive a relationship between the voltage across the membrane (i.e., E_m) and the current that flows through different kinds of ion channels that span the membrane; this is known as the *current–voltage relationship* (or diagram). We will accomplish this by developing a simple electrical model of a cell. Although this first model is unrealistic in many ways, it is helpful in an initial attempt to understand the electrical basis of the cardiac action potential. The model will then be refined to make it more realistic.

Membrane Conductance. Imagine an observer standing astride the thin membrane that separates the inside of the cell from the extracellular medium. He sees a 90-mV battery in series with a resistor; together they span the membrane such that the inside of the cell is electronegative. The battery represents the transmembrane potential difference (E_m) that is recorded when a microelectrode penetrates the cell's interior (see Figure 8-1). The E_m results from electrochemical forces acting across the membrane. The resistor corresponds to a channel that permits ions to enter or exit the cell. The battery and resistor, plus a pathway for return current that is hidden from view for the moment, constitute a circuit that is diagrammed in Figure 8-2A.

The observer's job is to count all the charges that flow through the membrane each second. Because the resistor is the only pathway through the membrane, the observer is actually measuring the current (number of charged particles/time) flowing through the cell's "ion channels." He measures the flow as 100 picoamperes (pA). Figure 8-2B contains a coordinate axis for plotting this observation. Current is plotted on the ordinate, and the battery voltage is plotted on the abscissa. In I/V relationships like this, electrophysiologists assign the lower (i.e., negative) limb of the y-axis to the flow of positive charge from the outside of the cell to the inside; they refer to such a flow as an *inward current*. By this same logic, negative charges exiting the cell also produce an inward current, but movement of anions does not play a dominant role in causing cardiac muscle action potentials. Because the inside of the cell is negative (corresponding to the left half of the coordinate plane), this first set of numbers resides in the *lower left quadrant* of Figure 8-2B, where it is marked using the symbol "o."

> The quantity of electric charge is measured in coulombs (C). A single electron (or an ion with one positive charge) carries a charge equal to 1.6×10^{-19} C. The rate of flow of electric charge (i.e., number of charged particles/time) is measured in amperes (A). An ampere is the amount of current that is produced by a potential difference of 1 volt (V) acting across a resistor of 1 ohm (Ω). Alternately, a coulomb is the amount of charge flowing in a current of 1 A in 1 second. Currents in physiologic systems are measured in milliamperes (mA; 10^{-3} A), microamperes (μA; 10^{-6} A), nanoamperes (nA; 10^{-9} A), or picoamperes (pA; 10^{-12} A).

Now suppose that the voltage of the battery is somehow decreased to 45 mV without changing its polarity (i.e., the inside of the cell is still negative). The vigilant spectator reports that 50 pA are now flowing through the membrane into the cell; this new information is recorded in Figure 8-2B with the symbol "●." Next, the battery's polarity is reversed, and the observer finds that a 50 pA current is now exiting the cell. This time, the symbol for this data point (■) is in the *upper right quadrant*, because the flow is in the opposite direction. The I/V relationship for this circuit is drawn by connecting the three observations, as is shown in Figure 8-2B.

FIGURE 8-2 ▶

Elementary Electrical Model of a Cell Membrane. (A) This figure shows a simple circuit representing some important electrical properties of the cell membrane. The resistor (R) corresponds to a channel that allows ions to enter or leave the cell. This element of the circuit may also be viewed as a conductor whose value, G, equals 1/R. The battery corresponds to the cell's transmembrane potential difference (E_m). For a nonselective membrane, E_m must equal zero. In reality, most resting cells have an E_m of about -90 mV because of the selectivity of the membrane to potassium. An observer positioned across the membrane is able to count the current flowing through the membrane, I_m, at any given instant. (B) This figure shows the current–voltage (I/V) diagram for this circuit. I_m, as recorded by the observer, is given on the ordinate with the flow of positive ions into the cell plotted in the lower (negative) axis. E_m is on the abscissa. The three sets of data given in the text are plotted on the coordinate axis. The ratio of current to voltage, or G, is constant for both inward and outward currents. (C) This figure shows the effect of placing a rectifier in the circuit that allows only inward currents to flow. As in panel B, the conductance for inward currents (G_i) is constant; conversely, the conductance for an outward current (G_O) is zero.

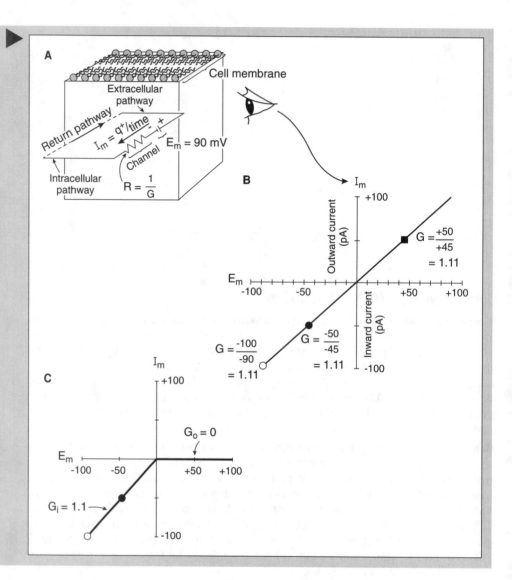

Just like fluids, currents always flow down an energy gradient. This gradient is expressed in terms of differences in "electromotive force," or volts. Alternatively, energy may be expended by a "pump" to move charged particles against an electrical energy gradient.

The electrical unit of conductance is the "mho," or "ohm" spelled backwards. More recently, the Siemen has been adapted as a standard unit. Ohm's law may be restated as I = EG.

A relationship like this is called "ohmic" because it follows Ohm's law: I = E/R. In this equation, E is actually the *voltage difference* between the two poles of the battery, and in this model, it equals the *transmembrane potential difference* maintained by the battery across the cell membrane. If the voltage of the battery were zero, there would be no energy gradient to drive a current flow, so the line passes through the origin of the coordinate system (see Figure 8-2B).

A membrane channel *allows* the flow of a given ion across the membrane. Therefore, it is often convenient to think in terms of a variable called the *conductance* (G), which measures how easily a circuit element passes current. G is defined as R^{-1} or 1/R. From now on, therefore, it is useful to refer to the resistor in Figure 8-2 as a "conductor." The conductance of an ion channel is related to its permeability to that ion. There are several valuable lessons from the relationship in Figure 8-2B.

- The I/V relationship for a circuit with a pure (ohmic) resistance—or conductance—is *linear* (i.e., a straight line).
- The ratio of current to voltage equals the conductance of the channel. Because this ratio is constant for a straight line, the conductance of the channel in Figure 8-2 is constant.
- It is essential to recognize whether the conductance of the channel or the current flow through the channel is being considered when analyzing the electrophysiologic function of any cell or ion channel. These two key variables describe different, although related, attributes of the system.

Rectification. There is an interesting and relevant variation of this model. The conductor in Figure 8-2 allows current to exit or enter the cell equally well. There are, however, circuit elements called *rectifiers* that allow current to flow in only one direction. It is possible, therefore, to incorporate a rectifier in series with the conductor to allow an inward current but inhibit the reverse flow. The I/V relationship for such a channel (assuming the rectifier works perfectly) is shown in Figure 8-2C. The conductance of the channel for an inward current—G_i—still has a constant, finite value; conversely, the conductance for an outward current—G_o—is zero (i.e., the line is flat along the abscissa). As it happens, some classes of potassium (K^+) channels in cardiac muscle allow flow preferentially in one direction compared to the other.

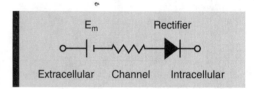

The model shown in Figure 8-2, even with the addition of a rectifier, is not a realistic representation of the cardiac myocyte in several significant ways. First, the conductance of many types of ion channels in cardiac muscle increases or decreases with changes in E_m. As a result, the I/V relationship for these *voltage-dependent* channels is not linear. The conductance of real channels also may change with time. Another weakness of the model of Figure 8-2B is that the conductor is not "ion selective"; that is, it conducts a current carried by any ion equally well. In reality, the ventricular myocyte's sarcolemma contains a category of channel whose conductance to K^+ exceeds its conductance to sodium ions (Na^+) or to calcium ions (Ca^{2+}), as well as another class that is more permeable to Na^+ than to K^+ or to Ca^{2+} (to name only two). As will be explained later, the I/V diagrams for ion selective channels do not pass through the origin of the graph. Moreover, the I/V relationship and time-dependence for the K^+ channel differ significantly from those of the Na^+ channel. The interplay of these and other channels ultimately accounts for the remarkable characteristics of the cardiac muscle action potential, as well as for the differences in action potentials recorded from different parts of the heart. Despite these weaknesses, the general principles that were developed in constructing Figure 8-2B are valid, and the I/V relationship is a very important descriptor of how real ion channels function.

IONIC BASIS OF THE RESTING MEMBRANE POTENTIAL IN VENTRICULAR MYOCYTES

The inside of a ventricular myocyte is approximately −80 to −90 mV electronegative with respect to the extracellular environment during electrical diastole. What accounts for this "resting" membrane potential? In this regard, the ventricular muscle cell is similar to skeletal muscle or to a nerve in that, for all three types of tissue, the resting membrane potential is approximately equal to the K^+ *equilibrium potential* (E_{K^+}). This statement means nothing, however, until one understands the basis of E_{K^+}.

The ionic basis of the resting E_m in atrial myocytes and in Purkinje fibers is similar to that of a ventricular myocyte. Conversely, there are marked differences in E_m during diastole in cells from the SA node and the AV node.

Potassium Equilibrium Potential (E_{K^+})

Figure 8-3A shows a hypothetical, electrically neutral cell. It contains 10 positively charged K^+, each of which is shown for instructional purposes as being associated with some negatively charged ion. There is no consistent orientation of the positively and negatively charged pairs within the cell. The "holes" in the cell membrane correspond to K^+-selective channels: they allow K^+ to pass with relative ease, but they do not conduct the negatively charged ions associated with K^+. The extracellular medium in Figure 8-3A

FIGURE 8-3 ▶

Development of the Potassium Equilibrium Potential (E_{K^+}). (A) The hypothetical cell is electrically neutral because the number of positive K^+ equals the number of negative charges carried by an ion or protein that cannot pass through the membrane. Positive and negative ions are shown as though they were loosely associated, for clarity. (B) This figure shows the state of the cell immediately after a single K^+, driven by the concentration gradient, has exited the cell through a channel. The membrane equilibrium (E_m) becomes faintly electronegative, because the negative charges cannot follow. However, E_m still exceeds E_{K^+}, so it is likely that additional K^+ will migrate out of the cell. (C) $E_m = E_{K^+}$, so the tendency for K^+ to exit (arrow 1) and enter (arrow 2) the cell are equal. The value of E_{K^+} in millivolts is given by the Nernst equation. Note that the extracellular positively charged K^+ and the excess intracellular negative charges are separated by the cell membrane. Their orientation across the membrane produces a dipole (shown by the shading for each ion pair). The membrane acts like a capacitor because of this ability to separate charge.

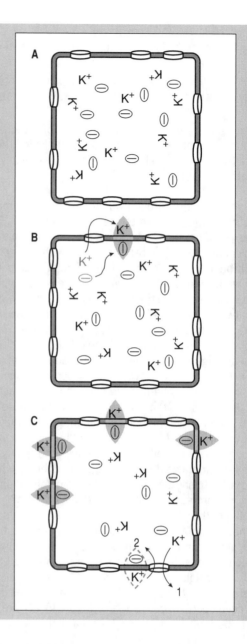

---

*The **permeability** of a membrane to a given ion is a measure of the ease with which the ion can pass through (i.e., permeate) the membrane. In actuality, the permeability of a myocyte's sarcolemma to K^+, or its P_{K^+}, depends on the conductance of the K^+ channels (i.e., G_{K^+}) and their total number. P_{K^+} is high in the resting ventricular myocyte, meaning that K^+ can cross the membrane with relative ease.*

*The separation of charge across the cell membrane means that the membrane acts like a **capacitor** (⊣ ⊢). As such, it "stores" charge.*

contains no ions. Although this latter feature is not realistic, the intracellular concentration of K^+ in real cells exceeds the extracellular concentration; that is, $[K^+]_i > [K^+]_e$. Another realistic feature is that many of the intracellular negative charges are "fixed" (i.e., trapped inside the cell) on large proteins or on ions that cannot permeate the membrane.

The situation shown in Figure 8-3A is physically unrealistic because of the large K^+ gradient across the cell membrane. Given this concentration difference, it is virtually inevitable that one of the K^+ will migrate out of the cell by virtue of its thermal motion. Figure 8-3B shows the state of the model immediately after the first K^+ has left the cell. The negatively charged ion that was previously associated with this K^+ is now left "unattended" inside the cell because it was unable to move through the K^+-selective channel. Therefore, the inside of the cell suddenly contained one excess negative charge and thus became slightly electronegative compared to the outside. The extracellular K^+ and the lone negative charge are separated by the cell membrane. By separating charge in this way, the cell membrane acts as a *capacitor*. This systematic orientation of the positive and negative charges across the membrane produces a *dipole*. Finally, there is another subtle difference between panel A and panel B: *the probability of K^+ moving in the reverse direction is no longer zero because there is now some extracellular K^+.*

The concentration gradient for K^+ is still very large, however, so it is likely that a second K$^+$ exits the cell. This second ion, however, must make a "choice." Because opposite charges attract, it must "decide" whether to migrate down its concentration gradient, like the first K$^+$, or remain inside, attracted by the newly available extra negative charge. But, as chance has it, the second ion does exit the cell, and negative charge continues to accumulate in the cell.

The process described above continues so that the inside of the cell becomes more and more electronegative relative to the outside. Eventually, *a negative intracellular potential is attained at which the tendency for an intracellular K$^+$ to exit the cell by migrating down its concentration gradient (Figure 8-3C, arrow 1) is exactly balanced by the tendency for an extracellular K$^+$ to enter the cell, despite the concentration gradient, because of the attraction of the excess negative intracellular charge (Figure 8-3C, arrow 2). The membrane potential at which this balance of forces is established is E$_{K^+}$.* This equilibrium state is shown in Figure 8-3C. Notice the following important points:

- The process that establishes this equilibrium does not require the expenditure of energy.
- The value of E$_{K^+}$ (mV) depends on the concentration gradient for K$^+$. For example, an increase in [K$^+$]$_i$ would make E$_{K^+}$ more negative because a larger intracellular negative charge would be required to offset the greater concentration gradient.
- The equilibrium requires the presence of the K$^+$-selective channels, but the value of E$_{K^+}$ does not depend on the permeability of the membrane to K$^+$ (P$_{K^+}$).
- The net flux of K$^+$ across the membrane at E$_{K^+}$ equals zero. This does *not* mean that no K$^+$ are able to cross the membrane. Instead, it means that, on the average, the number of ions moving into the cell over any given time equals the number leaving the cell.
- The positive and negative charges are separated by the membrane. The alignment of the "dipoles" across the cell membrane in panel C illustrates this separation of charge.

Nernst Equation

The value of the equilibrium potential for any given ion can be predicted using the *Nernst equation*. This equation is a mathematical statement of the conceptual relationships that were developed in Figure 8-3. Therefore, the "major players" in the equation for the prediction of E$_K^+$ should be [K$^+$]$_i$ and [K$^+$]$_e$. The following general statement of the Nernst equation bears this out:

$$E_{K^+} \approx -\frac{61}{z} \log_{10} \frac{[K^+]_i}{[K^+]_e}$$

Computing E$_{K^+}$ for K$^+$ becomes a simple chore. Using [K$^+$]$_i$ = 150 mM and [K$^+$]$_e$ = 4 mM, where the charge for the K$^+$ (i.e., z) is +1, then,

$$E_{K^+} = -61 \times \log 150/4 = -61 \times \log 37.5 = -61 \times 1.57 = -94 \text{ mV}$$

Consider carefully once more what information this computation provides. *When the inside of the cell is 94 mV negative to the extracellular medium, the tendency for K$^+$ to exit the cell because of diffusion down its concentration gradient is exactly offset by the electric field acting to retain (or attract) the positively charged ion, so the net flow of K$^+$ across the membrane is zero.*

At this moment three thoughts may have occurred to you. First, because the actual transmembrane potential for the cell is (only) −80 mV or −90 mV, *there must be some small, but continuous, leakage of K$^+$ from the cell.* This occurs because the intracellular electronegativity is not quite large enough to offset the K$^+$ concentration gradient totally. Second, there must be some mechanism to reclaim the lost K$^+$. Third, this mechanism must involve moving the K$^+$ from the extracellular medium to the intracellular medium against its concentration gradient. Therefore, the cell must expend energy to "pump" K$^+$ back into the cell. An explanation of this latter mechanism requires the development of a few more concepts regarding the role of Na$^+$ in the cell.

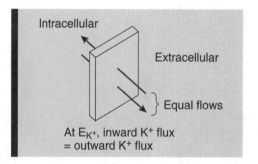

At E$_{K^+}$, inward K$^+$ flux = outward K$^+$ flux

I_{K1} Inward Rectifying Potassium (Kir) Channel

There are three broad classes of ion channels in cardiac myocytes. The classification is based upon the nature of the signal that causes the channel to open. The three classes are inward rectifiers, voltage-gated rectifiers, and ligand-gated rectifiers. Each channel is also categorized by the ion that it preferentially conducts. Important representatives of each class are encountered at appropriate points in the remainder of this chapter. One of the most important ion selective channels, and one of the most ubiquitous across species, is the potassium inward rectifier (Kir) channel, which carries a current known as I_{K1}. The Kir is considered first because it accounts in large part for the resting membrane potential in "working" myocardium (i.e., ventricular and atrial myocytes).

STRUCTURE OF KIR CHANNELS

The inward rectifier is structurally the least complicated of the known channels. Figure 8-4 is a schematic illustration of the subunit for the inward rectifier. By analogy with other channels, multiple (probably three or four) subunits are required to constitute a functioning Kir. The subunit is a peptide that consists of (only) two transmembrane helices: M_1 and M_2. M_1 and M_2 are connected by an extracellular loop known as H5 or the *pore region*. As is implied by the name, the H5 loops from each of the three or four subunits probably form the central pore through which ions move. Inward rectification might be due to a positively charged substance, perhaps magnesium ions (Mg^{2+}), that blocks the pore in a voltage-dependent manner, although other explanations are possible [2].

FIGURE 8-4 ▶

Proposed Subunit Structure of Potassium Inward Rectifier Channel. H5 is the chain of amino acids that links the putative α-helices, M_1 and M_2, that span the cell membrane. Multiple H5 loops contributed by cooperating subunits are thought to form the pore of the K^+ channel. C' and N' represent the carboxyl and amino terminals of the protein, respectively. Out = extracellular side of the membrane. In = intracellular side of the membrane. (Source: Reprinted with permission from Nichols CG, Mackhina EN, Pearson WL, et al: Inward rectification and implications for cardiac excitability. Circ Res 78:4, 1996.)

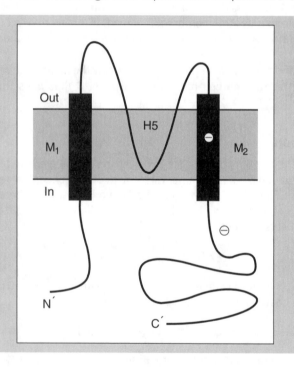

I_{K1} INWARD RECTIFYING CURRENT

The "observer" who counted the flow of charge, or current, across the membrane was a key agent in determining the I/V relationship in Figure 8-2. Several new biologic techniques have made the observer's task realistic for actual ion channels in living myocytes. As a result, it is now possible to determine the I/V relationship for the Kir and other channels.

Whole-Cell Patch-Clamp Preparation. Figure 8-5 illustrates one of these modern biologic techniques called the whole-cell patch-clamp preparation. In this process, a glass micropipette is attached by suction to a single myocyte. The membrane of the sarcolemma under the electrode is then treated in such a way as to place the interior of the cell in direct electrical continuity with the microelectrode. This allows two important measurements. First, the investigator is able to record the cell's E_m, and, in fact, one could simply measure the cell's action potential in this way. The second measurement, however, dramatically extends the usefulness of the preparation. The electrode is connected to a *voltage clamp*, which initially fixes, or "clamps," the cell's E_m at a *holding potential*. In this example, the holding potential is 0 mV (see Figure 8-5A). No matter what happens within the cell or its membrane, E_m remains at 0 mV as long as the voltage clamp is set at the holding potential. This experiment uses 0 mV because it is approximately equal to the voltage during the plateau phase of the action potential. The voltage-clamp amplifier measures the amount of current that it must inject (or withdraw) to hold the cell's E_m at 0 mV. This current must equal the sum of the currents through individual channels (i.e., $I_{total} = i_1 + i_2 + i_3 + ... + i_n$). In other words, because the investigator knows the current passing through the microelectrode, he or she also knows the current crossing the cell membrane through the channels (I_m). This is exactly the job performed by the observer in Figure 8-2. As shown in Figure 8-5A ("current recording"), at the holding potential there is a small outward current designated by an asterisk. Suddenly, the voltage clamp forces the cell's transmembrane potential to change to a new steady value chosen by the investigator; as before, it does this by injecting (or withdrawing) whatever charge is required at any given instant to render E_m at the desired value. The *voltage step*, or *command pulse* for this trial changed E_m to -120 mV. The current recording shows the charge/time (i.e., the current) that the voltage clamp had to withdraw from the cell to maintain the new value of E_m. Once again, *an equal number of charges/time had to enter the cell through the ion channels: this equals the membrane current, I_m.*

Why is the outward current at 0 mV so small, given the large electrochemical drive for K^+ to exit the cell? (Hint: Consider the implications of "inward rectification.")

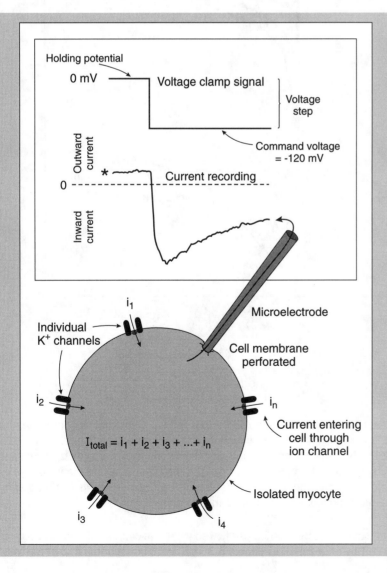

◄ **FIGURE 8-5**
Schematic Illustration of Whole-Cell Patch-Clamp Preparation. *The voltage clamp injects or removes by way of the microelectrode whatever charge is required to maintain the cell's membrane potential at a designated value. The voltage-clamp current is equal to the sum of the individual currents entering (or exiting) the cell through the ion channels (i_1 to i_n). The voltage clamp initially maintains membrane potential (E_m) at 0 mV and then suddenly causes a step change determined by the command voltage (inset, top tracing). The resulting current recording (inset, bottom tracing) equals the current through the cell's ion channels.*

Holding potential
0 mV
Voltage clamp signal
Voltage step
Command voltage = -120 mV
Outward current
*
Current recording
0
Inward current
Microelectrode
Cell membrane perforated
Individual K$^+$ channels
i_1
i_2
i_n
Current entering cell through ion channel
$I_{total} = i_1 + i_2 + i_3 + ... + i_n$
Isolated myocyte
i_3
i_4

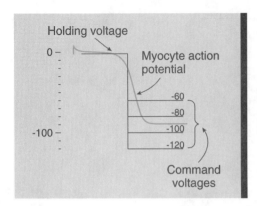

I_{K1} *Current–Voltage Relationship.* Figure 8-6 shows the I/V relationship for the I_{K1} inward rectifying current from an embryonic chick cardiac ventricular myocyte obtained using the whole-cell patch clamp. Two pieces of additional information are required before it is possible to analyze Figure 8-6. First, because neither the micropipette nor the bathing solution contained permeant ions besides K^+ (i.e., there was no Na^+ or Ca^{2+}), one can be confident that the currents that were recorded were carried only by K^+. Second, under the conditions of this experiment, E_{K^+} was approximately -54 mV. Figure 8-6A shows the actual currents when the cell's transmembrane voltage was shifted from the holding potential of 0 mV to -120 mV, -100 mV, -80 mV, and -60 mV (i.e., the command voltages at which the cell was clamped in the four tracings). Here, as always, *a negative recording indicates an inward current flow*. Because the ventricular myocyte's E_m is approximately 0 mV during the plateau, this experiment measures the I_{K1} current that flows through a ventricular myocyte cell membrane as it repolarizes. Repolarizing the cell caused the flow of an inward current that became larger as the cell was repolarized to a more negative potential.

FIGURE 8-6 ▶

Determination of the Current–Voltage (I/V) Relationship for I_{K1}. (A) This figure shows I_{K1} current measured in a 14-week-old chick embryonic ventricular myocyte using the whole-cell patch-clamp technique. The cell's membrane potential (E_m) was fixed at 0 mV (i.e., the holding potential) prior to each of the four voltage steps shown. The asterisk indicates the small outward current that flowed at the holding potential. The E_m was then suddenly changed to -120, -100, -80 or -60 mV (i.e., the command voltages). A downward deflection corresponds to the flow of positively charged ions into the cell. A 20-pA current and a 200-msec time calibration are shown at the lower right of panel A. The experiment determines the currents that flow in a ventricular myocyte when it repolarizes from the plateau (i.e., ≈ 0 mV) to various resting membrane potentials. (B) This figure shows the I/V relationship derived by plotting the peak currents recorded in panel A for the respective command voltages. The I/V curve for inward current is nearly linear and indicates that the I_{K1} channel readily allows K^+ to flow into the cell. Conversely, the conductance for outward currents is low. This inward rectification is an important characteristic of the I_{K1} channel. (Source: These data were provided courtesy of Dr. Jonathan Satin, Department of Physiology, University of Kentucky College of Medicine, Lexington, Kentucky.)

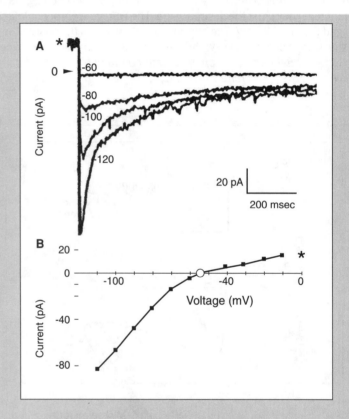

The data in Figure 8-6A, plus additional voltage steps that are not shown, allowed the investigator to construct the I/V relationship for the I_{K1} channel that is shown in Figure 8-6B. The peak current flow in response to each step voltage change is plotted on the ordinate; the abscissa gives the value of the corresponding command voltage. This I/V relationship describes some of the most important characteristics of the channel. The curve in panel B provides the following information:

• A small outward current (≈20 pA) flowed when the cell was clamped at 0 mV. This is indicated by an asterisk in panels A and B and corresponds to the relatively small outward flow of current during the plateau phase of a ventricular muscle action potential.

- The current flow across the membrane was zero when the cell was taken from the holding voltage to a command voltage corresponding to E_{K+} (-54 mV), which is shown in panel B by the symbol "○." This lack of net current flow conforms to the definition of the K^+ equilibrium potential.
- The I/V relationship is nearly linear for inward currents, indicating minimal voltage dependence for this type of channel, at least within a restricted range of E_m.
- The I/V relationship is notably flatter for outward currents than for inward currents, indicating that the conductance to inward currents exceeded the conductance to outward currents. This inward rectification (sometimes called *anomalous rectification*) is one of the defining characteristics of I_{K1}.

FUNCTIONAL SIGNIFICANCE OF INWARD RECTIFICATION

The relative flattening of the curve noted above is similar to Figure 8-2C. Although the rectification displayed by the I_{K1} is not as good as the perfect rectifier in the model in Figure 8-2C, it is physiologically significant. To understand why it is so important, note that the magnitude of the K^+ current flowing across the cell membrane (I_K) at any given moment is given by Ohm's law:

$$I_K = G_{K+} \times (E_m - E_{K+})$$

In this equation, the term "$E_m - E_{K+}$" is the potential *difference* driving the current flow; it is analogous to the potential difference created by a battery, although in many circuits the voltage of one "pole" of the battery is made to be 0 mV (i.e., "ground"). During the plateau phase, the difference between E_m and E_{K+} is large. This long potential difference would promote a large loss of K^+ from the cell. *Fortunately, therefore, the inward rectification, with the consequent decrease in outward K^+ conductance (G_{K+} above), minimizes the loss of K^+ and decreases the amount of energy the cell must expend to reclaim lost K^+.*

Goldman Field Equation and the Resting Membrane Potential

It is now possible to explain the small difference that exists between E_{K+} and the actual resting E_m in ventricular myocytes. The cell membrane also includes channels that are permeable to Na^+. In the resting state, the permeability of the membrane to K^+ (P_{K+}) far exceeds its permeability to Na^+ (P_{Na+}). This is because only a fraction of the Na^+ channels are in the open, or conducting, state at the diastolic E_m. Nonetheless, the concentration gradient acting to drive Na^+ into the cell is large, the negative potential inside the cell strongly attracts the positively charged Na^+, and a few channels permeable to Na^+ do conduct. Therefore, there is some inward leakage of Na^+ during electrical diastole. This small leakage of positive ions into the cell is called the *inward background current (I_b)*, and it causes the actual E_m to be slightly less negative than predicted by E_{K+}.

The actual value of E_m can be predicted using the *Goldman Field equation*, written below to include the most relevant ions:

$$E_m = -\frac{RT}{F} \ln \frac{P_{K+}[K^+]_i + P_{Na+}[Na^+]_i + P_{Cl-}[Cl^-]_e}{P_{K+}[K^+]_e + P_{Na+}[Na^+]_e + P_{Cl-}[Cl^-]_i}$$

Though this equation may look formidable, it is actually only a series of Nernst equations for each individual ion "weighted" by the relative permeabilities of the membrane for that ion. For example, suppose $P_{K+} >> P_{Na+}, P_{Cl-}$. In that case, one can virtually ignore all the terms except those relating to K^+, and the equation reduces to the Nernst equation for K^+ alone. Figure 8-7 shows another way to look at the Field equation. This "teeter-totter model" figuratively shows that E_m is determined by an interplay between the relative permeability of the membrane to K^+ versus Na^+. It ignores the contribution made by other ions, which is a reasonable first assumption in the resting state. When P_{K+} is much "heavier" than P_{Na+} (i.e., $P_{K+} >> P_{Na+}$), the pointer on the teeter-totter will fall

---

*Note that zero current flow occurs at ≈ -54 mV in Figure 8-6, not at 0 mV, as in Figure 8-2C. This is because Figure 8-6 shows flow through a K^+-**selective channel**, where a net zero current occurs at E_{K+}, not 0 mV. At what voltage will zero current flow occur for a Na^+-selective channel?*

The magnitude of the outward current at the holding potential of 0 mV in Figure 8-5 was small because of the inward rectification of the Kir.

Note the concentration designation—intracellular versus extracellular—is "flipped" for chloride (Cl^-) in the Goldman Field equation. This is because Cl^- carries a negative charge, which is easily accommodated in logarithmic notation by inverting the ratio. The R in the Field equation is the universal gas constant, T is the temperature in degrees Kelvin, and F is Faraday's constant.

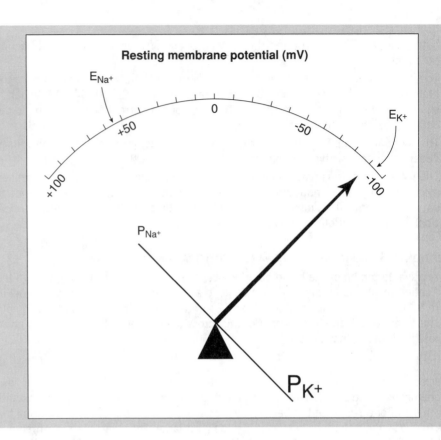

FIGURE 8-7 ▶

"Teeter-Totter" Model for Membrane Potential (E_m) in Resting Membrane. The value of the resting membrane potential is shown by the pointer as though it resulted from the relative "balance" between the permeability of the membrane to K^+ versus Na^+. The scale across the top represents the possible range of E_m. The equilibrium potentials for K^+ and Na^+, as determined by the Nernst equation, appear on opposite sides of this scale. In the resting state $P_{K^+} \gg P_{Na^+}$; this difference in permeability is represented by the relative size, or "weight," of each at either end of the balance beam. In the resting state, therefore, the pointer on the teeter-totter predicts an E_m that is only somewhat less negative than potassium equilibrium potential (E_{K^+}). This is a simple restatement of the Goldman Field equation, in which E_m is determined by a mathematical balance between the permeabilities of the membrane to the relevant ions.

nearly—but not quite—on E_{K^+}. Likewise, the Field equation predicts an actual E_m that depends on the relative "balance" between the two permeabilities.

Effects of Hypokalemia and Hyperkalemia on Resting E_m

Figure 8-8 shows how resting E_m changes as the extracellular concentration of K^+ increases (hyperkalemia) and decreases (hypokalemia) relative to the normal value of approximately 3.5–4.5 mM. The *solid line* shows E_{K^+} as predicted by the Nernst equation over the range of $[K^+]_e$ given on the abscissa. Using a logarithmic scale for the abscissa yields a linear plot. The *broken line* is the actual E_m measured by Page in cat papillary muscle [3]. For $[K^+]_e > 10$ mM, the actual E_m "tracks" E_{K^+} well, except that it remains somewhat less electronegative than predicted by the Nernst equation. This small difference is due to the inward leak of Na^+ described above. *Hyperkalemia* can be very dangerous, producing a weak heartbeat and, for severe elevations, even cardiac arrest. E_m also deviates noticeably from E_{K^+} in *hypokalemia* because of a decline in membrane conductance to K^+. In hypokalemia, therefore, even very small inward currents cause a relatively greater depolarization of the membrane and decreased stability of E_m. It is clear why physicians monitor plasma K^+ so carefully!

Sodium–Potassium Exchange (Na^+–K^+) Pump

Because K^+ continuously leaks out of the cell while Na^+ enters the cell, it is obvious that the cell must reclaim lost K^+ and expel the interloping Na^+. The sarcolemma possesses a *Na^+–K^+ exchange pump* powered by adenosine triphosphatase (ATPase). It is *electrogenic* because three Na^+ are expelled from the myocyte for every two K^+ that are reclaimed from the extracellular environment. The electrogenic action of the pump makes E_m more negative than it would be otherwise, but the difference is quantitatively small. The rate at which the pump works increases with a rise in $[Na^+]_i$ or an increase in $[K^+]_e$.

Stable Resting Membrane Potential in Ventricular Myocytes

In ventricular muscle cells, the inward leakage current, I_b, carried primarily by Na^+, is balanced by the outward leakage of K^+ plus the small net outward current produced by

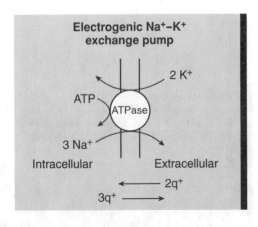

Electrogenic Na^+–K^+ exchange pump

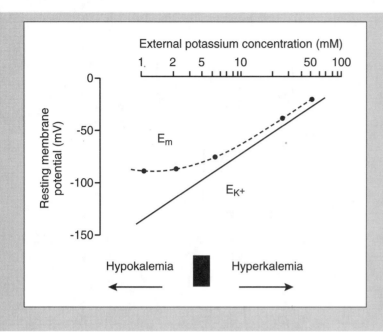

FIGURE 8-8
Effects of Extracellular K⁺ Concentration on the Resting Membrane Potential (E_m).
Experiments were performed in the cat by Page [3]. The solid line shows the electrical potential difference across the cell membrane (i.e., E_m) exclusively caused by the ratio of intracellular to extracellular K⁺ concentrations according to the Nernst equation (temperature is 27.5 C°, and $[K^+]_i = 200$ mM). The individual data points connected by the broken line are Page's actual experimental observations. For $[K^+]_e > 5$ mM, E_m followed the potassium equilibrium potential (E_{K^+}) fairly closely although E_m was always somewhat less negative because of inward "leak" currents. Hypokalemia or hyperkalemia can seriously disrupt the electrical stability of the cell. (Source: Adapted from Levick JR: An Introduction to Cardiovascular Physiology 2nd ed. Oxford, UK: Butterworth-Heinemann, 1995, p 32.)

the Na⁺–K⁺ exchange pump. As a result, the membrane potential in ventricular myocytes, as well as those from the atrium and Purkinje fibers, is normally stable during electrical diastole. The membrane potential in SA-nodal cells is *not* stable during diastole but depolarizes spontaneously until it reaches a *threshold* value and generates an action potential (see Sinoatrial (SA) Node and the Control of Heart Rate—Chronotropism).

VENTRICULAR MUSCLE ACTION POTENTIAL

Action potentials recorded from right and left ventricular muscle and Purkinje fibers characteristically have a rapid phase 0, a definite overshoot, and a long plateau followed by a rapid repolarization. The action potential for atrial fibers is generally similar except the plateau is less pronounced. These characteristics can be explained largely by the fast inward Na⁺ current (phase 0), the slow inward Ca²⁺ current (phase 2), and an interplay between decay of the slow inward current and a waxing outward K⁺ current (phase 3), respectively.

Rising Phase of the Ventricular Muscle Action Potential and the Na⁺ Channel

The *fast inward current* produces the rapid depolarization characteristic of phase 0 in ventricular myocytes. The dynamics of this current are determined by the *voltage-dependent and time-dependent characteristics* of the cardiac Na⁺-selective channel.

Structure of the Na⁺ Channel. The Na⁺-selective channel is structurally more complicated than the inward rectifying K⁺ channel described previously. (Recall, for example, that the inward rectifier is not voltage-dependent because it does not have a voltage-sensitive gating mechanism.) The voltage-dependent channels, whether for K⁺, Na⁺, or Ca²⁺, have a number of structural similarities. Figure 8-9 shows the proposed structure for the Na⁺ channel, which is a polypeptide with four repeating "motifs" labeled I–IV. Each motif, in turn, includes six membrane-spanning alpha-helices, usually designated S1–S6, that are connected one to another by intracellular and extracellular loops. The two-dimensional representation in Figure 8-9 can be misleading, however. For example, the helical portions of the motifs are not situated in a straight line within the cell membrane. Instead, they are snuggled close together to form an intimate three-dimensional structure. A three-dimensional representation of another voltage-dependent channel is described later (Figure 8-14B). A number of important features of the Na⁺ channel have emerged that are also broadly true of other voltage-gated channels:

Hodgkin and Huxley considered only a single type of Na⁺ channel and a single type of K⁺ channel in their classic experiments on the giant squid axon [4]. Similar structural forms of voltage-dependent channels have now been found in a variety of species for Na⁺ and Ca²⁺ as well as K⁺. Conversely, the variety of K⁺ channels across living systems amazes even the most seasoned investigator.

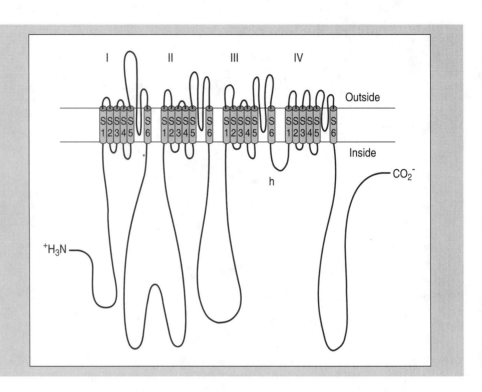

FIGURE 8-9

Proposed Two-Dimensional Structure of Na⁺-Selective Channel. The channel consists of four repeating motifs (I–IV). The fourth transmembrane α-helical segment in each motif (S4) endows the channel with the voltage-sensitive gating mechanism. The intracellular loop between III and IV confers the time-dependent inactivation. (Source: Adapted with permission from Catterall WA: Structure and function of voltage-sensitive ion channels. Science 242:55, 1988.)

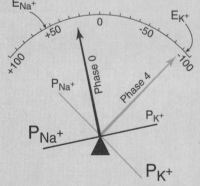

Membrane potential (mV)

The teeter-totter analogy shows how the change in the relative "weights" of P_{Na^+} and P_{K^+} during phase 0 causes the pointer to rotate away from E_{K^+} toward E_{Na^+}.

The current recorded with the whole-cell patch-clamp preparation, such as in Figure 8-6A and in Figure 8-12A, is the sum of all the currents through uncounted numbers of individual channels.

- The amino acid sequence for S4 is very similar across different types of channels (i.e., it is "highly conserved") and has a net positive charge. S4 probably confers the voltage sensitivity to the channel. It is thought that a change in the membrane potential causes a conformational change within S4 that opens the channel [5].

- The series of amino acids between S5 and S6 for each motif together probably compose the lining of the conducting pore.

- Once the membrane is depolarized, the intracellular loop that connects repeats III and IV (labeled h in Figure 8-9) is thought to swing with time into the mouth of the channel to interrupt further ion flow. This is known as the "ball-and-chain model" for *inactivation* (see also Figure 8-14).

Role of the Na⁺ Channel in Producing Phase 0. The traditional explanation of phase 0 of the ventricular muscle fiber's action potential is that depolarization of the cell beyond threshold activates a *positive feedback cycle*, which results in an explosive increase in G_{Na^+} (Figure 8-10). The electrochemical forces acting on Na⁺ dictate that this increase in Na⁺ *conductance* leads to an inward *Na⁺ current*. This fast inward current is responsible for the rapid depolarization of the ventricular muscle action potential.

The positive feedback concept is still useful for envisioning the genesis of the rapid upstroke, but the advent of patch-clamp techniques for measuring current flow through single channels affords another perspective. These experiments show that an individual Na⁺ channel converts from a nonconducting (sometimes called "closed") state to a conducting (sometimes called "open") state. Figure 8-11 is a record of the current through a single Na⁺ channel. These data were obtained using a patch-clamp preparation in which the membrane under the microelectrode remains intact; this patch of membrane may contain as few as one or two channels. Note that a single channel is either fully conducting or fully closed; there is no partially conducting state. At the point indicated by an asterisk (*), a second channel was momentarily conducting. *The probability for a given voltage-dependent Na⁺ channel to change from the nonconducting to the conducting state increases when the membrane depolarizes.* The progressive recruitment of more and more channels ultimately leads to the rapid depolarization of phase 0.

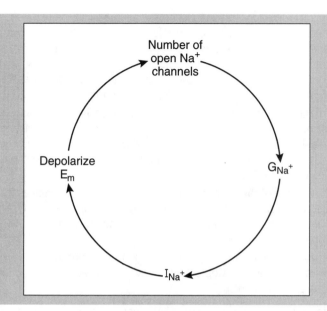

FIGURE 8-10
Positive Feedback Cycle Established When the Membrane Potential (E_m) Exceeds Threshold. *The increase in the number of Na+ channels in the conducting state causes the conductance of the membrane to Na+ (G_{Na+}) to increase. The resulting inward flow of positively charged Na+ (I_{Na}) causes E_m to depolarize even more. The cycle activates progressively more Na+ channels and is terminated only by their inactivation. This cycle is responsible for the "all-or-nothing" nature of many kinds of action potentials.*

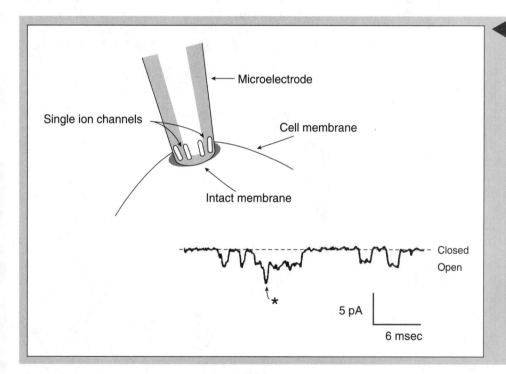

FIGURE 8-11
Patch-Clamp Recording of the Current Flow as a Result of the Opening of Single Na+ Channels in a Rat Ventricular Myocyte. *Each downward deflection resulted from the opening of one channel. At the point indicated by the asterisk, two channels were open simultaneously so that the currents from both channels superimposed. The scale at lower right shows the calibrations for current (in pA) and time (in msec). (Source: These data were provided courtesy of Dr. Jonathan Satin, Department of Physiology, University of Kentucky College of Medicine, Lexington, Kentucky.)*

I/V Relationship of the Na+ Channel. Figure 8-12 shows a whole-cell patch-clamp experiment in a single rat ventricular myocyte. The holding potential in this example was −100 mV, which is near the normal diastolic E_m. The individual tracings in Figure 8-12A show the *inward* currents that were elicited by step depolarizations (i.e., command voltages) ranging in 5 mV increments from −55 mV to −10 mV. Figure 8-12B shows the I/V relationship in which the peak currents in panel A (plus additional steps not shown in A) are plotted against the clamp/command voltage. Note the following specific points:

- Panel A shows that for most tracings the current increases very rapidly and then spontaneously decays because of time-dependent inactivation.
- The relationship shown in Figure 8-12B is highly nonlinear, unlike the I/V relationship for the simple model of Figure 8-2, or even for the I_{K1} channel in Figure 8-6B. The gating of the Na+ channel is not passive; instead, the channel's conductance varies dramatically with E_m.

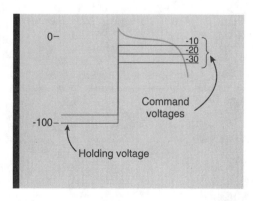

- The extreme left portion of the I/V relationship shows that the inward current is virtually nonexistent until the transmembrane voltage is changed from the holding potential to an E_m that is less negative than approximately -60 mV. *This is because the regenerative increase in G_{Na^+} does not occur until this threshold voltage is exceeded, which explains why $P_{K^+} >> P_{Na^+}$ at a normal resting E_m.*

- The peak magnitude of the inward current progressively increases when E_m is clamped within the range between approximately -50 to -35 mV; the dominant factor responsible for the increasing current within this range is the increasing number of channels recruited to the conducting state as E_m depolarizes more and more (i.e., as in Figure 8-10).

- The peak magnitude of the inward current progressively decreases as the membrane is depolarized to potentials less negative than approximately -35 mV. The dominant factor responsible for the decline in current within this range is the decreasing difference between E_m and E_{Na^+}.

- The current would have become zero had the membrane potential been clamped at a value equal to E_{Na^+}, and it would have converted to an outward current had E_m become more positive than I_{Na}.

Many students erroneously believe that the concentration gradient for Na^+ is reversed at the peak of the action potential compared to the resting state so that $[Na^+]_i > [Na^+]_e$. This is *not* the case. In fact, *although Na^+ does enter the myocyte during phase 0, and although the entering positive charges cause the inside of the cell to become slightly*

$$I_{Na} = G_{Na^+} \times (E_m - E_{Na^+})$$

$$E_{Na^+} \approx -61 \times \log_{10}\frac{[Na^+]_i}{[Na^+]_e} =$$

$$-61 \times \log_{10}\frac{15}{150} = +61\,mV$$

FIGURE 8-12 ▶
Determination of the Current–Voltage (I/V) Relationship for the Fast Inward Na^+ Current. (A) This figure shows a series of superimposed tracings of the whole-cell patch-clamp current flowing through Na^+ channels in a rat ventricular myocyte. Each recording began at a holding potential of -100 mV. The current at this holding potential approached zero (asterisk) because almost no channels were open (conducting) when the membrane potential (E_m) = -100 mV. The cell was then suddenly depolarized to a new steady level specified by the command voltage. Although the voltage steps are not shown here, each trace represents the current flowing during one such step. In general, an inward current (downward deflection) increased rapidly and then declined. The current declined because of the inactivation of the Na^+ channels, even though the command voltage did not change after the instantaneous transition from the holding potential. (B) This figure shows the I/V diagram derived from the data in panel A. Each data point gives the peak inward current that flowed during the step change from the holding potential plotted against the E_m specified by the command voltage. The current (nA) is given on the ordinate; the E_m specified by the command voltage is given on the abscissa. Unlike the results shown in Figure 8-6 for I_{K1}, this I/V diagram is highly nonlinear because of the strong voltage dependence of the cardiac Na^+ channel. (Source: These data were provided courtesy of Dr. Jonathan Satin, Department of Physiology, University of Kentucky College of Medicine, Lexington, Kentucky.)

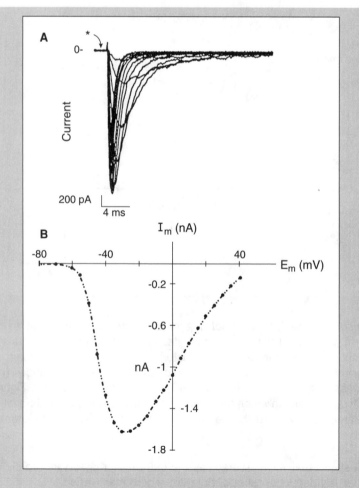

electropositive, even very sensitive instruments cannot detect a change in the relative concentrations of intracellular and extracellular Na+ over the course of a single action potential.

Time-Dependent Activation and Inactivation of the Na+ Channel. The recordings in Figure 8-12A clearly show that the fast inward current builds quickly to a peak and then decays rapidly to zero. This decay results from a spontaneous decline in G_{Na^+} and results from the *time-dependent* inactivation of the Na+ channel. In short, individual ion channels go through a series of transitions during the course of an action potential:

- At the beginning of an action potential, progressively greater numbers of membrane Na+ channels change from a closed (C), nonconducting (but responsive) state to an open (O), conducting state. As implied in Figure 8-10, this process accelerates dramatically as E_m becomes less negative.
- Once the action potential has peaked, the individual Na+ channels quickly progress to a nonresponsive or inactive (I) state.
- It is very unlikely that a channel returns directly from the open state to the closed state; instead, it passes through the inactive, nonresponsive state to regain the ability to open.

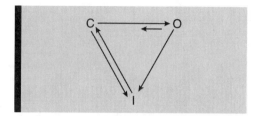

This last transition from state I to state C does not occur with any rapidity until the membrane repolarizes. As a result, the membrane cannot sustain another action potential until repolarization occurs and a significant percentage of the population of channels has again changed to the closed (C) configuration (i.e., from which they are able to open again). Additional details regarding the Na+ channel may be found elsewhere [5–7].

Ischemic cells are generally unable to maintain the normal E_m of -80 to -90 mV. Instead, they are partially depolarized so that a significant percentage of the Na+ channels are inactivated. As a result, the cell-to-cell conduction velocity in these myocytes is very slow, if they conduct at all. This may contribute to serious irregularities of rhythm, often because of a process called "reentry." Reentry is explained in more detail in the section on premature ventricular contractions.

Plateau Phase of the Ventricular Muscle Action Potential and the Role of Ca²⁺

Phase 0 of the action potential in ventricular muscle culminates in the *overshoot*. The short-lived, partial repolarization that follows (i.e., phase 1) is due to a transient outward current (I_{TO}). The identity of I_{TO} has been hotly debated, but the weight of evidence now attributes it to a K+ current (through a voltage-gated K+ channel). During the ensuing plateau phase, E_m remains near 0 mV for hundreds of milliseconds. Although P_{K^+} is relatively low during the plateau, it is not zero; therefore, some K+ exits the cell because of the large electrochemical driving force. Because E_m remains relatively constant during the plateau, one may logically infer that there is some inward current that offsets the outward K+ current.

Ca²⁺ Current. The inward current during the plateau is carried primarily by Ca²⁺. Two Ca²⁺-selective channels have been identified: the *L-type Ca²⁺ channel*, where *L* indicates the long duration of the channel's open state, and the transient, or *T-type, Ca²⁺ channel*. Of these two, the L-type plays the dominant role. A patch-clamp experiment to study these channels yields results generally similar to Figure 8-12 with three important differences:

- The rate of onset of the current (i.e., activation) is slower than in Figure 8-12A; the inward flow of Ca²⁺ through these channels is therefore sometimes called the "slow inward current."
- The current lasts longer (i.e., inactivates more slowly) than the fast inward Na+ current; this current therefore contributes to the long plateau phase of the ventricular muscle action potential.
- The depolarization required to activate the Ca²⁺ current is larger (i.e., to a less negative E_m) than for the Na+ channel. This is important for understanding the action potential in SA-nodal and AV-nodal cells (see SA Node and Initiation of the Heartbeat).

Ca²⁺ Current and the Control of Inotropism: Ca²⁺-Induced Ca²⁺ Release. Unlike skeletal muscle, extracellular Ca²⁺ is essential for myocardial contraction. Ca²⁺ binding to troponin C initiates a sequence of changes within the contractile proteins that shifts the position of tropomyosin and troponin I relative to actin. This shift "uncovers" the myosin-binding sites on actin, thereby allowing cross-bridge formation. In effect, Ca²⁺ switches active tension on and off. Figure 8-13 illustrates important features of this process that are unique to the heart. During the plateau (1) of the cardiac action potential Ca^{2+} enters the cell through L-type channels (2); this is known as "trigger Ca^{2+}." *The trigger Ca^{2+} controls (3) the amount of Ca^{2+} released from the sarcoplasmic reticulum (SR) and, therefore, the amount of free Ca^{2+} within the cytosol (4) that enables cross bridges to form.* The *upper left portion* of Figure 8-13 shows that activation of the β-receptor by norepinephrine increases the production of cyclic adenosine monophosphate (cAMP). The cAMP activates (5) a protein kinase (cAMP–PK) that phosphorylates (6) the Ca^{2+} channel, thereby increasing the inward flow of Ca^{2+}. *This increased influx of trigger Ca^{2+} by β-receptor activation is the basis for the increase in contractile force produced by cardiac sympathetic nerves. β-Receptor activation also shortens the duration of systole in two ways.* First, the protein kinase phosphorylates (7) another protein, *phospholamban*, which accelerates the rate of reuptake of Ca^{2+} from the cytosol into the SR (8). Second, the protein kinase also phosphorylates the inhibitory component of troponin (i.e., troponin I), which accentuates the latter's inhibitory effect (9) on Ca^{2+} binding by troponin C. This hastens the uncoupling of actin and myosin. These effects of β-receptor activation explain how an increase in contractility allows the muscle to perform more work, more quickly.[1]

Because Ca^{2+} enters the cell with each action potential, it is essential that over the course of time an equal amount be removed from the cell. A sodium–calcium (Na^+–Ca^{2+}) exchange pump (10), powered by the Na^+ concentration gradient across the cell membrane and an adenosine triphosphate (ATP)–driven Ca^{2+} pump (11), accomplish this task. The classic explanation for the therapeutic action of digitalis is that it poisons the Na^+–K^+-ATPase (12), thereby increasing $[Na^+]_i$. This decreases the rate of removal of Ca^{2+} from the cell by the Na^+–Ca^{2+} exchange pump. More recent data show that long-term digoxin therapy results in significant increases in parasympathetic activity and decreases in sympathetic activity in patients with CHF, both of which would be advantageous [9].

Several different classes of drugs have been developed that block the Ca^{2+} chan-

---

[1] A recent discovery shows that G proteins also play a role in L-channel regulation. It is thought that a stimulatory G protein (G_s) acts via cAMP on the channel to increase the probability of its being in an open state. In addition, the G protein βγ-subunit acts directly on the Ca^{2+} channel. These actions increase the inward flow of Ca^{2+} [8].

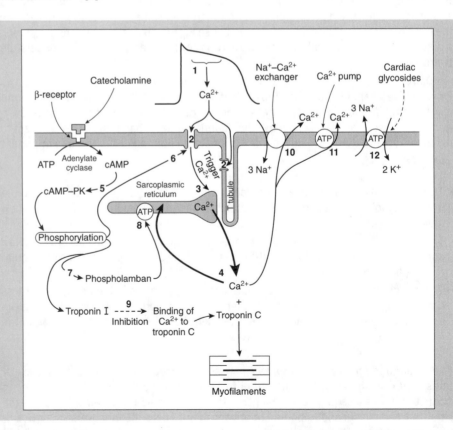

FIGURE 8-13

Summary of the Role of Ca^{2+} in Excitation–Contraction Coupling and Regulation of Inotropism in Cardiac Muscle. *There are three important concepts embodied in this figure. First, activation of the β-receptor enhances contractility by increasing the inward flow of trigger Ca^{2+} (3) that controls the release of Ca^{2+} from the sarcoplasmic reticulum (SR); this increases the amount of Ca^{2+} available to activate cross bridges between myosin and actin (4). Second, activation of the β-receptor also shortens the duration of the action potential by increasing the rate at which Ca^{2+} is resequestered into the SR (8) and by potentiating the action of troponin I (9). Troponin I diminishes the affinity of troponin C for Ca^{2+}. Third, the amount of Ca^{2+} entering the cell must eventually be removed by membrane pumps (10, 11); this assures a constant (i.e., homeostatic) level of intracellular Ca^{2+}. Cardiac glycosides inhibit the Na^+–K^+ exchange pump (12), which results in intracellular Na^+ accumulation, thereby slowing the Na^+–Ca^{2+} exchange pump.* (Source: Adapted with permission from Berne RM, Levy MN: Physiology, 3rd ed. St. Louis, MO: Mosby Year Book, 1993, p 402.)

nels. These include verapamil and its derivatives, diltiazem, and the dihydropyridines (e.g., nifedipine). Their therapeutic effects are clinically very important. For example, patients whose coronary vessels are barely able to supply adequate amounts of oxygenated blood at rest typically experience myocardial ischemia during exercise or stress. Placing these patients on a Ca^{2+} channel-blocking agent blunts the increase in $M\dot{v}o_2$ that would otherwise be caused by increased cardiac β-adrenergic stimulation (see Chapter 10, Figure 10-6).

Repolarization Phase

Inactivation of the inward Ca^{2+} current helps terminate the plateau phase. However, the rapid repolarization of phase 3 also requires that an outward current asserts itself toward the end of phase 2. This outward current is known as I_K.

Voltage-Dependent K^+ Channels. It is difficult to summarize the characteristics of myocardial voltage-dependent K^+-selective channels because at least six different types exist in the heart. The I_K channel has a number of structural similarities to the voltage-dependent Na^+ channel described previously. It consists of four subunits (Figure 8-14A), but unlike the motifs of the Na^+ channel, there is no covalent link from subunit to subunit, and the structure of each of the four units is generally similar. However, there are some variations called isoforms. The fact that the subunits are not covalently bound potentially allows the assembling of different subunit isoforms. This "mix-and-match"

> I_K **is different from** I_{K1}**.** For example, the channels that carry the latter current do not have an S4 segment; therefore, they are **not** voltage dependent. In addition, the I_{K1} current shows an inward rectification; the I_K current shows an outward rectification.

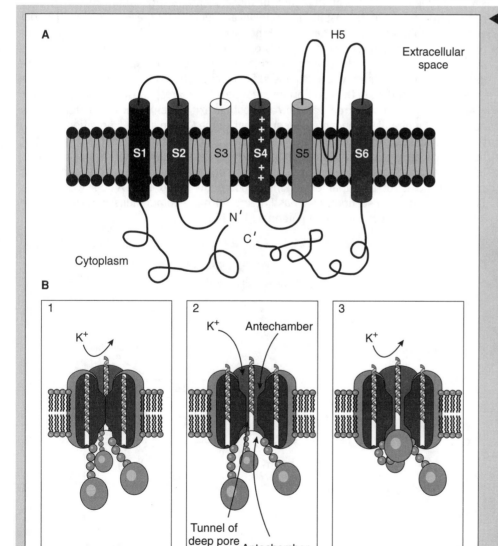

◀ **FIGURE 8-14**
Structure of Voltage-Dependent K^+ Channel. (A) S1–S6 represent membrane-spanning α-helices. S4 has a net positive charge, is highly conserved across species, and probably serves as the channel's voltage sensor. The model also shows the intracellular and extracellular loops. The loop between S5 and S6 (H5) probably forms the pore in conjunction with a similar loop provided by each of the remaining three (or more) subunits. (B) "Ball-and-chain" model for K^+-selective voltage-dependent delayed rectifier channel. The most anterior subunit of the tetramer has been removed to reveal the channel's pore, tunnel, and antechamber. The ribbon-like helices are the S4 voltage sensor. The channel is nonconducting in 1, conducting in 2, and inactivated by the ball's obstructing the channel's pore in 3. (Source: Adapted with permission from Taglialatela M, Brown AM: Structural correlates of K^+ channel function. News Physiol Sci 9: 170–171, 1994.)

option seems to account for the almost bewildering variety of K+ channels. Figure 8-14B shows an artist's conception of the tetramer assembly for a K+ channel. (The fourth unit has been removed to reveal the central pore.) When the pore is closed, the conductance of the channel is low. With appropriate changes in E_m, the channel's voltage sensitivity allows unobstructed movement of ions through the pore. With the passage of time, one of the intracellular loops is thought to change its position to block access to the mouth of the pore. This *ball-and-chain model* is compatible with the *time-dependent inactivation* of the channel.

Delayed Rectification and I_K. The voltage-dependent character of the delayed rectifier causes this channel to *activate progressively during the plateau* phase. Moreover, this channel acts like an outward rectifier. The resulting outward current (I_K) swells during the latter part of the plateau, and this progressively accelerating exit of positively charged K+ assists repolarization. The inward rectification of I_{K1} wanes as the cell's membrane potential nears its resting value toward the end of phase 3, which adds a final assist to the repolarization process.

Summary of the Ionic Basis of the Ventricular Muscle Action Potential

Most medical texts include a representation of the ionic events of the action potential similar to Figure 8-15A. The depiction of these events is very simplified, but it does capture the process at its most fundamental level. Figure 8-15B revisits the initial model of the cell in Figure 8-2. This new model, however, contains multiple pathways through the membrane, which represent the individual ion-selective channels. Each channel is shown as a variable conductor/resistor; this depicts the time-dependent and voltage-dependent characteristics of the channels. Each conductor is connected in series with a battery corresponding to the equilibrium potentials for the respective ions. The circuit is also complete because currents are now able both to exit and enter the cell. In reality, this portion of the circuit is conceptually equivalent to the Goldman Field equation. Finally, the capacitor (C_m) reflects the ability of the membrane to separate charge. No attempt has been made to incorporate an electrogenic pump in this model. Table 8-1 summarizes the properties of several major ion channels contributing to the resting membrane potential and action potential for working myocardium and for the SA node (see below). See Coraboeuf and Escande as well as Fozzard for more comprehensive reviews of the ionic events of the cardiac action potential [10, 11].

FIGURE 8-15 ▶

Summary of Electrophysiology of the Cell Membrane. (A) A simplified summary of the genesis of the ventricular muscle action potential. The events are expressed as changes in membrane conductance, not as current flows. Each tracing, and especially that for G_{K+}, is the overall conductance change for that ion; this plot often represents the summated effect of changes in individual channel types, each with unique characteristics. The G_{K+} graph indicates times at which changes in I_{K1} (inward rectifier), I_{TO} (transient outward), and I_K (delayed rectifier) are most obvious. ↓I_{K1} = decrease in I_{K1}. (B) A model of the cardiac cell membrane incorporating variable conductances, shown as resistors (R = 1/G), for K+-, Na+-, and Ca^{2+}-selective channels. The batteries represent the equilibrium potentials for each ion. C_m, a capacitor, represents the cell membrane's ability to separate charge. The values of individual resistors change during the course of an action potential as shown in panel A.

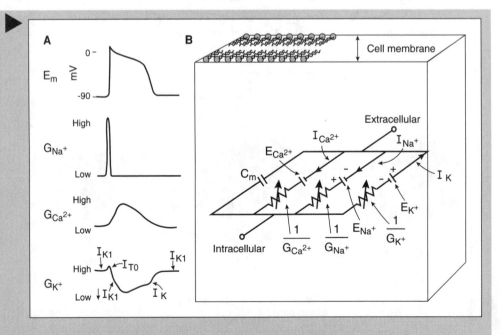

Channel Name	Current Name	Comments
Potassium ion (K+)		
Inward rectifier	I_{K1}	Sometimes called the background current because it is responsible for high-membrane permeability during diastole in working myocytes. Accounts for strongly negative *phase 4* diastolic potential. Not present (or present in low concentration) in SA and AV nodes. Inward rectification limits outward flow of K+ during plateau. Not voltage dependent.
Delayed rectifier	I_K	Characterized by outward rectification. Voltage-dependent channel slowly activated by depolarization. Helps terminate action potential (*phase 3*). Slowly deactivates with repolarization; gradual inactivation during diastole decreases G_{K+} and contributes to pacemaker potential in nodal cells.
Transient outward	I_{TO}	Voltage dependent; activated by depolarization. Significant contribution to *phase 1*.
I_{K-ACh}	Muscarinic-K+-channel	Ligand ACh-activated channel. Activation accounts for increased negativity of pacemaker potential as result of parasympathetic nervous activity. Decreases HR. Shows modest inward rectification.
I_{K-ATP}	ATP-sensitive K+ channel	Increases G_{K+} when intracellular ATP is low, as during ischemia. Terminates action potential early and reduces contractility, thereby limiting metabolic demand. Shows weak inward rectification.
Sodium ion (Na+)		
I_{Na}	Fast inward Na+	Voltage and time-dependent gating. Responsible for rapid depolarization (*phase 0*) in ventricular, atrial, and Purkinje fibers. Absent or low concentration in nodal cells.
I_b	Background	Passive background current. Explains why $E_m \neq E_{K+}$ in working myocytes.
I_f	Pacemaker current	"Funny" current contributes to diastolic depolarization in nodal cells. Channel conducts both Na+ and K+. Increased by β_1-receptor activation to increase HR; decreased by muscarinic receptor activation to decrease HR.
Calcium ion (Ca²⁺)		
L-type Ca²⁺	Slow inward current	Voltage- and time-dependent gating; threshold is less negative than for Na+ channel. Activates more slowly than Na+ channel. Responsible for inward current during plateau (*phase 2*). Increased by β_1-receptor activation; Ca²⁺-induced Ca²⁺ release phenomenon explains positive inotropism from sympathetic stimulation.
T-type Ca²⁺	Transient Ca²⁺	Voltage- and time-dependent gating. Inactivates quickly. May be responsible for final "kick" as pacemaker potential approaches threshold.

Note. ACh = acetylcholine; ATP = adenosine triphosphate; AV = atrioventricular; E_{K+} = potassium equilibrium potential; E_m = membrane potential; G_{K+} = outward conductance of potassium; HR = heart rate; SA = sinoatrial.

SINOATRIAL (SA) NODE AND CONTROL OF HEART RATE— CHRONOTROPISM

The inherent automaticity of the heart makes the heart transplant procedure possible. The donor's heart—not the recipient's nervous system—is responsible for initiating the heartbeat.

The heart continues to beat regularly after being removed from the body, provided it is given adequate metabolic support, because it possesses an *inherent automaticity. The autonomic nervous system can increase heart rate (HR) [a positive chronotropism] or decrease heart rate (negative chronotropism), but it is not responsible for initiating the beat.*

SA Node and Initiation of the Heartbeat

An action potential recorded from a *pacemaker cell (P cell)* within the SA node differs greatly in appearance from that of a ventricular muscle. In fact, the myocytes within this region do not look like ventricular muscle cells. Small, round cells within the node that have relatively few organelles and myofibrils are thought to be the P cells. Figure 8-16 compares action potentials recorded from a ventricular myocyte and a SA-nodal cell. Note the following specific characteristics of the SA-nodal recording as compared to the ventricular recording:

- The diastolic membrane potential is less electronegative.
- The membrane potential spontaneously depolarizes during diastole; this is called the *pacemaker potential*, diastolic depolarization, or phase 4 depolarization.
- As a result of the pacemaker potential, E_m eventually attains threshold and produces an action potential. This action potential initiates the next heartbeat by propagating to all parts of the heart via the electrical coupling between cardiac myocytes.
- The rate of rise of the action potential is relatively slow. As a result, the velocity of the conduction of the action potential within the SA node is relatively slow (≈ 0.01 m/sec).

FIGURE 8-16 ▶

Comparison of Action Potentials from a Ventricular Myocyte and a Pacemaker Cell within the Sinoatrial (SA) node. During electrical diastole, the SA node's membrane potential (E_m) spontaneously depolarizes to threshold. This pacemaker potential accounts for the automaticity of the heartbeat. The diastolic potential is more negative, and phase 0 is more rapid in the ventricular recording.

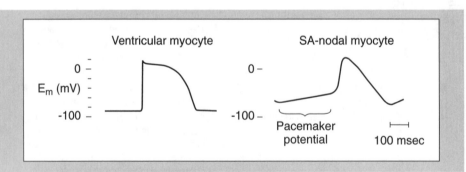

Ionic Basis for the SA-Nodal Action Potential

The channels responsible for the inward rectifier that are so characteristic of the sarcolemma of the ventricular myocyte do not exist in the SA-nodal cell membrane. As a result, there is no I_{K1}. Recall that I_{K1} is the major factor responsible for the resting membrane potential's being close to E_{K+} in ventricular muscle. The "resting" membrane potential is much less electronegative because of the lack of the inward rectifier in the SA node. In addition, Na^+ channels either do not exist or are very sparse within the SA node; those that may exist would be inactivated because of the low E_m. Therefore, *the SA-nodal action potential is carried primarily by the slow inward Ca^{2+} current.* This dependence on the slow inward current accounts for the low dV/dt during the upstroke of the SA-nodal action potential. But what accounts for the pacemaker potential?

There are three key factors responsible for the phase 4 depolarization. First, SA-nodal cells have a definite inward background current (I_b), which, by its very nature, tends to depolarize the cell. Second, although there is no I_{K1}, these cells do possess the channels that carry I_K. Recall that this voltage-dependent current *activates during the plateau* and then *inactivates during diastole*. Finally, the T-type Ca^{2+} channels activate during the latter portion of the pacemaker potential; this additional inward current provides a final "push" to bring the membrane to threshold. In simple terms, therefore, the progressively decreasing outward current, coupled with I_f and growing inward Ca^{2+} flow results in the pacemaker potential. Details of these ionic mechanisms may be found in a recent review by Irisawa and colleagues [12].

There is another inward current known as I_f; the "f" stands for "funny." I_f is a major factor in causing the diastolic depolarization and is therefore often called the pacemaker current.

Autonomic Control of Heart Rate

The rate at which the heart beats in the absence of neurohumoral influences is called the *intrinsic HR*. The heart in a cardiac transplant patient beats at or near the intrinsic rate of approximately 90–95 beats/min. The heart beats at a much lower rate than this in the healthy, resting adult. This difference is attributed to the lack of an effective autonomic control of the SA node in the transplanted heart.

The cardiac *parasympathetic preganglionic innervation of the SA node* is primarily via small branches of the tenth cranial nerves (i.e., the left and right vagi). The parasympathetic ganglia reside at the heart and project axons to the SA node. Increased cardiac parasympathetic nervous activity slows heart rate—a *negative chronotropism*—by hyperpolarizing the pacemaker cells of the SA node or by slowing the rate of their phase-4 depolarization (Figure 8-17A). The acetylcholine (ACh) released from the vagal nerve endings interacts with a *muscarinic receptor* on the SA-nodal cell membrane. The muscarinic receptor is linked to an inhibitory G protein (G_i). Activation of G_i has two effects. First, it suppresses intracellular levels of cAMP, which, in turn, decreases the inward I_f current. Second, it activates a K^+ channel (I_{K-ACh}), increasing the conductance of the cell membrane to K^+. Together, these actions explain the changes in the action potential shown in Figure 8-17A.

Vagus or vagi? The word "vagus" is singular, as in "the right vagus nerve." "Vagi," in which the "g" is pronounced as a "j" and rhymes with "magi," is plural, as in "the left and right vagi."

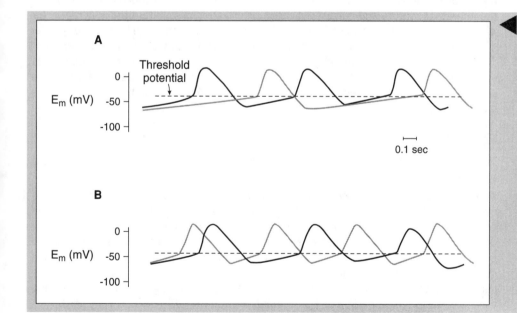

◀ FIGURE 8-17

Nervous Control of Heart Rate (HR). *(A) A series of sinoatrial (SA) node action potentials at normal resting levels of cardiac parasympathetic nervous activity (heavy line) and at elevated vagal tone (light line). The broken line designates the threshold potential at which an action potential initiates. Increased parasympathetic activity also hyperpolarizes the diastolic membrane potential (not shown) and slows the pacemaker potential so that the membrane potential (E_m) takes longer to attain threshold, and HR slows. (B) The dark line is identical to the resting data in panel A. The light line shows the increased slope of the pacemaker potential caused by increased cardiac sympathetic nervous activity. Threshold is attained more rapidly, and HR increases.*

Healthy individuals at rest generally have an ongoing vagal tone and, therefore, a relatively low resting heart rate. Withdrawal of this normal resting activity allows pulse rate to increase toward the intrinsic HR. Exercise training accentuates parasympathetic nervous activity at rest, thereby producing the well-known *bradycardia* in conditioned athletes.

Resting HR accelerates during inspiration and slows with expiration. This cyclic change in HR originates in the SA node (i.e., the sinus) and thus is called the *respiratory sinus arrhythmia*. It is mediated by changes in cardiac parasympathetic activity, and its disappearance is among the earliest signs that the body is being challenged by stress or

The major direct effects of the parasympathetic nervous system on the heart are at the SA and AV nodes, which slow heart rate and AV conduction, respectively. Increased parasympathetic activity also depresses atrial contractility, but the functional impact of this negative inotropism is modest. Increased parasympathetic tone indirectly depresses ventricular inotropism by presynaptically inhibiting the release of neurotransmitter from the cardiac sympathetic nerves.

an incipient disease process. The tachycardia or bradycardia caused by decreases or increases in parasympathetic nervous activity, respectively, occur almost immediately after the change in nervous input to the SA node. Some individuals suffer *vagal syncope*, or fainting, because of sudden, often unexplained, increases in cardiac parasympathetic nervous activity.

The *sympathetic innervation to the SA node* and other parts of the heart is primarily via nerves branching from the left and right middle cervical and stellate ganglia. Increasing sympathetic nervous activity exerts its positive chronotropism by increasing the rate of the phase 4 depolarization in the SA node (Figure 8-17B). L-type $I_{Ca}v2+$, I_K, and I_f and the Na^+-K^+ exchange pump current are all affected by β-adrenergic agonists. In particular, the β-receptor is linked to a stimulatory G protein (G_s), which increases intracellular cAMP; this increases the probability that the I_f channel is open and increases the inward pacemaker current. Sympathetically mediated changes in HR are expressed somewhat more slowly than changes in vagal activity. Under extreme circumstances, increased sympathetic nervous activity can produce a tachycardia exceeding 200 beats/min.

ATRIOVENTRICULAR (AV) NODE AND CONTROL OF AV CONDUCTION—DROMOTROPISM

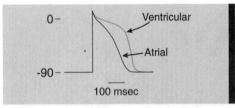

A-N = atrial-nodal
N = nodal
N-H = nodal-His

The depolarization originating within the SA node is conducted throughout the left and right atria. The atrial action potential is similar in many respects to that of the ventricular myocyte, although the overshoot is less marked, and the plateau phase is less pronounced. The next step in the highly coordinated sequence of electrical events leading to the depolarization of the entire heart involves the *AV node*. The AV node is situated within the interatrial septum and consists of three different regions. Within the *A-N region* (or *junctional region*), the cytologic features of the cells gradually change from those of atrial muscle to those of the *nodal region* itself. The N-region cells anatomically and functionally resemble those of the SA node in many respects. In particular, action potentials recorded from cells within the N region look like those of the SA node, except that the slope of the pacemaker potential is slower than for the SA node. Finally, the N-H region is a transition between the AV node and the *bundle of His*.

Four Functions of the AV Node

The AV node has four important functions, which are determined by the anatomic and electrophysiologic properties of the nodal cells.

A "Conduction Bridge" Between the Atria and Ventricles. The AV node is normally the only pathway whereby the supraventricular depolarization originating in the SA node is conducted through to the ventricles. This aspect of its function is analogous to a border crossing between countries. Just as a specified border checkpoint allows authorities to control the flow of goods and information between countries, passing the electrical depolarization through the narrow confines of the AV node allows the autonomic nervous system to have precise control over the electrical coupling between the atria and ventricles (see Sympathetic and Parasympathetic Control of AV-Nodal Function).

Induction of a Delay Between Atrial and Ventricular Depolarization. One of the notable similarities between the action potentials of the SA and AV nodes is the low rate of change of voltage during phase 0. As a result, the conduction of the electrical depolarization through the AV node is slow ($\approx$ 0.05 m/sec), just as it is within the SA node. This introduces a delay between the depolarization of the atria and the depolarization of the ventricles, which allows time for atrial contraction to contribute to ventricular filling.

A "Backup" Pacemaker. Cells within the AV node, especially in the junctional region, have a pacemaker potential that can, under appropriate circumstances, attain threshold and sustain an action potential. In particular, if the SA-nodal pacemaker fails to initiate a heartbeat in a timely manner, the "junctional pacemaker" can assume the role of cardiac pacemaker. There are two important points to remember about this function.

- The rate of the phase 4 depolarization in the AV node is slower than in the normally functioning SA node; therefore, the SA node is normally the dominant pacemaker.
- The HR in persons with a junctional rhythm is relatively low (e.g., 40 beats/min) compared to a normal sinus rhythm because the phase 4 depolarization of these cells is slow. They may consequently feel lethargic and complain of lassitude. Physicians often opt to implant an artificial pacemaker that maintains a higher HR.

AV-Nodal Block: Protective or a Sign of Disease. Even a perfectly healthy AV node is incapable of extremely rapid conduction. Therefore, if the atria are beating very rapidly (atrial tachycardia), the AV node may not pass every atrial depolarization through to the ventricles. This AV-nodal block protects the ventricles from attempting to fill and eject blood more rapidly than they are effectively capable of doing. In other—often pathologic—cases, the AV node does not conduct every impulse even when the atria are beating at normal rates. AV-nodal block is classified as first, second, or third degree.

Sympathetic and Parasympathetic Control of AV-Nodal Function

The autonomic nervous system closely coordinates the *chronotropic* and *dromotropic* functions of the heart. Parasympathetic nervous activity slows AV conduction, which is a negative dromotropism. Low levels of vagal activity merely tend to slow AV-nodal conduction velocity (*first-degree block*). Somewhat higher intensity stimulation may allow only every other atrial depolarization to be conducted (a 2:1 *second-degree block*) or perhaps only every third (a 3:1 *second-degree block*). More intense parasympathetic activity may cause a complete block (*third-degree block*) in AV conduction. Conversely, sympathetic stimulation increases the rate of AV-nodal conduction (a positive dromotropism). These specific examples may give a false impression, however, of the role of the nervous regulation in "policing" the flow of information across this border between the atria and ventricles. In reality, the nervous system typically acts to ensure that increases in the rate at which the SA node initiates a heartbeat are matched by increases in the rate at which the AV node conducts each beat through to the ventricles. Therefore, during exercise, the AV node normally conducts 1:1 (i.e., every atrial beat) although the rate of atrial depolarization is quite rapid. This is another example of how an increase in sympathetic nervous activity, coupled with a withdrawal of parasympathetic activity, allows the heart to perform more work, more rapidly.

> The most rapid pacemaker suppresses the rate of the pacemaker potential in other cells, such as a potential AV-nodal pacemaker. This "overdrive suppression" assures that the SA node, with its more rapid phase 4 depolarization, normally does not have to compete with other dormant pacemakers for dominance in control of HR.

> *Common "isms" of Cardiology*
> Chronotropism: modification of HR (from Greek chronos [time])
> Dromotropism: modification of conduction rate, primarily of the AV node (from Greek dromos [a running])
> Inotropism: modification of muscle contractility (from Greek in [fiber])

BUNDLE OF HIS AND THE RAPID SPREAD OF DEPOLARIZATION THROUGHOUT THE VENTRICLES

The *bundle of His* originates from the N-H region of the AV node and consists of muscle fibers (*not* nerves) that are specialized for rapidly conducting electrical depolarization from cell to cell. These specialized cells are called *Purkinje fibers*. Their rapid conduction velocity (1–4 m/sec) is due in part to their large diameter (70–80 μ compared with 10–15 μ for ventricular myocytes). The action potential recorded from the Purkinje fiber is similar to that from a ventricular myocyte except that, in these specialized cells, the rate of rise of E_m during phase 0 is even more rapid, and the plateau lasts even longer.

The bundle of His divides into the *left and right bundle branches*, which project down the left and right sides of the interventricular septum, respectively. The bundle branches *arborize* by breaking into multiple smaller branches that carry the depolarization rapidly to the ventricular free walls. The normal syncytial conduction from cell to cell then ensures that the depolarization ultimately passes to every muscle fiber within the heart. However, the myocytes within the ventricles do not, in fact, depolarize simultaneously. The actual pattern of depolarization has been determined in detail, originally in painstaking experiments by Scher and Young, in which they mapped the spread of excitation throughout the canine ventricles [13]. Briefly, the first areas to depolarize are the middle to apical regions of the interventricular septum and the papillary muscles. The endocardial surfaces of the ventricles follow, with depolarization spreading in the epicardial direction. The wave "breaks through" to the epicardial surfaces of the thin walls of the right ventricle earlier than for the thicker left ventricle. The last regions to depolarize are toward the basal regions of the left ventricle and septum. The movement of these "waves" of depolarization through the heart can be represented by a vector that changes continuously in direction and magnitude. These dynamic changes in the heart's electrical vector explain the nature and shape of the waves of the ECG.

INTRODUCTION TO THE ELECTROCARDIOGRAM

Figure 8-18 shows an illustrative ECG for a single heartbeat. Recordings such as this have almost become the symbol for the practice of medicine to the general public, and, in fact, the ECG has been a mainstay for the diagnosis of many forms of heart disease for nearly a century. The beginning medical student may, therefore, understandably wish to launch directly into a study of its clinical use before comprehending its physiologic basis. This, however, is not only unwise but also impractical. Instead, the student must learn first what the ECG is (and is not). Only then will it be practical to take the first steps toward using the ECG as a diagnostic tool. Accordingly, the remainder of this chapter is intended, first, to explain the fundamental concepts of how the ECG is recorded, and, second, what information that recording can provide about the normal electrical activity of the heart. Examples of pathologic conditions are given when they advance these two major goals. Finally, the ECG is used to help demonstrate the effects of several different types of irregular rhythms on the pumping action of the heart. Other sources should be consulted for details of clinical electrocardiography [14–16].

FIGURE 8-18 ▶

Electrocardiogram (ECG) for a Single Heartbeat. The "waves" of the ECG are indicated along with important time intervals. The P wave is due to atrial depolarization. The QRS complex is produced by depolarization of the right and left ventricles. In effect, then, the QRS complex demarcates the end of diastole and the beginning of systole. The T wave is caused by repolarization of the ventricles. The intervals shown below the recording (e.g., PR) fall within a normal range in the healthy heart (see Table 8-2). The sequence of waves repeats within each heartbeat.

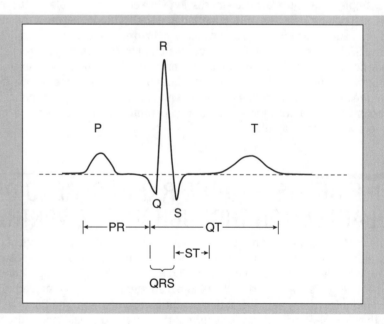

ECG Leads

Without exception, the electrical signals presented thus far in this chapter have been transmembrane action potentials. *The ECG is not a transmembrane action potential.* Instead, *the ECG is an electrical signal recorded on the surface of the body that results from the depolarization and repolarization of countless atrial and ventricular muscle fibers.* The depolarization and repolarization of the multitudes of myocytes that comprise the heart produce cyclic changes in the electric potential on the body's surface that can

*The ECG does **not** result from **contraction** of heart muscle fibers. Instead, it results from the **electrical field** created by the summed electrical events within the individual myocytes.*

be recorded using metal tabs (electrodes) attached to the skin surface. The shape of the recorded signal differs according to the anatomic location of an electrode with respect to the heart. Actually, an electrode on a certain area of the skin records the projection of the cardiac signal on that particular surface area. A given electrode, therefore, provides a restricted piece of the whole picture of cardiac electrical activity. It is a view from one "window" at a three-dimensional structure—the heart. A given viewpoint on the overall electrical activity of the heart is called a *lead* of the ECG. Simultaneous recordings of the heart's electrical signal, using multiple leads arranged in several standardized locations around the heart, provide a comprehensive image of the heart's activity.

Ten electrodes are attached to the body to record the conventional ECG: one on each of the four limbs, and six on the anterior chest wall. The one on the right lower limb serves as a ground electrode to decrease electrical noise, and the other nine are used for recording the electrical potential at their respective locations. From these nine electrodes, cardiologists have twelve distinct views (i.e., leads) of the electrical activity of the heart. The first to be recorded (historically) measured the potential *difference* between *pairs* of electrodes on the limbs. These *bipolar limb leads* are still the first to be recorded in the sequence of the 12-lead ECG in the clinic. They are named leads I, II, and III. The remaining nine leads are recorded relative to a single point that is theoretically not influenced by the heart's electrical signal. They are called *unipolar leads*. The three bipolar leads and the nine unipolar leads together form the conventional 12-lead surface ECG that "looks" at the heart in both the *frontal* plane that passes through the center of the heart parallel to the body surface and the *horizontal plane* that passes through the heart perpendicular to the chest wall (see Figure 8-22.)

The moment-by-moment electrical activity of the myocardium can be represented by a vector originating in the heart. The amplitude of the vector and the direction in which it points vary continuously during the cardiac cycle, as determined by the spread of the wave of depolarization across the myocardium (see Bundle of His and the Rapid Spread of Depolarization Throughout the Ventricles). This process creates an ever-changing electrical field on the body surface that appears as a potential (i.e., voltage) difference between any *two* points on the skin. Figure 8-19 illustrates the simplest method for recording the bipolar leads of the ECG. Electrodes are placed on both of the patient's arms and on the left leg. The potential difference recorded between the electrodes on the person's left arm (LA) and right arm (RA) is called *lead I* of the ECG. This small voltage difference can be recorded by attaching the wires from the electrodes to the input of a high-gain amplifier. By convention, the amplifier is connected so that an upward pen deflection results when the voltage at the left arm is more positive than at the right arm. The other *limb leads* are recorded between the right arm and left leg (lead II) and left arm and left leg (lead III).

Although the electrodes are connected near the patient's hands and feet, the recording would not be appreciably different if the recording locations were at the shoulders and near the umbilicus. This is because the limbs, unlike the torso, behave as linear conductors that transmit the electrical signal without any significant alteration in polarity. The result of figuratively moving the location of the electrodes is a triangle, known as *Einthoven's triangle*, after the scientist who first recorded the ECG. The heart lies at the center of this triangle; the vector representing the summed electrical activity of the myocytes at any given instant is visualized as originating at the center of the heart and triangle. Einthoven's triangle itself lies on the two-dimensional space that constitutes the frontal plane. Figure 8-20 shows how Einthoven's triangle is formed by lead I across the top with leads II and III comprising the two sides. The plus sign (+) and minus sign (−) designations at the corners of the triangle designate the conventional polarity for each bipolar lead.

The instantaneous size and angular direction of the vector determine the ECG recording in each lead. Because the direction and size of the vector change continuously during the cardiac cycle, the situation shown in the figure must correspond to some particular instant in time. In fact, the vector shown would be recorded at the instant when the largest number of ventricular myocytes are in the process of depolarizing. Imagine that there is a light bulb just below the bottom pole of the triangle, as shown. The vector at the heart would cast a "shadow" on lead I of a certain size. *The amplitude of the ECG recording at any given instant in lead I is proportional to the length of this shadow.* The

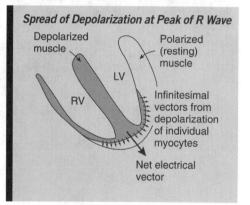

The different leads of the ECG are something like looking at an automobile from different perspectives. The "image" provided by lead I is analogous to viewing the car from the front. The perspective from lead II is akin to looking at the car from its right rear. All 12 leads provide a nearly encompassing impression of the car/heart.

Spread of Depolarization at Peak of R Wave

Depolarized muscle

Polarized (resting) muscle

LV

RV

Infinitesimal vectors from depolarization of individual myocytes

Net electrical vector

The ECG is recorded using either single- or multichannel devices. A single-channel device records one lead at a time, so that the operator has to switch 12 times to complete the recording. In some multichannel recorders, the electronics are such that no switching is required, and a virtually complete 12-lead ECG is printed out automatically.

FIGURE 8-19 ▶

Recording Procedure for Leads I, II, and III of the Electrocardiogram (ECG). *These three bipolar leads are recorded from electrodes placed on the patient's right (RA) and left arms (LA) and left leg (LL), as shown. Electrically, this is equivalent to electrodes figuratively placed at the shoulders and near the umbilicus to form an equilateral triangle, Einthoven's triangle, with the heart at its center. The electrical depolarization and repolarization of myriads of individual myocytes produce an electrical field that can be represented by a vector within the heart. The electrical field, as represented by the vector, changes continuously during the cardiac cycle. The changing electrical field produces minute voltage differences between any two points on the body surface. In practice, standard locations on the body are used to record the potential difference. Amplifying the potential difference between the right arm and left arm produced by this electrical field yields lead I of the ECG. Switching the input leads to the amplifier to RA/LL and LA/LL yields leads II and III, respectively.*

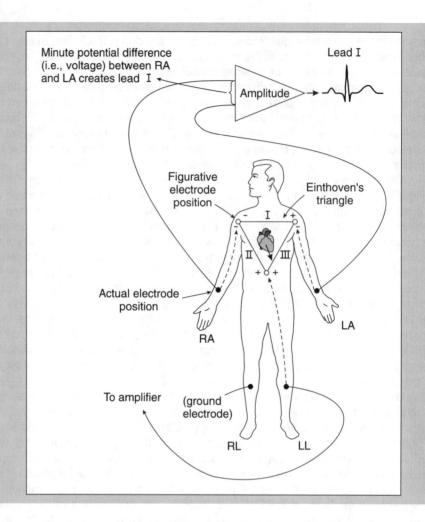

FIGURE 8-20 ▶

Determination of Size of the Deflection in Leads I, II, and III at Any Moment during the Cardiac Cycle. *The heart is centered within Einthoven's triangle. The vector shown originating at the center of the heart results from the net electrical activity at that moment summated across countless individual myocytes. The shadows cast by the vector on each limb of the triangle determine the amplitude of each lead of the electrocardiogram. A vector in lead I pointing toward the left arm (LA) yields a positive deflection (*). Likewise, vectors pointing toward the left leg (LL) in leads II and III give upright deflections. The isoelectric line is designated at the left of each limb lead reconstruction.*

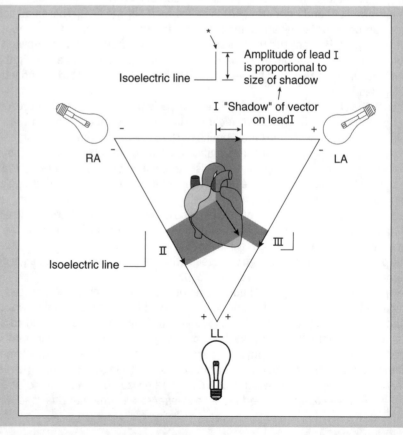

size of the shadow (i.e., the reflection of the vector on lead I) changes—and with it the amplitude of the lead I recording—as the wave of depolarization that creates the vector sweeps over the heart. Likewise, if the vector were illuminated by a light at the upper left corner of the triangle, it would cast a shadow of a given amplitude on lead II. In this example, the amplitude of this shadow and the resultant size of the momentary deflection in lead II exceed that of lead I. Finally, a light at the right arm would cast its shadow on lead III and yield a small recording. Consider one other snapshot in time. During electrical diastole, the magnitude of the vector would be zero because no myocytes are in the process of depolarizing and no currents are flowing within the heart. This explains the *isoelectric line.*

Convention and ease of analysis have prompted cardiologists to use a different representation of Einthoven's triangle in which the three leads "collapse" into the geometric center of the triangle, without changing their angular orientation with respect to each other. The single point at which the three leads intersect after this implosion corresponds to the electrical center of the heart. Much like a compass, the points around this new axis are assigned angular values: 0° corresponds to "east" on a compass. The heart's electrical vector is visualized as originating at the intersection of these axes, which corresponds with the center of Einthoven's triangle. The vector has a magnitude and a direction in degrees relative to the axis.

To review quickly, leads I, II, and III are called bipolar leads because each measures the potential difference between two electrodes on the body surface. In the remaining nine leads, the signal is recorded between a body surface electrode and an *indifferent electrode.* The names of the unipolar leads start with "V" followed by the anatomic location of the sensing electrode. For example, "VR" means the unipolar lead in the right arm; it measures the "absolute" change in electrical potential measured at the right arm caused by cardiac electrical activity. VL and VF are the other two unipolar limb leads on the left arm and left foot, respectively. Actual clinical practice differs slightly from the process just described: a change in the electrical wiring of the indifferent electrode results in the "augmented" unipolar leads (i.e., aVR, aVL, aVF), which are preferred because the amplitude of the signal in these leads is larger than in the original configuration. In total, the six limb leads nearly surround the heart in the frontal plane, as shown in Figure 8-21.

In addition to the six limb leads, there are six unipolar chest leads that are numbered from V1 to V6 starting from right to left in the fourth and fifth intercostal spaces that view the heart from the anterior and left lateral parts of the horizontal plane. The potential at each chest position is, once again, measured against the indifferent electrode. Figure 8-22 summarizes the location of the limb leads on the frontal plane and the precordial leads on the horizontal plane. In this representation, the position of each lead is represented at the appropriate angular position on the circumference of the circles.

Recording the ECG

It is essential to have standard recorder settings to calculate meaningful durations and voltage amplitudes of the ECG components. The recording paper is printed with a grid of vertical and horizontal lines that are 1 mm apart. Every fifth line is printed in bold so that each small square is 1 mm × 1 mm, and each big square is 5 mm × 5 mm. The standard paper speed used in clinical settings is 25 mm/sec; therefore, each thin vertical line designates 0.04 second, and the time between the heavy-print lines is 0.2 second (i.e., 5 × 0.04). The machine is calibrated so that a 1 mV potential difference displaces the writing pen 1 cm from the baseline. By adhering to these standardized settings, it is easy to calculate the duration and the voltage amplitude of the various components of the ECG. Consequently, it is possible to define a normal range of values for each component. Knowing the electrophysiologic basis and the quoted normal range for each component allows the identification of various cardiac syndromes that alter cardiac electrical activity. Figure 8-23 shows a modern ECG recording of the 12 standard leads and a short series of beats from 3 selected leads.

Components of the ECG

Table 8-2 describes the normal components of the ECG (left) and some important pathologic changes (right). The latter list is not intended to be exhaustive but should help the student to understand how underlying changes in cardiac electrophysiology alter the ECG.

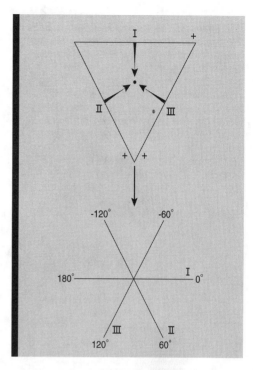

*The indifferent electrode is formed by connecting the individual limb electrodes at a common terminal. Electrically speaking, this common terminal acts as though it were isolated from the electrical activity in the heart, that is, "indifferent" to the heart's presence. It can be regarded as having an invariant potential of 0 mV, against which the potential at the body surface electrode is measured. In a sense, therefore, the unipolar leads measure the "absolute" potential **at** the specified electrode on the body surface, as opposed to the potential **difference** between two locations, as in the bipolar leads.*

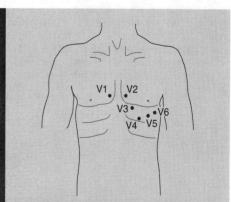

Leads V1 and V2 are located on the fourth intercostal space on the right and left sides of the sternum, respectively. Leads V4, V5, and V6 are located on the left fifth intercostal space on the midclavicular, anterior axillary, and midaxillary lines, respectively. Lead V3 is placed between V2 and V4.

FIGURE 8-21 ▶

Six Leads of the Limb Electrodes, Their Names, and Angular Degree Assignments. *The plus sign (+) designates the conventional polarity assignments; a shadow of the cardiac vector pointing in the "+" direction yields an upward deflection in that lead. The positive pole of lead I is designated 0°. The angle advances in the clockwise direction in 30° intervals so that the positive pole of the augmented unipolar limb lead on the left leg (aVF) is at +90°, and the negative pole of lead I is at 180°. The positive pole of the augmented unipolar limb lead on the left arm (aVL) is assigned −30°, and so forth.*

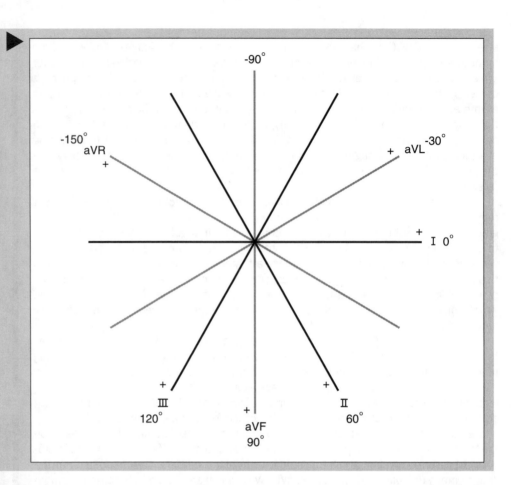

FIGURE 8-22 ▶

Frontal and Horizontal Planes Formed by the Electrocardiogram Leads. *The three bipolar (I, II, III) and the three unipolar (aVF, aVL, aVR) limb leads create the frontal plane that passes through the center of the heart parallel to the anterior and posterior surfaces of the body. The positions of each lead are shown at an appropriate point on the circumference of a circle. The chest leads create the horizontal plane that also passes through the center of the heart but in a direction perpendicular to the frontal plane. Again, the locations of V1–V6 are shown on the circumference of a circle residing within the horizontal plane.*

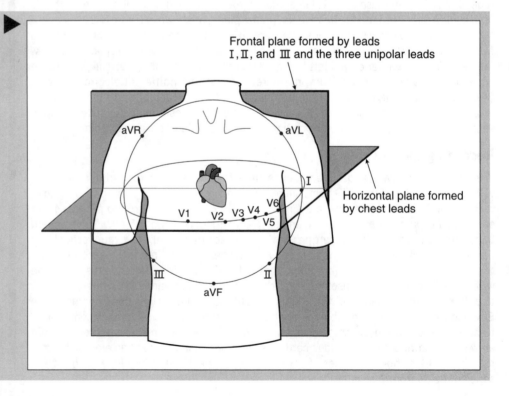

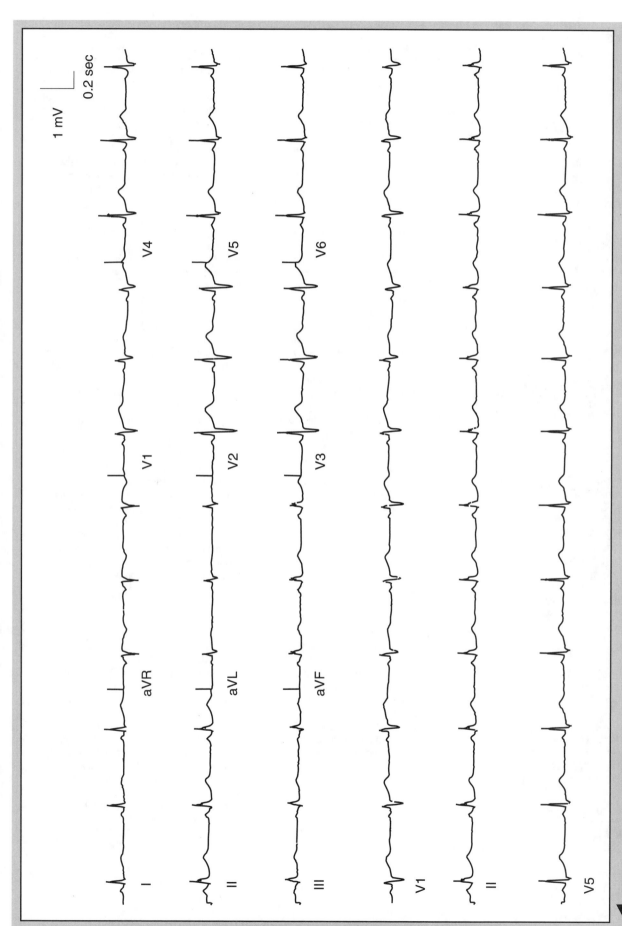

FIGURE 8-23

Modern 12-Lead Electrocardiogram Recording from a Healthy Adult. *The top three lines show a series of three heart beats from each of the 12 leads, as identified at their lower left margin. The bottom three lines show a longer recording of V1, II, and V5; the longer recording interval allows the physician to examine the rhythm. This person's heart was beating in a normal sinus rhythm.*

TABLE 8-2 ▶

Electrocardiogram (ECG)

Normal ECG Components	Pathophysiologic Changes
The *P wave* is due to *atrial depolarization*. Its amplitude is small because of the small muscle mass of the atria. Normally it does not exceed 0.12 second in duration (i.e., 3 mm on the chart recording) or 3 mm in height. Its axis is approximately 60° so that it appears positive in leads I, II, and aVF and negative in aVR.	Prolongation or peaking of the P wave usually results from atrial enlargement: the increase in electrical "power" from the depolarization of an increased atrial mass results in a larger electrical signal on the body surface. Reversal of the deflection (i.e., being positive in aVR and negative in I, II, and aVF) means that the electrical axis has reversed, usually because the atria are being depolarized from below upwards, as in an AV-nodal rhythm.
The *QRS complex* is produced by *ventricular depolarization*. It is the dominant wave of the ECG. Its duration should be between 0.06 and 0.1 second. Its mean axis in the frontal plane (i.e., as calculated from limb leads) should lie between −30° and +90°. This is because the *mean electrical axis* is normally pointing toward the thicker left ventricle. In precordial leads, the QRS complex is mainly negative in V1 (with a small initial positive wave signifying depolarization of the interventricular septum) and mainly positive in V5 and V6; leads V2–V4 show a gradual transition in the deflection. The voltage amplitude varies in different leads but should be generally below 30 mm (adding both positive and negative components).	Prolongation of the QRS complex indicates an intraventricular conduction delay either in one of the two AV bundle branches or, less frequently, in their smaller, distal branches. Increased voltage implies ventricular hypertrophy—either left, right, or biventricular—depending on the site of the relative projection of the augmented electrical vector on different leads. Right ventricular hypertrophy is usually associated with augmented positive waves in leads V1 and V2. Conversely, abnormally high positive waves in left-sided leads, exceedingly deep negative waves in the right ones, or both suggest left ventricular hypertrophy.
Ventricular repolarization produces the *T wave*. Its axis generally follows that of the QRS complex. Its amplitude should not exceed 5 mm in the limb leads or 10 mm in the precordial leads.	A change in the shape or polarity of the T wave indicates a disordered ventricular repolarization caused by either myocardial ischemia or other, less frequent, nonischemic causes. The T wave is notoriously labile because it is affected by a variety of cardiac and noncardiac conditions (e.g., ischemia, electrolyte disturbances, some drugs). It can be either inverted, flat, or peaked. Thus, it has poor specificity.
The *PR interval* is the time from the beginning of the P wave to the start of the QRS complex (see Figure 8-18). It normally lasts from 0.12 to 0.2 second. It has two components: the P wave itself, which is due to atrial depolarization, and the portion of the isoelectric line between the end of the P wave and the beginning of the QRS complex (PR segment) during which the electrical impulse is making its way through the AV node.	Prolongation of the PR interval (i.e., > 0.2 second) indicates abnormally delayed AV conduction, a condition called first-degree heart block (see Figure 8-26). A PR interval shorter than 0.12 second means that AV conduction does not experience the normal physiologic delay. This situation is usually encountered in a condition called pre-excitation syndrome in which there is an *accessory* AV pathway made of non-nodal cardiac muscle fibers (i.e., ordinary myocytes) connecting the atria and the ventricles. This pathway does not impose the electrical delay that is characteristic of the specialized AV-nodal cells.

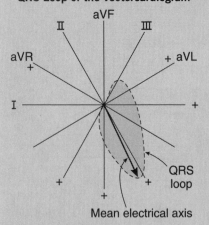

QRS Loop of the Vectorcardiogram

Mean electrical axis

*Depolarization of the ventricles, as signaled by the QRS complex, produces a continuously changing electrical vector; a plot of the position of the tip of this electrode yields a "loop" within the frontal plane. The **mean electrical axis** is the average electrical vector that is created by this loop. It is oriented within the range of −30° and +90° in the frontal plane. This is useful diagnostically because the orientation of this **electrical axis** changes, for example, in a person with right or left ventricular hypertrophy.*

The electrical activity resultant from AV-nodal depolarization is so weak that it cannot be detected by an electrode on the skin. AV-nodal activity can be recorded, however, by introducing a catheter, with a bipolar electrode at its tip, through a large vein into the lower right atrial region, where it is physically near to the AV node. This is often called a bundle of His recording.

Normal ECG Components	*Pathophysiologic Changes*
The *QT interval* extends from the beginning of a QRS complex to the end of the ensuing T wave (see Figure 8-18). It begins with ventricular depolarization and ends with ventricular repolarization. Its duration varies inversely with heart rate (HR) and is probably affected by gender. Normally, it should not exceed 0.47 second in females or 0.45 second in males after correction for HR.	Prolongation of the QT interval generally indicates an abnormal delay in ventricular repolarization (see Resolution of Clinical Case).
The *ST segment* begins at the end of the QRS complex and extends to the beginning of the T wave (see Figure 8-18). The normally functioning ventricles are completely depolarized during the time represented by that segment; there is consequently no potential difference between any points within the ventricles, so there is no current flow during this interval. As a result, this segment lies upon the isoelectric line.	Displacement of the ST segment in either the positive or negative direction indicates an abnormal current flow because of some regions within a ventricle that are not at the same electrical potential as the rest of the ventricular myocardium. This abnormal current is commonly created when a part of the myocardium is rendered ischemic by severe coronary insufficiency. ST displacement can be up in some leads and down in others in the same patient, depending on the relative projection of the vector produced by the injury current on different leads (Figure 8-24).
The *T-P segment* lasts from the end of the T wave to the beginning of the next P wave. During this phase, the whole heart is completely polarized. It is considered the standard isoelectric line in the electrical cardiac cycle.	

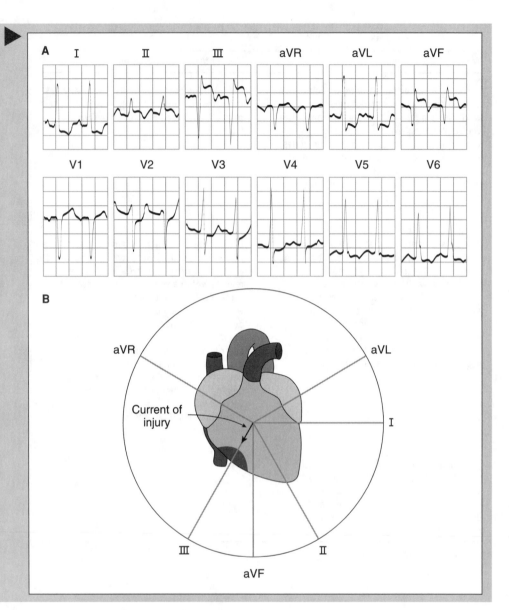

FIGURE 8-24

An Electrocardiogram Recording from a Patient Suffering an Acute Myocardial Infarction of the Apical (Inferior) Portion of the Heart. (A) This figure shows a definite ST-segment elevation in leads III and aVF, with a smaller elevation in lead II. Leads I and aVL show a ST-segment depression. There is no noticeable elevation or depression in the ST segment in lead aVR. In the horizontal plane, leads V2–V4 show ST-segment depression. There are abnormal Q waves in leads III and aVF, which indicate that the ischemia has progressed to infarction, at least in some muscle fibers. (B) This figure is an analysis in the frontal plane to determine the location on the heart of the ischemic region. The ST-segment changes are attributed to a "current of injury" flowing between regions of the myocardium that are at different potentials during the plateau phase of the action potential. The ST deflection is zero in lead aVR, indicating that the vector produced by this current flow is nearly perpendicular to this lead (i.e., it "casts no shadow" on lead aVR). Conversely, the vector casts a large shadow in the positive direction of leads III, aVF, and, to a lesser degree, lead II. Finally, it is negative on lead aVL. This type of analysis, plus a similar appraisal in the horizontal plane, allows the cardiologist to diagnose the presence of affected muscle (shaded area) on the inferior portion of the heart. (Source: ECG recording adapted with permission from Chou TC, Knilans TK: Electrocardiography in Clinical Practice Adult and Pediatric, 4th ed. Philadelphia, PA: W. B. Saunders, 1996, p 126.)

TEMPORAL RELATIONSHIP BETWEEN WAVES OF THE ECG AND ACTION POTENTIALS FROM DIFFERENT REGIONS OF THE HEART

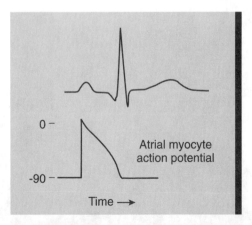

Because the QRS complex is attributed to ventricular depolarization, it should have a demonstrable relationship in time with phase 0 of a typical ventricular muscle action potential. Figure 8-25 shows the two signals juxtaposed in time, but it is important to recognize that the two are fundamentally different types of recordings. In any case, the rising phase of the action potential indeed occurs during the QRS complex. Moreover, the repolarization phase of the ventricular muscle action potential occurs during the T wave. The exact timing of the action potential with respect to the QRS complex and T waves depends on the precise region of the ventricle from which the action potential originates. By this same logic, phase 0 of an atrial action potential would occur during the P wave. There is usually no deflection in the ECG attributable to atrial repolarization because the QRS complex overwhelms any manifestation of the atrial event. Likewise, the mass of the SA-nodal cells responsible for the initiation of the heartbeat is so small that this event is not seen in the ECG, although it obviously would occur noticeably in advance of the P wave.

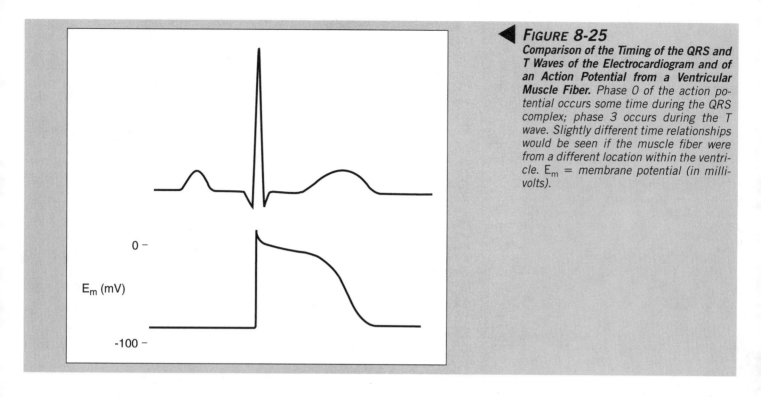

◀ FIGURE 8-25

Comparison of the Timing of the QRS and T Waves of the Electrocardiogram and of an Action Potential from a Ventricular Muscle Fiber. *Phase 0 of the action potential occurs some time during the QRS complex; phase 3 occurs during the T wave. Slightly different time relationships would be seen if the muscle fiber were from a different location within the ventricle.* E_m = *membrane potential (in millivolts).*

EXAMPLES OF DISTURBANCES OF NORMAL ELECTRICAL RHYTHM

From among the many different disease categories that alter the ECG, some examples of rhythm disturbances were chosen to be discussed below because they illustrate the effects of alterations in the normal sequence of myocardial electrical activation. The student should take care to understand the electrophysiologic basis for the observed changes in the ECG during the various conditions presented below.

AV-Nodal Block

The *top tracing* of Figure 8-26 shows a normal sinus rhythm: each QRS complex is preceded by a P wave; the PR interval is within the normal range. Conduction velocity through the AV node is slowed as a result of a first-degree AV-nodal block, which produces an abnormally long (> 200 msec) PR interval, as shown in the *second tracing* of Figure 8-26. In second-degree block, the AV node conducts some of the supraventricular depolarizations but not others. Consequently, some P waves are followed by a QRS complex, whereas others—those for which the AV node fails to conduct—are not. The *third tracing* of Figure 8-26 gives an example of a 3:2 second-degree AV-nodal block. Note that there are three P waves for every two QRS complexes; that is, a 3:2 ratio. Other ratios are possible, such as 2:1. Finally, in third-degree block there is complete electrical block between the atria and ventricles because the AV node fails to conduct any signals. Notice, therefore, in the *bottom tracing* of Figure 8-26 that there is no discernable coupling between the electrical activity of the atria and ventricles.

Premature Ventricular Contractions (PVCs)

The heartbeat normally originates within the atria (specifically, within the SA node) "above" the ventricles; this is called a *supraventricular rhythm.* However, there may be abnormal situations, such as acute myocardial ischemia, when the heartbeat originates within either the left or right ventricle. These ventricular beats disturb the normal rhythm of the heart (i.e., arrhythmias) and can have very serious consequences, even *sudden cardiac death* (see Ventricular Fibrillation). One important example of these arrhythmias are the PVCs. Figure 8-27 shows arterial blood pressure, left ventricular

FIGURE 8-26 ▶

Electrocardiogram Recordings during Normal Sinus Rhythm and First-, Second-, and Third-Degree Block of the Atrioventricular (AV) Node.

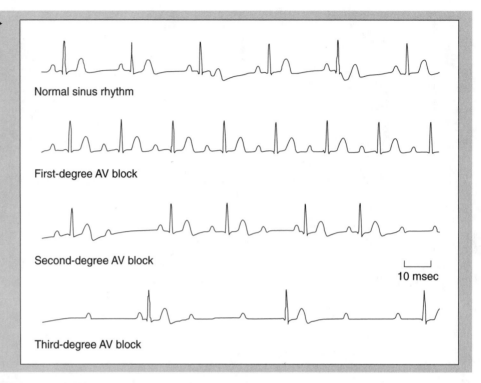

Normal sinus rhythm

First-degree AV block

Second-degree AV block

⊢ 10 msec

Third-degree AV block

FIGURE 8-27 ▶

Effects of a Premature Ventricular Contraction (PVC) on Left Ventricular Pump (LVP) Performance. The third beat with a peculiar (i.e., "bizarre") QRS waveform occurred prior to the next expected ventricular depolarization (arrow), that is, prematurely. The premature ventricular ectopic beat yielded lower left ventricular and arterial systolic blood pressures. The "compensatory pause" following the premature beat allowed a longer filling time, so the next beat was unusually strong (i.e., post–extrasystolic potentiation). Patients with PVCs often feel this "pounding" beat. ECG = electrocardiogram; BP = blood pressure.

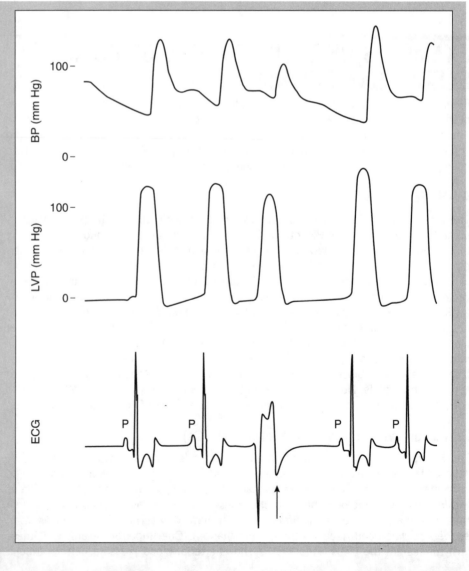

pressure, and an ECG for two normal (or sinus) beats followed by a PVC and then two more normal sinus beats. For clarity, the P wave has been denoted for each of the four supraventricular beats. Note the following unique characteristics of the ventricular beat:

- This beat was *not preceded* by a P wave, indicating that it does not have a supraventricular origin.
- If the rhythm had been regular, the next QRS complex would have been expected at the point indicated by the *arrow*; therefore, the ventricular beat was *premature*.
- The shape, amplitude, and duration of the QRS complex for the PVC was markedly different (i.e., "bizarre") from those of the normal sinus beats, indicating that the wave of depolarization did not sweep over the heart via the conducting network in the normal fashion.
- Ventricular systolic pressure was noticeably decreased for the premature beat, as was arterial pressure. This is explained in part by the decreased filling time (and thereby decreased preload) caused by the prematurity and in part by the less efficient contraction attributable to the irregular electrical activation.
- The diastolic interval following the PVC is inordinately long while the heart "waits" for the next sinus beat. This *compensatory pause* allows increased filling time for the next beat. As a result of the increased preload, the stroke volume for this beat is usually large, giving rise to a high systolic pressure. Patients who experience PVCs often notice this "pounding" beat.

> The left ventricle may not develop a pressure sufficiently high in a PVC to open the aortic valve, so the stroke volume is zero. If so, there is no sign whatever in arterial pressure of the beat's having occurred.

There are several possible electrophysiologic explanations for ventricular ectopic beats (VEBs), another name given to this type of arrhythmia. Under certain pathologic conditions, of which myocardial ischemia is the most common, the membrane potential of cells in specifically affected myocardial regions can exhibit oscillations during the course of repolarization. These oscillations result in temporary shifts in E_m to a more depolarized state and are called *after depolarizations*. They are designated either early, if they occur during the plateau phase of the action potential, or late, if they appear during phase 3. If they are strong enough to reach the threshold potential, a premature beat is initiated from the affected (i.e., ectopic) area. This process is called *increased automaticity*.

Another explanation invokes a concept called *reentry*. This term means that an impulse, of whatever origin, reenters a segment of myocardial fibers to depolarize them again. Under normal physiologic conditions, this situation can never happen because the wave of depolarization enters and depolarizes all of the fibers in a uniform manner. Therefore, every wave of depolarization normally depolarizes the whole heart just one time and then vanishes prior to the initiation of the next beat. This is not so with a reentrant beat.

A reentrant rhythm requires two conditions: a unidirectional block and retrograde decremental conduction. The *top portion* of Figure 8-28 pictures a small region of a healthy heart with two branching pathways (perhaps some trabeculae). A normal wave of depolarization entering this region of myocardium from "a" would be conducted through both pathways (b and c), if the myocardium were healthy, and would emerge approximately simultaneously at "e" and "f"; the waves through "b" and "c" would mutually excite the segment at "d" and then self-extinguish. The *lower panel* envisions a reentrant scenario in this same microdomain where the lower conducting pathway is ischemic (*shaded region*). As before, a wave of depolarization enters at "a," but the normal forward conduction through the lower pathway is now blocked at "c" because the ischemic tissue cannot be excited. The wave of depolarization originating at "a" enters the other pathway ("b") and propagates to "e," as before. Now, however, it conducts through "d," and impinges on the other side of the ischemic region. Instead of blocking, however, the impulse conducts in the retrograde (i.e., "backward") direction—but only slowly—through the depressed, ischemic tissue. (Note that this tissue blocks conduction in one direction, but allows conduction, albeit only slowly, in the other; this constitutes the *unidirectional block*.) When this wave emerges from the ischemic region, the tissue at "g" will have repolarized sufficiently so as to no longer be refractory. A new wave of excitation throughout the heart arises from this *reentrant* process. This VEB is often called a "coupled" beat because it owes its origin to the original depolarization at "a." VEBs may "devolve" into much more serious ventricular rhythms such as ventricular tachycardia (Figure 8-29A) or even ventricular fibrillation (Figure 8-29B), where cardiac output falls immediately to zero.

Ventricular Fibrillation (VF)

VF is the ultimate disturbance of cardiac rhythmicity, and the patient dies unless the fibrillation is reversed within a few minutes of onset. The "signature" of VF is an ECG

FIGURE 8-28 ▶

Origin of Reentry Ectopic Beat. *(A) In the normal heart (top), a wave of depolarization enters a small region of the myocardium from point "a" and flows smoothly to exit at "e" and "f." The small bridge of tissue at "d" is invaded from both sides by waves "b" and "c" that then mutually extinguish. (B) A region of ischemia (shaded area) blocks transmission of the incoming impulse at "c." However, the signal does conduct slowly within the ischemic area (zig-zag line) in the retrograde direction. The delay in conduction allows this wave to emerge at "g" when this muscle is no longer refractory. Therefore, a new wave of depolarization results and produces another heartbeat. Because this second beat is produced by the original beat, it is often called a "coupled beat."*

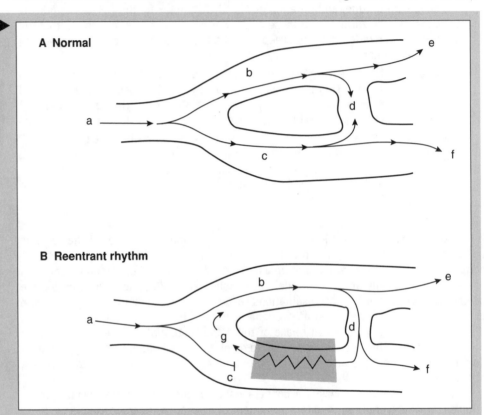

A Normal

B Reentrant rhythm

FIGURE 8-29 ▶

Electrocardiogram (ECG) Recordings of Ventricular Dysrhythmias. *(A) This figure illustrates a bout of ventricular tachycardia (V-tach). The first four beats originated in an atrial pacemaker, probably the sinoatrial node, as evidenced by the presence of a P wave. A run of nonsustained V-tach followed. The signature of V-tach is the absence of a P wave and the bizarre shape of the QRS complex. A supraventricular rhythm was re-established during the last four heartbeats. (B) In this figure, the four initial sinus beats are followed by a short run (four beats) of V-tach, which devolves quickly into ventricular fibrillation. Small deflections on the time scale = 1 sec; large deflections = 5 sec.*

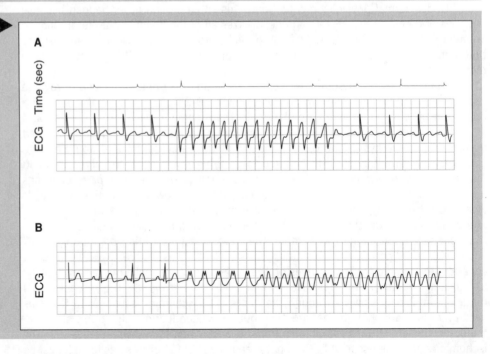

A

ECG   Time (sec)

B

ECG

that shows no obvious structure: there are no P waves, QRS complex, or T waves. Instead, the ECG consists of irregular fluctuations with no fixed pattern (Figure 8-29B). This lack of pattern occurs because there is no temporal coordination of depolarization and repolarization of the muscle fibers. Therefore, although each fiber is depolarizing, contracting, and consuming energy, there is no consistent electrical or mechanical rhythm. VF is often triggered by an ectopic beat or a run of ventricular tachycardia. The moment it occurs, the heart stops pumping and starts to swell because of venous blood accumulating within the chambers. Anyone who has seen a heart in fibrillation remembers the uncoordinated writhing of the muscle composing the ventricular wall, often described as looking like a "bag of worms." VF can be reversed by a process known as *counter shock* in which a current from a *defibrillator* is passed across the chest. This depolarizes all muscle cells in unison. A new electrical synchrony can arise if a dominant pacemaker assumes control of the rhythm. Figure 8-30 shows the hemodynamic consequences of VF.

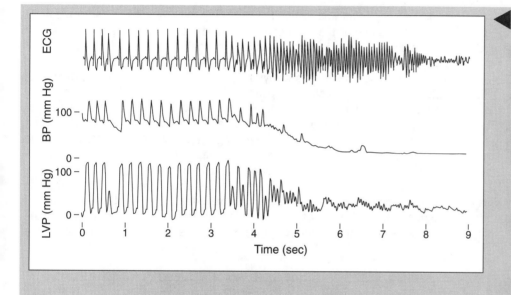

FIGURE 8-30
Hemodynamic Consequences of Ventricular Fibrillation (VF). *The recordings were made during a short episode of myocardial ischemia produced by sudden occlusion of a coronary artery in a dog. The first three beats were supraventricular, as evidenced by a clear P wave in the electrocardiogram (ECG) and a definite atrial kick in left ventricular pressure (LVP). The fourth beat was a premature ventricular contraction (PVC); note that the pressure developed by the ventricle was so small that there is barely a hint of the beat in arterial blood pressure (BP). The rhythm was normal again until approximately 3.5 seconds when it converted to a ventricular tachycardia. The left ventricle was able to develop a reasonable pressure during the first few ventricular beats, but by shortly after 4 seconds, there was no longer a coordinated beat. Arterial pressure dropped precipitously until by 8 seconds it was near 0 mm Hg, and the ECG clearly registered a pattern indicative of VF.*

SUMMARY

The etiology of the resting membrane potential and the nature of the action potential can be explained on the basis of the electrochemical properties of the cell. The shape of the action potentials recorded from different regions of the heart can differ markedly. These differences result from the blend of ion channels within the membranes of the various myocytes. The nature of each channel can be expressed in terms of its time-dependence and voltage-dependence, or lack thereof. The pacemaker potential of the SA node, which endows the heart with automaticity of heartbeat, and the rapid rate of depolarization and of conduction velocity in the Purkinje fibers are only two examples of the coupling of unique electrophysiologic and functional properties. The ECG results from the moment-to-moment summated electrical activity across the heart, and it is a useful tool for diagnosing disturbances of electrical rhythm and other cardiac pathologies.

RESOLUTION OF CLINICAL CASE

The quoted upper limit for the duration of the normal QT interval, corrected for HR, is 460 msec for men and 470 msec for women. Correction for HR is made using **Bazette's formula**: $QT_c = QT/\sqrt{RR}$, *where RR is the time between R waves (the RR interval).*

The woman described at the beginning of the chapter has a condition called *long QT syndrome* (LQTS). In patients with LQTS, the action potential duration, at least for some myocardial fibers, is abnormally long, as manifested by the prolonged QT interval. In a way that is not yet clear, this prolonged action potential predisposes to attacks of a characteristically labile ventricular tachycardia (V-tach). The woman's syncopal episode, therefore, was due to a run of that V-tach, during which her cardiac output fell to a very low level because of extreme shortening of ventricular filling time and inefficient coordination of muscle contraction. This produced a temporary, but profound, hypotension and loss of consciousness. The previous occasions when her pulse disappeared were also probably caused by runs of V-tach that were not long enough to produce syncope. Her description of a pounding heartbeat after a skipped beat reflects the hemodynamic changes occasioned by PVCs.

The woman's physician was justified in excluding the possibility of ischemic heart disease because it is one of the most common causes of ventricular arrhythmias. The LQTS is one example of nonischemic, neurally mediated V-tach. These episodes of polymorphic V-tach have the well-known French name "torsades des pointes." Figure 8-31 shows an ECG typical of this arrhythmia; compare this recording with that of Figure 8-29A to see the "twisting of points." This is a potentially life-threatening arrhythmia because it often disintegrates or "devolves" to ventricular fibrillation. Mortality among symptomatic, untreated patients is nearly 50% within 10 years of the first syncopal episode. The syndrome can be either congenital, as in this patient, or acquired because of conditions like hypokalemia, hypomagnesemia, hypocalcemia, atrioventricular block, or the unwanted side effects of certain drugs.

Polymorphic V-tach is a common clinical designation meaning that the appearance of the QRS complex is not constant for every beat. The polymorphism occurs because the focus of origination of the ectopic beats changes. Torsades des pointes means "twisting of points." The term was used by Dessertenne in 1966 in his report of a patient with syncope and marked QT prolongation because it described a characteristic cyclic change in shape (a time-dependent change in the electrical axis) of the aberrant QRS complexes.

The study of the LQTS is especially interesting in contemporary medicine because its electrophysiologic basis is becoming clear. Its basic feature is a disturbed balance of the ionic currents during the plateau phase of cardiac action potential that leads to the abnormal prolongation of the QT interval. In fact, all of the symptoms of this patient are

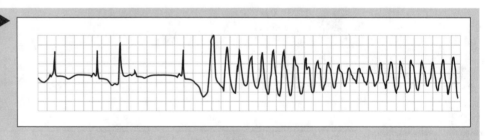

FIGURE 8-31 ▶

Episode of Torsades des Pointes Ventricular Tachycardia in a Patient with Long QT Syndrome on Electrocardiogram. The T waves are "inverted" in this recording. The first and second heartbeats have a P wave. The third beat is premature and is followed by a long pause. Notice the change in waveform during the ventricular tachycardia. Compare this figure with Figure 8-29A.

Congenital LQTS is primarily a disease of the ion channels in myocytes caused by an error in encoding their protein molecules. Structural alterations in channel proteins can change the protein's spatial orientation within the membrane; this, in turn, alters the natural gating action of membrane voltage changes or ligand effects. Genetic and clinical studies of families affected by this syndrome show a heterogeneity of the syndrome so that different channels can be affected among different families. However all variations ultimately lead to a prolongation of the plateau phase.

attributable to an upset in the delicate ionic balance during the plateau phase of the cardiac action potential. Molecular genetics studies have identified four human chromosomal locations that appear to cause different varieties of LQTS. One location is in gene *SCN5A*, on chromosome 3, which encodes the cardiac Na+ channel. Another site is in the *HERG* gene, on chromosome 7, which is responsible for the synthesis of the delayed rectifier K+ channel's protein. The other two locations on chromosomes 4 and 11 have not yet been linked to specific ionic channels. The first mutation results in defective Na+ channel inactivation, and the second one produces a decreased outward K+ current. The result is a decrease in the net outward positive current so that the duration of the plateau phase is increased. Although the molecular mechanisms of the polymorphic V-tach are not yet completely understood, it appears that depolarizing oscillations in the membrane potential during repolarization occur more frequently as the plateau becomes more prolonged. These afterdepolarizations may occur either during the plateau phase itself or during phase 3. They may be strong enough to reach the threshold potential and trigger a premature action potential. Occurrence of this triggered activity in multiple sites in ventricular myocardium at different rates could give rise to the characteristic torsades des pointes V-tach. For details of the molecular basis of the LQTS and other abnormalities of ion channel function see references [7] and [17–20].

The woman experienced her syncopal episode while driving, which is a situation that may be sometimes associated with nervous stress. Patients with the congenital type of LQTS commonly develop their episodes of V-tach during periods of adrenergic stimulation, such as psychologic or physical stress. Moreover, β-blockers, by limiting the effects of stress-related increases in cardiac sympathetic activity, can decrease the frequency of the episodes of arrhythmia and syncope in these patients. The underlying molecular mechanisms of that adrenergic dependence are not yet fully understood, but sympathetic stimulation increases the L-type Ca^{2+} current and the K^+ repolarizing currents. This increases HR and shortens action potential duration. It may be that patients with LQTS fail to shorten their QT interval appropriately during adrenergic stimulation. The cause could be either altered response of one of the above currents or different behavior of the mutant channels under adrenergic stimulation. This case clearly illustrates the clinical relevance of the fundamental concepts of electrophysiology presented in this chapter.

The patient has been healthy on β-blocker therapy.

REVIEW QUESTIONS

Directions: For each of the following questions, choose the **one best** answer.

1. Which one of the following statements regarding the cardiac action potential is correct?

   (A) Depolarization of a sinoatrial (SA)-nodal pacemaker cell is due to a fast inward Na^+ current

   (B) The plateau phase of a Purkinje fiber action potential is of short duration and is terminated by a decrease in I_{K1}

   (C) Phase 0 of a Purkinje fiber action potential occurs slightly in advance of the QRS complex

   (D) Conductance of Ca^{2+} through the membrane of the sarcolemma is high during electrical diastole in ventricular myocytes

   (E) An increase in the permeability of the sarcolemmal membrane to K^+ tends to depolarize the cell

2. The membrane potential of a ventricular myocyte is closest to the potassium equilibrium potential (E_{K^+}) during

   (A) phase 0 of the action potential

   (B) phase 2 of the action potential

   (C) phase 3 of the action potential

   (D) phase 4 of the action potential

   (E) the effective refractory period

3. Increased cardiac parasympathetic nervous activity tends to increase the

   (A) conductance of the sinoatrial (SA)-nodal pacemaker cell to K^+

   (B) slope of the pacemaker potential in the SA node

   (C) velocity of conduction through the atrioventricular node

   (D) inward flow of Ca^{2+} during phase 1 of a ventricular muscle fiber

   (E) inward flow of K^+ during phase 4 of a SA-nodal pacemaker cell

4. The cell-to-cell conduction velocity of an action potential is slow within the atrio-ventricular (AV) node. Which one of the following scenarios results?

   (A) The PR interval in the ECG is shorter than would otherwise be the case

   (B) There is adequate time for atrial contraction to assist in ventricular filling

   (C) The AV node is the only myocardial tissue that depends on a muscle end-plate potential to initiate depolarization

   (D) The bundle of His/Purkinje fiber system is excited before the atrial muscle

   (E) The AV valves close before atrial contraction

5. The slow inward current in a ventricular myocyte is

   (A) carried primarily by Na^+ ions

   (B) decreased by phosphorylation of the T-type Ca^{2+} channel

   (C) increased by increased cardiac parasympathetic nervous activity

   (D) responsible for phase 1 of the action potential

   (E) sometimes called the "trigger Ca^{2+} current" because it activates release of Ca^{2+} from the sarcoplasmic reticulum

6. Repolarization of a ventricular myocyte

    (A) occurs during the P wave of the electrocardiogram

    (B) is synchronous with phase 1 of the action potential

    (C) is largely due to a decrease in the inward Ca^{2+} current and progressive increase in the delayed rectifier current

    (D) is largely due to decline of the fast inward current

    (E) is delayed by increased cardiac sympathetic nervous activity

7. Which one of the following statements is correct regarding the current–voltage (I/V) relationship shown below for a cardiac ion-selective channel?

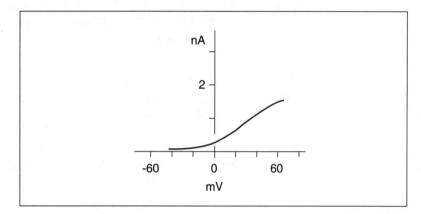

    (A) This channel shows outward rectification

    (B) The channel must be a Na^+-selective channel

    (C) The channel must be a Ca^{2+}-selective channel

    (D) The equilibrium potential for the ion carried by this channel is 0 mV

    (E) This channel would carry a large current during electrical diastole

8. The P wave of the electrocardiogram (ECG) is best described by which one of the following statements?

    (A) It results from depolarization of the pacemaker cells within the sinoatrial (SA) node

    (B) It occurs shortly after SA-nodal depolarization

    (C) It occurs slightly after depolarization of the Purkinje fibers in the bundle of His

    (D) It is caused by right and left atrial contraction

    (E) It starts at a membrane potential of −60 mV

9. During a second-degree block of the atrioventricular (AV) node, which one of the following situations occurs?

    (A) There is a P wave, but there is no atrial contraction

    (B) All heartbeats originate from a focus within the ventricle

    (C) The QRS complex is seen in leads I and III but is absent in lead II

    (D) Some, but not all, P waves are linked to a subsequent QRS complex

    (E) There is never a consistent temporal association between the P wave and the QRS complex

10. During an episode of ventricular tachycardia (V-tach), which one of the following situations occurs?

   (A) There are no action potentials in the ventricular muscle fibers

   (B) The PR interval is longer than 0.2 second

   (C) There is no P wave, and the shape of the QRS complex is bizarre

   (D) The patient's blood pressure tends to be unusually high

   (E) The rate of ejection of blood from the left and right ventricles during systole is more rapid than normal

11. A patient's ECG shows an upright P wave of normal amplitude prior to each QRS complex, but the QRS complex lasts 0.16 second, and its shape is abnormal. The most reasonable diagnosis on the basis of these data alone is that the patient's heart

   (A) is in a ventricular rhythm

   (B) is in a nodal rhythm

   (C) has a marked atrial hypertrophy

   (D) has an unstable pacemaker that shifts periodically into the right ventricle

   (E) has a bundle branch block

12. The figure below shows a simultaneous recording of the ECG and an action potential from some region of the heart. The action potential was probably recorded from which one of the following locations?

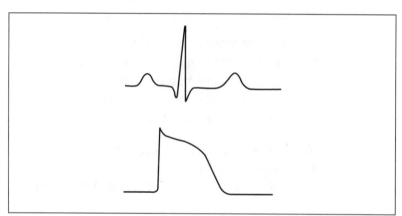

   (A) The right or left atrium

   (B) The right atrium only

   (C) The bundle of His

   (D) The left or right ventricle

   (E) The left ventricle only

ANSWERS AND EXPLANATIONS

1. The answer is C. Depolarization of the Purkinje fibers in the bundle of His and the bundle branches precedes depolarization of the mass of the ventricular musculature that generates the QRS complex. The Purkinje fiber has a very rapid upstroke and long plateau phase (B). The SA-nodal action potential is carried primarily by the slow inward current (A).

2. The answer is D. During electrical diastole, or phase 4, the membrane potential (E_m) is approximately equal to the potassium equilibrium potential (E_{K^+}) in the ventricular myocyte.

3. The answer is A. Increased cardiac parasympathetic nervous activity tends to hyperpolarize the SA node via an increase in the outward conductance of potassium (G_{K+}). Elevated parasympathetic tone decreases the slope of the pacemaker potential (B) and has a negative dromotropic effect (C).

4. The answer is B. One of the important functional consequences of the time delay introduced by the slow conduction velocity within the AV node is that atrial contraction can contribute to ventricular filling. There is no equivalent to an end-plate potential in any cardiac muscle (C).

5. The answer is E. This is the basis of a positive inotropism produced by sympathetic nervous system activation of the β-receptor, subsequent phosphorylation of the L-type Ca^{2+} channel, and a consequent increase in inward Ca^{2+} current.

6. The answer is C. The delayed rectifier current corresponds to I_K; the progressive increase in this outward current during the latter portion of the plateau acts in synergy with the decay in the inward current of (I_{Ca}) to restore resting membrane potential. Increased sympathetic nervous activity shortens the action potential by truncating the plateau and speeding repolarization (E).

7. The answer is A. This I/V relationship is for I_K, the delayed rectifier that conducts outward currents better than inward currents. In ventricular myocytes, this outward current assists in repolarization. Answers B and C cannot be correct because at positive membrane potentials, these currents would be inward, not outward as shown. There is an outward current flowing at 0 mV, so this cannot be an equilibrium potential (D). Finally, the I_K current is low during diastole (E) when the membrane potential (E_m) is electronegative.

8. The answer is B. It is important to learn the relative timing of electrical events at various locations within the heart and the waves of the ECG. Do not be fooled into attributing the P wave (or QRS complex or T wave) to a mechanical event (e.g., contraction, option D; or, for the T wave, relaxation) or confusing the characteristics of the ECG with those of a transmembrane potential recording (i.e., option E).

9. The answer is D. In second-degree block, some, but not all, supraventricular depolarizations are conducted through the AV node and result in ventricular depolarization. Answer E would be correct for third-degree block when there is no consistent temporal association between the P waves and QRS complexes.

10. The answer is C. The beat originates in a focus within the ventricle (i.e., no P wave) and spreads abnormally across the heart (i.e., the bizarre shape of the QRS complex). Stroke volume and the rate of ejection are low [or zero (E)], and blood pressure tends to be low (D).

11. The answer is E. The fact that the P wave is normally shaped and is regularly associated with a QRS complex rules out options A through D. A bundle branch block would prolong the process of depolarizing the ventricles and cause the QRS complex to be unusually shaped (because the wave of depolarization does not sweep over the heart in the normal pattern) and prolonged (because the conduction velocity is lower through the abnormal pathways).

12. The answer is C. The upstroke of the action potential occurs too late with respect to the P wave to have been recorded from either atrium (and it is not possible to discriminate between the right and left atrium with these data). Moreover, unlike an atrial action potential, this recording has a very long and definite plateau, which is characteristic of the Purkinje fibers comprising the bundle of His. Finally, the upstroke of the action potential occurs before the beginning of the QRS complex, when the bundle of His is activated, but before ventricular muscle depolarization.

REFERENCES

1. Hille B: *Ionic Channels of Excitable Membranes*, 2nd ed. Sunderland, MA: Sinauer Associates, 1992.
2. Nichols CG, Makhina EN, Pearson WL, et al: Inward rectification and implications for cardiac excitability. *Circ Res* 78:1–7, 1996.
3. Page E: The electrical potential difference across the cell membrane of heart muscle: biophysical consideration. *Circulation* 26:582–595, 1962.
4. Hodgkin AL: *The Conduction of the Nervous Impulse*. Springfield, IL: Charles C. Thomas, 1964.
5. Papazian DM, Bezanilla F: How does an ion channel sense voltage? *News Physiol Sci* 12:203–210, 1997.
6. Nilius B: Gating properties and modulation of Na+ channels. *News Physiol Sci* 4:225–230, 1989.
7. Ackerman MJ, Clampham DE: Ion channels: basic science and clinical disease. *N Engl J Med* 336:1575–1586, 1997.
8. Robishaw JD, Foster KA: Role of G proteins in the regulation of the cardiovascular system. *Ann Rev Physiol* 51:229–244, 1989.
9. Krum H, Bigger JT, Goldsmith RL, et al: Effect of long-term digoxin therapy on autonomic function in patients with chronic heart failure. *J Am Coll Cardiol* 25:289–294, 1995.
10. Coraboeuf E, Escande D: Ionic currents in the human myocardium. *News Physiol Sci* 5:28–31, 1990.
11. Fozzard HA: Ion channels and cardiac function. In *Molecular Cardiovascular Medicine*. Edited by Haber F. New York, NY: Scientific American, 1995, pp 211–224.
12. Irisawa H, Brown HF, Giles W: Cardiac pacemaking in the sinoatrial node. *Physiol Rev* 73:197–227, 1993.
13. Scher AM, Young AC: Ventricular depolarization and the genesis of the QRS. *Ann NY Acad Sci* 65:768–778, 1957.
14. Catalano JT: *Guide to ECG Analysis*. Philadelphia, PA: J. B. Lippincott, 1993.
15. Stein E: *Electrocardiographic Interpretation: A Self-Study Approach to Clinical Electrocardiography*. Philadelphia, PA: Lea and Febiger, 1991.
16. Dubin D: *Rapid Interpretation of EKGs: A Programmed Course*, 5th ed. Tampa, FL: Cover Publishing, 1996.
17. Roden DM, Lazzara R, Rosen M, et al: Multiple mechanisms in the long-QT syndrome: current knowledge, gaps, and future directions. *Circulation* 94:1996–2012, 1996.
18. Splawski I, Timothy KW, Vincent GM, et al: Molecular basis of the long-QT syndrome associated with deafness. *N Engl J Med* 336:1562–1567, 1997.
19. Sanguinetti MC, Keating MT: Role of delayed rectifier potassium channels in cardiac repolarization and arrhythmias. *News Physiol Sci* 12:152–157, 1997.
20. Lehmann-Horn F, Rüdel R: Channelopathies: their contribution to our knowledge about voltage-gated ion channels. *News Physiol Sci* 12:105–112, 1997.

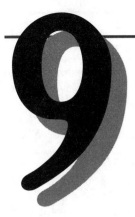

THE CARDIAC CYCLE

CHAPTER OUTLINE

INTRODUCTION OF CLINICAL CASE

A 26-year-old woman in her third trimester of pregnancy presented to the outpatient clinic because of shortness of breath. She stated that her *dyspnea* first occurred about 2 months previously and had progressively worsened. She now feels dyspneic at the slightest effort. She also reported that she had an attack of acute rheumatic fever when she was 12 years old. During a routine medical checkup at the age of 16, she was told that she had a *cardiac murmur* but had thought nothing of it since then. On physical examination, her heart rate (HR) was 94 bpm (beats per minute); her arterial blood pressure was 130/65 mm Hg; and her respiratory rate was 22/min. On *auscultation* (with a stethoscope), an accentuated S_1 heart sound, an opening snap (OS), and a mid–diastolic murmur with presystolic accentuation were heard over the apex of the heart. In addition, an early diastolic murmur was detected over the second right space and propagated down the left sternal border.

Echocardiography revealed a mild left atrial and left ventricular dilatation with thickening and restriction of motion in both the mitral and aortic valves (Figure 9-1). A color-coded ultrasound and Doppler study of the flow across the mitral valve showed a mild degree of *mitral stenosis*: the cross-sectional area of the valve was 1.7 cm² (normal: 4–6 cm²), and the computed mean diastolic pressure gradient across the valve was

Echocardiography uses a beam of high-frequency oscillations, or ultrasound, emanating from a probe placed on the patient's skin. These oscillations reflect from internal structures back to the surface, much as a sonar wave reflects from underwater objects. The anatomy and movement of the internal structures are displayed on a screen in real time. In the Doppler and flow color-coded modes, when the ultrasound beam deflects from flowing blood, the frequency of the reflected sound wave is Doppler-shifted in proportion to the velocity of the blood flow. The magnitude of the change in frequency between the incident and reflected ultrasound, proportional to flow direction and velocity, can be color-coded to allow rapid visualization of the areas of abnormal flow.

7.1 mm Hg (normal: <5 mm Hg). The aortic valve showed a moderate-to-severe degree of *incompetence* (valve leakage during diastole) with a nearly normal systolic pressure gradient.

The patient was admitted to the hospital. She was placed on a salt-restricted diet and given digitalis and a mild diuretic. Her condition improved. She was released and subsequently had a normal vaginal delivery.

The patient presented again 6 months later with palpitations and shortness of breath that had begun only a few hours previously. She had felt well prior to the sudden onset of dyspnea, even after she stopped taking her medication. She was admitted to the hospital. An electrocardiogram (ECG) showed atrial fibrillation with a ventricular rate of 122 bpm.

FIGURE 9-1 ▶

Single Frame of an Echocardiograph during Diastole, Showing the Heart of a Patient with Mitral Stenosis. In this non–color-coded mode, left ventricular (LV) and right ventricular (RV) cavities, as well as the lumen of the aorta (A), are black because there is less reflection of the ultrasound from the blood within them. The narrow orifice of the mitral valve can be visualized using this technology. The left ventricle and left atrium (LA) are dilated in this patient in left heart failure. (Source: Adapted with permission from Wada T: Basic and Advanced Visual Cardiology. Philadelphia, PA: Lea & Febiger, 1991, p 353.)

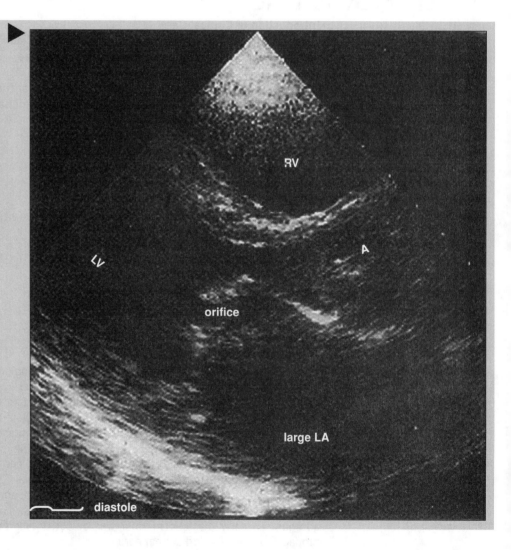

RELATIONSHIP BETWEEN MYOCARDIAL FUNCTION AND CARDIAC PUMP PERFORMANCE

Chapter 3 focuses on the fact that fundamental principles of physics underlie many aspects of cardiopulmonary function. Chapter 4 centers on the premise that a solid foundation in the fundamental nature of the development of force and muscle shortening is essential to understand the normal function of the heart and respiratory system. This chapter and Chapter 10 unite these two themes to explain the sequence of events that constitute the heartbeat and thereby endow the organ with the ability to pump blood.

RECAPITULATION: PRESSURE, FLOW, PRELOAD, AND AFTERLOAD

Pumps are encountered in many different settings. For example, a gauge on the instrument panel of almost any automobile monitors the pressure generated by the engine oil pump. This pump must circulate an adequate volume of oil through the motor each minute (the oil *flow*), or the engine will quickly fail. Like virtually any other pump, this one must obey a simple equation reminiscent of Ohm's law:

$$\dot{Q} \text{ (q/min)} = \text{oil pressure (lbs/in}^2)/\text{resistance}$$

If the system is functioning properly, the motor's resistance to the flow of oil remains essentially constant. Therefore, one can infer that an engine is receiving an adequate rate of oil *flow* (i.e., $\dot{Q}$) by monitoring oil *pressure: flow and pressure are tightly linked* in this, or any other, pump. Accordingly, the oil pressure would drop precipitously if the pump were to fail. As Chapter 3 explains, however, fluid always flows down a *pressure gradient*. The simple equation given above assumes that the oil pressure on the input side of the pump is always zero and may consequently be ignored in computing this gradient. This assumption is not valid for the heart. This seemingly simple difference between the two pumps actually probes some of the most fundamental issues contained in this chapter and in Chapter 10. By way of warning, the logic is a bit circuitous (literally).

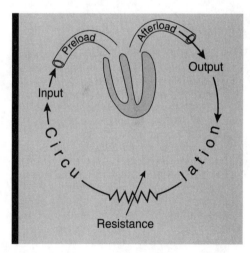

A mechanical oil pump is not very dynamic, except that it changes its output with changes in the engine's throttle setting. The heart, in marked contrast, must constantly adapt its pumping capacity to the changing *demands* of the organism for blood flow. There are two fundamental aspects of "demand." First, the blood that the heart ejects must eventually return to be pumped again. This *venous return* to the heart contributes significantly to the overall demand on the pump: an increase in the volume of blood returning to the heart with each beat (i.e., a *flow*) concomitantly increases the volume of blood inside the ventricle immediately prior to the next heartbeat. This, in turn, increases the stretch on the muscle fibers composing the chamber. As Chapter 4 demonstrates, this stretch refers to the length of the ventricular muscle fibers immediately prior to their contraction: the *preload*. Preload is analogous to the initial load, P, on the muscle shown in Chapter 4, Figure 4-4.

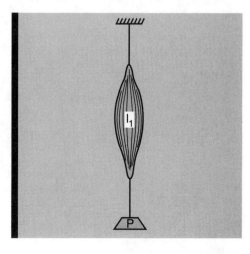

The second aspect of demand on the heart is *afterload*. In Chapter 3, the resistance to the ejection of blood is represented by the variable called "total peripheral resistance" (TPR). In living organisms, this variable is extraordinarily labile; for example, it decreases markedly during heavy rhythmic exercise and can increase during sustained isometric exercise. As a result, arterial blood pressure may increase strikingly during isometric exercise as a consequence of increased cardiac output (CO) without a corresponding decrease in systemic vascular resistance. An increase in pressure while maintaining resistance to flow would "demand" that the heart eject its stroke volume (SV) against a higher *afterload*. This is analogous to increasing the afterload of the muscle in Figure 4-4, which must lift from the lighter weight (A) to the heavier weight (B).

EVENTS OF THE CARDIAC CYCLE: THE WIGGERS DIAGRAM

If it is not immediately obvious that resistance falls during rhythmic exercise, consider that many additional vascular beds have to be perfused; the resistance to flow in each of these beds, such as the exercising muscle, will decrease. Using the equation for the resistance to flow in parallel circuits from Chapter 3, one can show that in such a situation, the TPR must decrease. In isometric exercise, the sustained contraction of the skeletal muscle increases the pressure in the interstitium outside the blood vessels, thereby decreasing the transmural pressure. Consequently, the diameter of these vessels decreases, so that their resistance to flow increases.

This chapter develops two diagrams that portray the events occurring during a heartbeat: the Wiggers diagram and the pressure–volume loop. In addition to relating changes in ventricular pressure and volume, each diagram allows the observer to determine the preload and afterload on the heart. The initial focus of this chapter is on the left ventricle/systemic circulation, followed by a brief consideration of the right ventricle/pulmonary circulation.

Events of Left Ventricular Cardiac Cycle and Arterial Blood Pressure

Chapter 3 explains that the *heart expends energy to develop a blood pressure (potential energy) and to eject blood (kinetic energy).* Panel A of Figure 9-2 focuses upon the first of these aspects of cardiac function, showing pressure recordings from inside the aorta (*top*) and inside the left ventricle (*middle*) for two heartbeats. The calibrations in mm Hg given immediately to the left of each channel are identical. The *bottom tracing* is an ECG. Look first at the ECG signal. Chapter 8 explains that the QRS complex demarcates the end of *diastole* and the beginning of *systole*. The myocardium is relaxed during the

FIGURE 9-2 ▶

(A) Schematic illustration of the heart (left) and pressure recordings from the aorta (upper right), left ventricle (middle), and electrocardiograph (ECG) [bottom]. The calibrations for both pressure channels (at left of each recording) are identical. The broken line through the arterial pressure recording indicates mean arterial blood pressure (MAP). Ventricular pressure during diastole is close to 0 mm Hg; conversely, arterial pressure never falls to near zero because of the action of the aortic valve. (B) The two pressure recordings have been plotted against a common scale to demonstrate that during the ejection phase, aortic and ventricular pressures are essentially identical. A = aorta; IVC = inferior vena cava; LA = left atrium; LV = left ventricle; M = mitral valve; PA = pulmonary artery; PV = pulmonary vein; RA = right atrium; RV = right ventricle; T = tricuspid valve; SVC = superior vena cava.

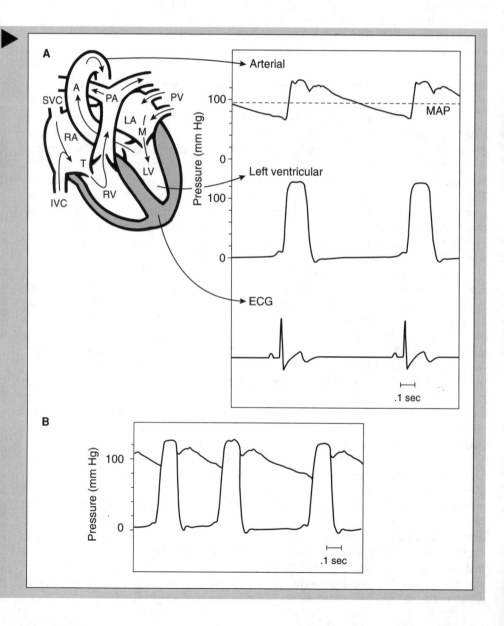

diastole, so the pressure *inside* the ventricle is very low; indeed, Figure 9-2A shows that the ventricular pressure recording prior to the QRS complex never exceeds ≈ 10–15 mm Hg above atmospheric pressure.

Careful examination of the ventricular pressure recording reveals a small increase in the pressure very shortly before the large, rapid upswing. The *mitral valve* is *open* during diastole, so that the left atrium and the left ventricle effectually constitute a single chamber. Therefore (although atrial pressure is not shown in Figure 9-2), during diastole atrial pressure must be esentially identical to ventricular pressure. The P wave occurs shortly before this small increase in ventricular pressure. The contraction of the left atrium immediately after the P wave explains the small "atrial kick" in the left ventricular pressure recording. Atrial contraction generates only a small increase in the atrial/ventricular pressure because its muscle mass is small.

Ventricular pressure starts to rise rapidly almost immediately after the QRS complex is inscribed. Systole has begun. This rise in ventricular pressure quickly produces a pressure gradient between the ventricle and atrium that causes the *mitral valve to close*. The turbulence from this closure produces the *first heart sound* (S_1)—the "lub" of the "lub dub." As a result of this closure, left ventricular pressure and left atrial pressure differ markedly until the mitral valve opens again. The *aortic valve opens* as soon as left ventricular pressure rises just above the pressure inside the aorta. Toward the end of systole, the T wave is inscribed (seen here as a biphasic deflection), and the myocardium starts to relax; as a result, ventricular pressure falls. The *aortic valve closes* as soon as pressure inside the left ventricle falls below aortic pressure. This closure produces the *second heart sound* (S_2). The *atrioventricular (AV) valve opens* once the pressure inside the relaxing ventricle falls below atrial pressure, and a new cardiac cycle starts with ventricular filling.

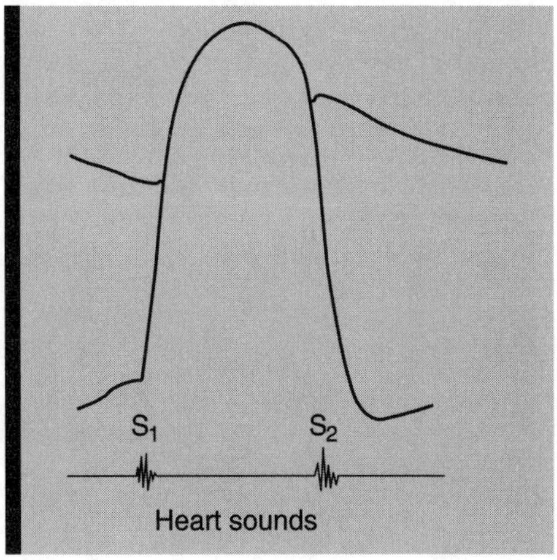

The *top tracing* of Figure 9-2A shows that arterial pressure increases and decreases with every beat of the heart; however, unlike ventricular pressure, it never falls to venous pressure levels. What accounts for this markedly different pressure profile? Once the aortic valve opens, blood moves rapidly from the heart into the aorta during the *ejection phase* of the cardiac cycle. This bolus of blood must be temporarily stored in the root of the aorta because it cannot flow instantaneously into the peripheral vessels. The physical expansion of the aorta to accommodate the SV leads to a peak arterial pressure known as arterial *systolic blood pressure* (SBP). In healthy, young *normotensive* individuals, SBP averages about 120 mm Hg, with a range of about 100–130 mm Hg (Table 9-1). With advancing age, SBP generally rises principally as a result of a decrease in aortic compliance. The ensuing closure of the aortic valve physically isolates the heart from the arterial system. The resulting reverberation of blood flow produces a small oscillation in pressure known as the *dicrotic notch*, or *incisura*. Blood is unable to "fall" back into the low-pressure reservoir inside the left ventricle; the valve closure causes physical isolation of the ventricle from the aorta. Instead, the blood that filled the aorta and major arterial vessels during systole gradually drains into the periphery. As a result, arterial pressure falls progressively during diastole, attaining its lowest value, arterial *diastolic blood pressure* (DBP), immediately prior to the onset of the next ejection phase. Human DBP is generally around 80 mm Hg (Table 9-1). The difference between SBP and DBP is the *pulse pressure* (ΔP). The amplitude of the ΔP is related to the stroke volume (ΔV) and the compliance of the arterial vessels (C_a), according to the relationship given in Chapter 3:

$$\Delta P = \frac{\Delta V}{C_a}$$

Finally, the average or *mean arterial blood pressure* (MAP) can be estimated by adding one-third the value of ΔP to DBP:

$$MAP \approx DBP + \frac{SBP - DBP}{3}$$

MAP is indicated in Figure 9-2A by a *broken horizontal line* through the pressure tracing.

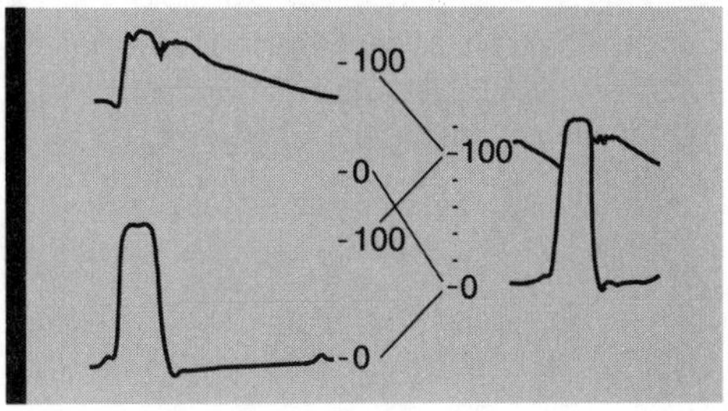

Panel B of Figure 9-2 shows a different perspective on the relationship between arterial and left ventricular pressures, plotting them on a common axis. Left ventricular

TABLE 9-1 ▶
Normal Hemodynamic Values in Adult Subjects in the Basal State

Variable	Units	Mean[a] (± 2 SD)[b]
Heart rate	bpm	71 (53–89)
Blood flow		
Cardiac output	L/min	6.50 (3.6–9.4)
Cardiac index	L/min/m^2	3.63 (2.0–5.2)
Stroke volume	mL	93 (53–133)
Blood pressures,[c] systemic		
Ao, S/D	mm Hg	122/83
Ao, mean	mm Hg	97 (80–114)
Ao, pulse	mm Hg	39 (24–54)
Large vein[d]	mm Hg	8 (4–12)
Right atrium, mean	mm Hg	5 (0.2–9)
Blood pressures,[c] pulmonic		
MPA, S/D	mm Hg	22/11
MPA, mean	mm Hg	14.6 (10–19)
MPA, pulse	mm Hg	11.4 (6–17)
Terminal vein, mean	mm Hg	8 (4–12)
Left atrium, mean	mm Hg	7.9 (2–12)
Vascular bed resistance		
Pulmonic	dyn sec/cm^5	70 (20–120)
Systemic	dyn sec/cm^5	1070 (660–1480)

Note. Ao = ascending aorta; S/D = systolic/diastolic; MPA = main pulmonary artery.
Source: Adapted with permission from Milnor WR: *Cardiovascular Physiology.* New York, NY: Oxford University Press, 1990, p 33.
[a] For male subjects aged 30 years, weight 68 kg, height 175 cm, surface area 1.80 m^2.
[b] The standard deviation (SD) is a measure of the variation of a given variable, such as mean arterial blood pressure (MAP), above and below its average value within a population. If the values for the variable are "normally distributed" (i.e., in a bell-shaped curve), 68% of the individuals in the population have a value within ± 1 SD, and 95% lie within ±2 SD. For example, MAP is given here as 97 mm Hg, and the SD is 8.5 mm Hg. Therefore, 95% of the population will have a resting MAP between 80 and 114 mm Hg (97 ± 2 × 8.5 mm Hg).
[c] Direct measurements through catheters.
[d] For example, brachial or femoral.

Muscle: Heart
The isometric phase of contraction *used to derive the force–velocity curve (Chapter 4, Figures 4-4 and 4-5) is analogous to iso-*volumic contraction *in the cardiac cycle. The* isotonic phase of contraction *is analogous to the* ejection phase *of the cardiac cycle.*

and aortic pressures are essentially identical during systole. This makes sense from a hydraulic perspective; the ventricle and aorta constitute a single chamber while they are connected via the patent orifice of the aortic valve.

Equal in importance to the hydraulic events of the cardiac cycle are the changes in ventricular volume. Figure 9-3, a Wiggers diagram (named after the American physiologist Carl J. Wiggers), includes these changes, along with other important information. In the young adult, there is only a small increase in ventricular volume resulting from atrial contraction; in older people, the contribution of atrial contraction to ventricular filling is more significant. During heavy exercise, the atria may contribute as much as ≈ 30% of ventricular filling, even in healthy young subjects. Also, there is *no change* in ventricular volume between the time the mitral valve closes and the aortic valve opens, even though ventricular pressure rises dramatically. This interval (demarcated by *solid, parallel lines* in Figure 9-3) is called *isovolumic contraction.* Ventricular volume decreases rapidly during the *early ejection phase*; in fact, *ejection is almost complete during the first half of systole.* Finally, there is no change in volume between the closure of the aortic valve and the opening of the mitral valve; during this *isovolumic relaxation* (*broken parallel lines*), ventricular pressure falls rapidly.

During ventricular systole, blood cannot move from the right atrium into the right ventricle because the tricuspid valve is closed. Therefore, blood returning from the periphery accumulates within the right atrium. Likewise, blood returning from the lungs gathers in the left atrium. This temporary storage of blood is an important function of both atria. With the opening of the AV valve, the accumulated blood rushes rapidly from the engorged atrium into the ventricle during the *rapid filling phase* of diastole. As a result, *ventricular volume increases rapidly early in diastole such that minimal additional filling*

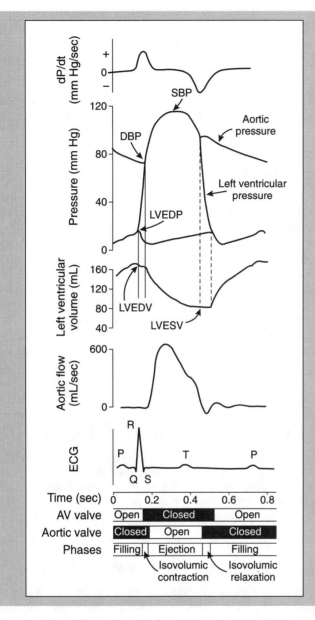

FIGURE 9-3
Wiggers Diagram of the Left Ventricle Showing Recordings for Aorta and Left Intraventricular Pressure, Ventricular Volume, and ECG. The dP/dt and flow recordings show the rate of change of left ventricular pressure and left ventricular volume, respectively. Events are simplified for ease of comprehension. The positions of the aortic and mitral valves are shown along with the phases of the cardiac cycle at the bottom of the figure. DBP = diastolic arterial blood pressure; LVEDP = left ventricular end diastolic pressure; LVEDV = left ventricular end diastolic volume; LVESV = left ventricular end systolic volume; SBP = systolic arterial blood pressure AV = atrioventricular valve. (Source: Adapted with permission from Randall WC (ed): Neural Regulation of the Heart. New York, NY: Oxford University Press, 1977, p 50.)

occurs during late diastole. That portion of the ventricular volume trajectory during late diastole is often called *diastasis.*

The Wiggers diagram also shows the *rate of change* of ventricular pressure (dP/dt, given in mm Hg/sec) and the rate of change of ventricular volume (given in mL/sec); note that this latter variable is *aortic flow,* which equals the rate at which the heart ejects blood. These variables provide insight into the *rapidity* with which the heart performs its important functions of developing pressure and ejecting blood.

Several specific points in the Wiggers diagram have been labeled in Figure 9-3. Two of these, the left ventricular pressure at the very end of diastole (*left ventricular end diastolic pressure, LVEDP*) and the volume of the left ventricle at the end of diastole (*left ventricular end diastolic volume, LVEDV*), are important indices of the *preload* on the ventricular myocardium (see Ventricular Preload below). The *left ventricular end systolic volume* (*LVESV*) is also indicated in the figure. The position of the valves and the names of the individual phases of the cardiac cycle are indicated below the flow tracing. Other important lessons from the Wiggers diagram include the following:

• SV is equal to the difference between end diastolic and end systolic volume.

• The heart does not completely empty with each beat (i.e., end systolic volume ≠ 0); the *ejection fraction* (SV divided by end diastolic volume) ranges from ≈ 50%–60% in the healthy human.

- Within limits, SV would not be severely compromised even if the duration of systole and diastole were noticeably decreased, as during an increase in heart rate (HR) [*tachycardia*]; this is because of the rapid initial ejection and rapid early filling.

Finally, note that CO (mL/min) can be computed by multiplying SV (mL/beat) times HR (bpm). In humans, CO at rest is about 5½–7½ L/min (see Table 9-1).

Events of Right Ventricular Cardiac Cycle and Pulmonary Arterial Blood Pressure

A Wiggers diagram for the right ventricle and pulmonary arterial pressure would be almost identical to Figure 9-3 with a single, remarkable exception: *typical pulmonary arterial systolic and diastolic pressures would be only ≈ 25 mm Hg and ≈ 10 mm Hg, respectively.* The explanation for the large difference between systemic and pulmonary pressures is simple: the resistance to the flow of blood through the pulmonary circulation is much lower than that of the peripheral circulation, so that less energy is required to perfuse the lungs with blood. Conversely, *the SVs of the right and left ventricles, on the average, are virtually identical.* In other words, the outputs of the left and right ventricles are equal to each other, even though they operate at very different pressures. The explanation for this phenomenon is given in Chapter 10. Table 9-1 provides some normal values (±2 standard deviations, SD) for some important cardiovascular variables.

PRESSURE–VOLUME RELATIONSHIPS

The ability to generate pressure and the ability to move volume are two key performance parameters for any pump. In studying the pumping ability of the heart, it is helpful to combine these two attributes in a single diagram. The *pressure–volume* loop does exactly this. The diastolic component of the loop depends upon the passive properties of the myocardium, whereas the systolic component reflects the active contractile properties of the muscle.

Pressure–Volume Relationship during Diastole

Figure 3-2 was derived by measuring the volume and the pressure inside a balloon as it was progressively inflated. Now suppose the same experiment were performed for the left ventricle while the muscle is relaxed (i.e., during diastole). Plotting the measured pressure on the ordinate and the volume on the abscissa would yield a *left ventricular diastolic pressure–volume relationship*. Comparable data for the right ventricle would be conceptually identical to those for the left.

These data are available directly from the Wiggers diagram. All that is necessary is to pick some starting point, such as the opening of the AV valve, and read the left ventricular pressure and the corresponding left ventricular volume directly from the diagram at successive times during diastole. For example, in panel A of Figure 9-4, both the pressure and volume are low at time 1 on the pressure and volume curves; these two values correspond to point 1 on the graph in Figure 9-4B. By time 2, the volume has increased noticeably, although the pressure is only modestly elevated; this point appears on the axis in panel B and likewise for time 3. Plotting a large number of samples during diastole would generate the solid portion of the graph shown in panel B. Although it is not possible to make any actual measurements from this beat for pressures lower than that for point 1 or higher than that for point 3, the relationship actually extends above and below the *solid line*, as indicated by the *dashed line*. Chapter 10 explains why this additional information is valuable.

The pressure and volume during diastole must conform to this relationship, although for any given heartbeat, some values may lie on the *broken line* below point 1, or on the extension above point 3. *This line provides information about the diastolic pressure–*

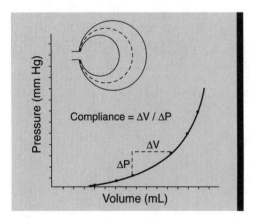

Pressure (mm Hg) vs Volume (mL)

Compliance = ΔV / ΔP

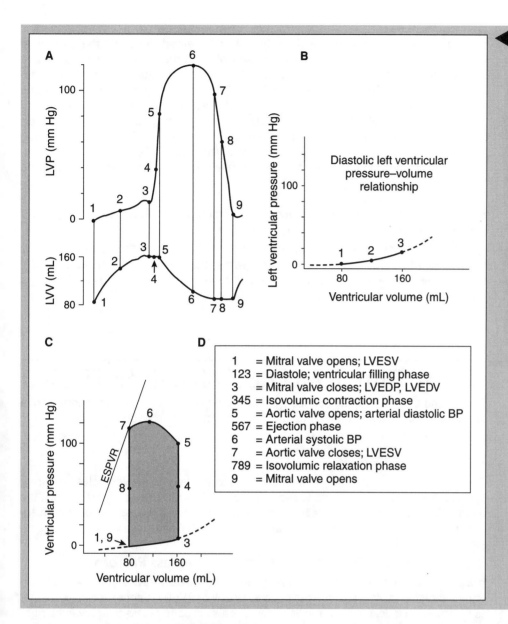

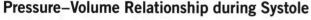

Derivation of Left Ventricular Pressure–Volume Loop from Wiggers Diagram. (A) *Recordings of left ventricular pressure (top) and left ventricular volume (bottom) are taken from the Wiggers diagram. Points 1–9 in each curve represent simultaneous values for pressure and volume at selected times during the cardiac cycle.* (B) *Plot of points 1, 2, and 3 from panel A, where the ordinate is ventricular pressure and the abscissa, ventricular volume. The resulting curve is the left ventricular diastolic pressure–volume relationship, from which the passive ventricular compliance may be calculated. Broken lines to the left and right of points 1 and 3, respectively, are extensions of the relationship that could not be determined directly from the tracings in panel A.* (C) *Complete left ventricular pressure–volume loop. The area within the loop (shaded) is stroke work. The curve abuts the end systolic pressure–volume relationship (ESPVR) at point 7.* (D) *Definitions of points 1–9.*

volume properties of the heart. This relationship does not change measurably from moment to moment, or even from day to day. In Chapter 3, Figure 3-2 helps to illustrate the concept of compliance. Over the *long term*, the compliance of any of the heart's chambers *can* change as a result of certain disease processes and thereby shift the position of the curve on the axes. *These long-term changes in compliance can significantly alter the heart's ability to fill, and consequently can have profound effects on its ability to pump blood.*

Finally, observe that the passive length–tension curve for a muscle is analogous to the diastolic pressure–volume relationship of the ventricle in Figure 9-4B. In fact, *the diastolic pressure–volume relationship results from the passive length–tension characteristics of the myocardium.* This is one example of how cardiac pump function can be understood and interpreted in terms of the functional characteristics of the heart muscle.

Pressure–Volume Relationship during Systole

Ventricular systole begins at point 3. Simultaneous assessment of the ventricular pressure and ventricular volume curves in the Wiggers diagram from 3 onward shows the large increase in pressure for points 4 and 5 of Figure 9-4C. The time between points 3 and 5 corresponds to the isovolumic contraction phase of the cardiac cycle; it is represented by the vertical line connecting points 3, 4, and 5 in panel C. By the time indicated by point 6

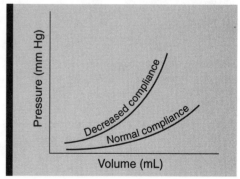

The ESPVR can be determined by setting a preload and then making the heart contract against an infinitely high afterload so that ejection never occurs (e.g., clamping the aorta closed). For any given preload, ventricular pressure will rise to a peak value that lies on the ESPVR. In effect, this contraction is a pressure–volume loop that has been compressed to zero "thickness" (i.e., $\Delta V = 0$). The shape and slope of the ESPVR can be determined by testing peak isovolumic pressure over a range of preloads. The diagrams in this chapter simplify the shape of the pressure–volume loop and ESPVR somewhat for ease of explanation. Finally, although the pressure–volume loop does not contain any element of time, time is required to "sweep" out the loop. If one were to view the loop on an oscilloscope, the point of light on the screen would move around the loop with each heartbeat.

during the ejection phase, ventricular volume has decreased along with the continuing pressure increase. Point 7 represents the closure of the aortic valve and the beginning of isovolumic relaxation. In panel C, the "shoulder" of the pressure–volume loop corresponding to point 7 abuts an obtuse line labeled ESPVR (end systolic pressure–volume relationship). Chapter 10 shows how this ESPVR demarcates the size of the SV and depends upon the inotropic state of the heart. Finally, a new cycle starts at point 9 with the opening of the AV valve and the onset of filling.

The points in Figure 9-4A were chosen to illustrate the information inherent within the pressure–volume relationship. Their identities are given in Figure 9-4D. Note the following:

- SV can be read directly from the loop by subtracting end diastolic volume (points 3–5) from end systolic volume (points 7–9).
- The stroke work equals $P \times \Delta V$ (see Chapter 3, or $W = \int P dV$); the energy expended by the heart for this beat equals the area within the pressure–volume loop (*lightly shaded* in Figure 9-4C). Alternatively, HR times SBP, the *double product*, is a useful estimate of the work being performed by the heart.

VENTRICULAR PRELOAD AND AFTERLOAD

Preload and afterload can be defined specifically with respect to the events portrayed in the Wiggers diagram and in the pressure–volume loop. *Both concepts are central to the practice of cardiology.*

Ventricular Preload

Preload is the length of a muscle fiber prior to contraction. As the ventricles fill during diastole, the muscle fibers constituting their walls are stretched progressively. Thus, the volume of the chamber just prior to the onset of systole is a direct reflection of preload. The relevant volumes for ventricular function are LVEDV and right ventricular end diastolic volume (RVEDV).

USING VENTRICULAR END DIASTOLIC PRESSURE TO ASSESS PRELOAD

It is usually impractical to measure ventricular volume directly, so clinicians typically use some indirect assessment of preload such as LVEDV or RVEDV. *Central venous pressure*, as measured in a deep vein or the vena cava, is also used to assess the prevailing right ventricular filling pressure. How can an intraventricular *pressure* be used to assess ventricular *volume*? The answer is quite simple: the diastolic pressure–volume curve (see Figure 9-4B) depicts the obligatory relationship between ventricular pressure and volume. This relationship depends only upon the compliance characteristics of the chamber and holds for end diastolic volume/end diastolic pressure as well as for any other point on the curve. Thus, end diastolic pressure is normally a valid estimate of preload. Either end diastolic volume or end diastolic pressure may be read directly from the Wiggers diagram or the pressure–volume loop.

USING PULMONARY CAPILLARY WEDGE PRESSURE TO ASSESS LEFT VENTRICULAR PRELOAD

LVEDP normally cannot be directly recorded in the clinical setting. Fortunately, *pulmonary capillary wedge pressure*, an indirect assessment of left ventricular preload, can be measured using a flow-directed, "balloon" catheter, first described in 1970 by Drs. H. J. Swan, W. Ganz, and colleagues [1] (Figure 9-5A). The physician inserts the catheter into a peripheral vein; when the balloon is inflated, the catheter is carried by the blood flow—or "floated"—into the right atrium (Figure 9-5B). The pressure recording and cardiac electrogram (similar to an ECG) at the *lower left* show the changes in the pressure wave as the tip moves from the atrium to the ventricle. Advancing the catheter eventually places its tip in the pulmonary artery (position 2 to 3; recordings at *upper left*). The balloon is then temporarily deflated, and the tip of the catheter is advanced into a smaller pulmonary artery (position 4). The balloon is reinflated and "wedged" against the wall of the artery. The inflated balloon completely obstructs the vessel at a point behind the tip, thereby blocking the flow of blood and, thus, the transmission of the pulmonary arterial pressure (PAP) through to the tip. Once the catheter is positioned in this way, it records the pressure "in front of" its tip—left atrial pressure or, more precisely, the pulmonary capillary wedge pressure. In the healthy individual, average left atrial/wedge pressure is about 8 mm Hg (see Table 9-1). The recordings in Figure 9-5 were taken from a patient with a higher-than-normal PAP and a markedly elevated wedge pressure resulting from congestive heart failure (CHF).

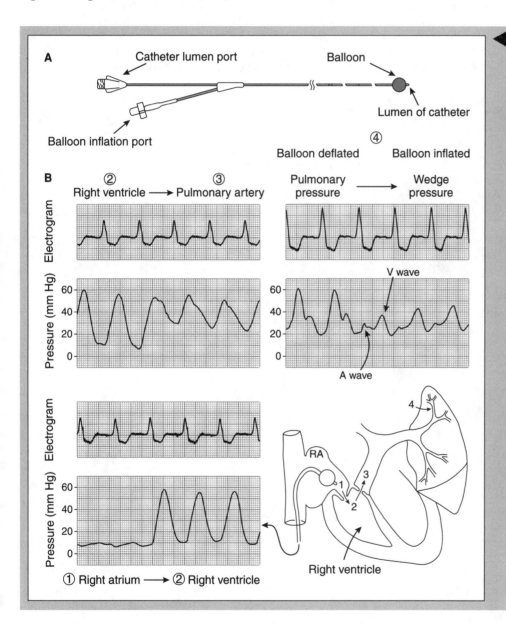

FIGURE 9-5

Determination of Pulmonary Capillary Wedge Pressure Using a Flow-Directed Catheter. *(A) The two ends of a Swan-Ganz catheter. The catheter is filled with saline, and a pressure transducer is coupled to the lumen port. The balloon is inflated and deflated through the inflation port. Although the recorded pressure signal will be somewhat distorted as a result of imperfect transmission through the catheter and transducer, it does provide useful recording of pressure at the catheter tip. The catheter may have additional "ports" and be used to determine cardiac output (CO) by thermodilution. (B) The heart and left lung, showing a flow-directed catheter, with balloon inflated, as its tip is about to move from the right atrium (position 1) into the right ventricle (position 2). The recording at the lower left shows the electrograph and the change in pressure waveform upon entering the right ventricle. Likewise, the recordings at the upper left show the transition from the right ventricle (position 2) into the pulmonary artery (position 3). If the tip of the catheter is advanced into the smaller vessel (position 4), inflating the balloon changes the recorded pressure wave from pulmonary arterial pressure to pulmonary capillary wedge pressure (upper right). Capillary wedge pressure was elevated in this patient with congestive heart failure. (Source: Recordings provided courtesy of Dr. Peter Sapin, Division of Cardiology, University of Kentucky College of Medicine, Lexington, Kentucky.)*

Ventricular Afterload

In contrast to preload, there is no distinct point or set of values on the Wiggers diagram or pressure–volume loop that corresponds precisely with the afterload (weight A hung on the muscle in Figure 4-4). Fortunately, arterial diastolic pressure is a useful estimate of left ventricular afterload and is quite adequate in most applications. For example, elevated arterial pressure that occurs during isometric exercise markedly increases the work of the heart, just as would increasing the afterload on the muscle in Figure 4-4.

EFFECT OF INCREASED SYMPATHETIC NERVOUS SYSTEM ACTIVITY ON THE WIGGERS DIAGRAM: A POSITIVE INOTROPISM

Chapter 4 explains that increased sympathetic nervous system (SNS) activity increases the contractility of cardiac muscle via activation of β_1-adrenergic receptors. The present chapter concludes by determining how this change in *muscle function* manifests itself in terms of cardiac *pump function* (i.e., the Wiggers diagram). The *solid lines* in Figure 9-6 are essentially the same as those in Figure 9-3. This can be considered a "control" beat for which SNS activity is relatively low. Conversely, the beat shown in a broken line would be recorded if SNS activity were elevated. The following list relates the similarities and

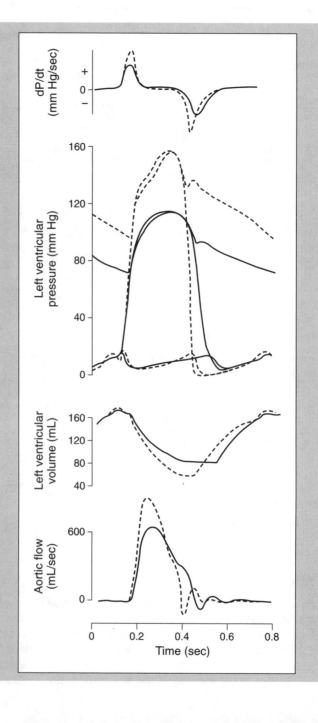

FIGURE 9-6 ▶

Wiggers Diagram for Heartbeat at Rest (solid line) *and during Increased Sympathetic Nervous System (SNS) Activity. Positive inotropism resulting from sympathetic activation allows the heart to do more work, as evidenced by increased pressure generation and increased stroke volume. The rate of performing the work, or power, is also increased, as evidenced by the elevated rate of rise and fall of ventricular pressure and rate of ejection of blood into the aorta (flow).*

Some of the simplifications included in the original Wiggers diagram for ease of interpretation no longer occur in this figure. For example, there actually are measurable pressure gradients between ventricular and arterial pressures during early systole and between ventricular and atrial pressure in early diastole. This is because fluids actually flow from a region of higher energy to lower energy; the kinetic energy of the blood during early ejection contributes to the energy gradient, leading to movement of blood from inside the ventricle to the aorta. (Source: Adapted with permission from Randall WC (ed): Neural Regulation of the Heart. New York, NY: Oxford University Press, 1977, p 50.)

differences in pump function between these two beats to the effects of a positive inotropism (or increase in contractility) on myocardial contraction or on the electrical properties of heart muscle.

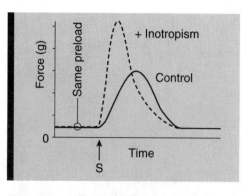

Comparisons of Cardiac Pump Function in Control vs. Positive Inotropism

- Preload does not differ between the two beats, as indicated by unaltered LVEDV and LVEDP.

- SV is increased.

- Ventricular and arterial systolic pressures are increased.

- Duration of systole decreases, rate of pressure rises and falls (peak +dP/dt and peak −dP/dt) increases, and rate of blood ejection increases.

Principles of Myocardial Muscle Function

- *An increase in contractility acts to increase muscle work and power without an increase in preload.*

- An increase in contractility acts to increase muscle shortening (ΔL) without an increase in preload; increased myocardial shortening augments SV.

- An increase in contractility allows the myocardium to develop greater force and to perform more work without an increase in preload; an increased SV, tachycardia, and augmented arteriolar vasoconstriction resulting from elevated sympathetic drive increase pressure:
$$BP = SV \times HR \times TPR.$$

- Sympathetic stimulation decreases duration of ventricular muscle action potential; the rate of force generation and maximal rate of shortening (V_{max}) increase with positive inotropism.

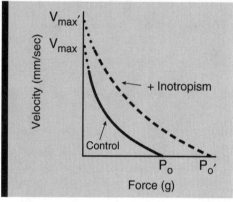

The changes in the Wiggers diagram associated with the increased sympathetic drive reflect the important axiom that a *positive inotropism allows the heart to do more work, more quickly without an increase in preload.* This is analogous to the increase in the work and power output of an engine's oil pump resulting from the increased rate of fuel consumption when the throttle setting is increased. The following formal definition of an increase in contractility is worth memorizing. *An increase in contractility occurs when the heart performs more work than before starting from the same, or smaller, end diastolic volume.*

Chapter 10 explains how these changes are reflected in the heart's ability to pump blood around the circulation.

SUMMARY

The cardiac cycle consists of a series of events triggered by the wave of cellular depolarization that sweeps across the myocardial functional syncytium. These events, particularly including a sequence of changes in atrial and ventricular pressures and volumes, are outlined in the Wiggers diagram. The two key parameters of pump function are combined in the pressure–volume loop. This loop consists of both diastolic and systolic components; an understanding of each component is critically important to the practice of medicine. Cardiac pump function can be understood best in terms of the underlying muscle physiology. Key attributes of myocardial function include its preload, afterload, and inotropic state; each of these is reflected in the pressure–volume loop. Chapter 10 explains (1) how the heart responds as a pump to changes in the amount of blood delivered to it (i.e., preload), the pressure against which it must eject (i.e., afterload), and changes in neurohumoral drive (i.e., contractility); and (2) how these responses depend upon the contractile properties of the myocardium.

RESOLUTION OF CLINICAL CASE

The woman in the case study presented at the beginning of the chapter experienced an attack of acute rheumatic carditis when she was 12 years old. Unlike the pathologic consequences in other organs, rheumatic cardiac lesions tend to heal by *fibrosis*, which usually causes permanent valvular distortion and dysfunction. This woman had a mild *stenosis* of the mitral valve (narrowing of the valve orifice) and a moderate-to-severe aortic valve *incompetence* (failure to close completely, with resultant leakage). Each type of valvular lesion distorts the normal patterns of flow through the valve and produces a characteristic murmur. To understand the differences in timing, tone, and nature of the various murmurs, it is necessary to identify the exact phases of the cardiac cycle during which the disturbed flow pattern occurs.

The *phonocardiogram* is a useful clinical tool for recording the timing and length of the heart sounds and murmurs that occur during the cardiac cycle. In this test, a microphone is placed on the patient's chest; an ECG is usually recorded simultaneously. Figure 9-7 shows a phonocardiogram of the heart sounds from the patient. The *top tracing* is an ECG. The remaining channels are recordings from the microphone tuned for the mid- (M_1) and high-frequency (H) sounds. *Each sound can be explained on the basis of the events of the cardiac cycle.*

In the recording taken at the level of the second rib at the left sternal border (2LSB), the physician would expect to hear sounds best that originate from the pulmonary and aortic valves. As expected, each heartbeat produces two heart sounds, S_1 and S_2, that are detected in both the mid- and high-frequency recordings. The high-frequency recording of S_2 actually shows an early component resulting from closure of the aortic valve (A_2) and a slightly later sound (P_2) resulting from closure of the pulmonary valve. These two components can usually be distinguished even in healthy persons. However, the P_2 in this clinical case is followed by a lower-amplitude murmur that continues throughout early diastole. These sounds are transmitted down to the microphone positioned at the fifth rib and left sternal border (5LSB). The patient's physician heard an early diastolic murmur (early-DM) over the second right space, and it was propagating down along the left sternal border. This sound results from the incompetence of the aortic valve. Immediately after the S_2, blood starts to flow from the higher pressure in the aorta, through the incompetent valve, into the lower pressure of the left ventricle. This abnormal flow produces the abnormal early-DM.

The mid- and high-frequency recordings from 2LSB and 5LSB also show an *ejection murmur* (ej-M) following S_1 that results from turbulent blood flow through the aortic valve. This murmur can often be heard in patients with an incompetent aortic valve, even in the absence of a true or genuine aortic stenosis. The patient's physician did not report this sound from the physical examination, but it can be seen rather easily in the phonocardiogram.

The lowest two recordings are from the apical region of the heart; sounds originating from the mitral valve are usually heard most clearly in this region. They show a "rumbling" murmur during mid-diastole with a "presystolic accentuation" (i.e., occurring during late diastole). These sounds are attributable to the stenosed mitral valve. When this valve opens, the blood that has accumulated in the left atrium flows rapidly into the ventricle; this rapid flow through the narrowed valve yields the mid-diastolic sound. Flow velocity and the intensity of the sound gradually decrease until the final "atrial kick," when velocity increases for a short period. The relative contribution of atrial contraction to ventricular filling increases in cases of mitral stenosis, so this late diastolic (or presystolic) flow is relatively accentuated.

One puzzle remains: the "accentuated heart sound, S_1" and the "opening snap (OS)" described by the patient's physician. These findings are due to the decreased compliance of the fibrosed mitral valve. Fibrosed valves open with a sharp sound, which can be detected in all the sound recordings shown in Figure 9-7. Normal valves open without making any sound.

Valve lesions such as these impose a hemodynamic burden upon the heart that varies according to the severity, number, and type of valvular lesions. By calling upon

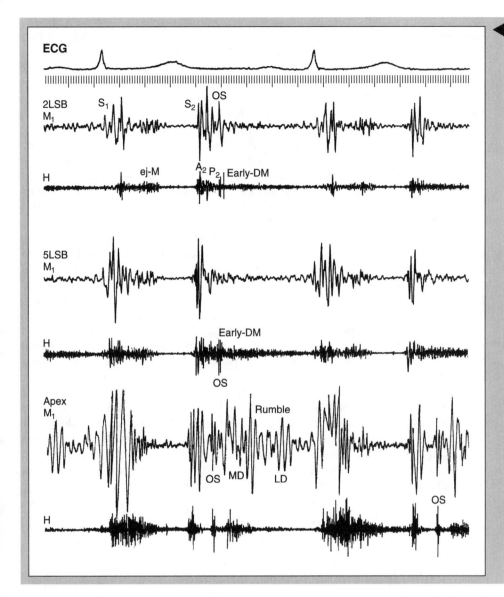

FIGURE 9-7

Phonocardiogram from the Patient with Stenoses of the Mitral Valve and Aortic Incompetence. The microphone is tuned for mid- (M_1) and high- (H) frequency sound. The apex recording (bottom) shows a mid-diastolic (MD) rumbling murmur with presystolic (i.e., late diastolic, or LD) accentuation; these sounds originate from the stenosed mitral valve. The fibrosis of this valve also produces the sharp sound known as an "opening snap" (OS). The top set of recordings taken at the level of the second rib at the left sternal border (2LSB) and the next set from the fifth rib at the left sternal border (LSB) show aortic (A_2) and pulmonary (P_2) contributions to the second heart sound. They also show a systolic ejection murmur (ej-M) and early diastolic murmur (early-DM) from the incompetent aortic valve. (Source: Adapted with permission from Wada T: Basic and Advanced Visual Cardiology. Philadelphia, PA: Lea & Febiger, 1991, pp 41 and 352.)

its compensatory reserve mechanisms, the heart can tolerate mild-to-moderate lesions of one or two valves for many years without obvious symptoms. Pregnancy places yet another hemodynamic burden upon the heart, in part because of excess retention of salt and water resulting from the high estrogen levels. At term, maternal blood volume is elevated by about 40%, which aids in meeting the increased metabolic demands of the mother and developing fetus. Unfortunately, the heart may not be able to maintain adequate function under the totality of these burdens. In this patient, decompensation or pump failure had progressed to the extent that she felt dyspneic whenever she increased her activity even modestly above normal levels (such as exercise).

An increase in end diastolic muscle fiber length is one of the myocardium's major compensatory mechanisms. In Chapter 10, this engorgement is discussed in terms of the Frank–Starling law of the heart. An increase in SNS activity also helps to maintain CO and would, along with a corollary decrease in parasympathetic activity, also account for this patient's elevated HR. The rapid respiratory rate was another compensatory mechanism to maintain arteriolar oxygen content.

The salt restriction and the mild diuretic the patient received in the hospital decreased the total amount of fluid in her body, thereby reducing her total blood volume and the hemodynamic load on her heart. The physician needed to ensure that the patient's decrease in blood volume did not decrease to the extent that uteroplacental perfusion was compromised. Digitalis was given for its positive inotropic effect. This drug works by poisoning the adenosine triphosphatase (ATPase) that powers the sarcolemmal sodium/potassium (Na^+/K^+) exchange pump. As a result, $[Na^+]_i$ increases.

This decreases the concentration gradient for Na^+ across the cell membrane. This Na^+ concentration gradient powers the calcium/sodium (Ca^{2+}/Na^+) exchange pump. As a result, intracellular Ca^{2+} levels increase, which has a positive inotropic effect. (The therapeutic range of digitalis and related drugs is narrow; care must be exercised in its use.) This balanced approach helped the patient complete her pregnancy. After delivery, the extra fluid and elevated hemodynamic load was removed, and the woman's heart was able to maintain adequate CO during her daily activities.

The patient's hospital admission 6 months later was due to her atrial fibrillation. This condition results when there is no longer any dominant supraventricular (i.e., atrial) pacemaker; coordinated atrial electrical activity and coordinated atrial contraction are therefore lost. Ventricular rate is then governed by the rate at which the AV node is excited at its junctional border and conducts this impulse. The rapid ventricular rate reflects this interplay between atrial fibrillation and AV nodal function.

The normally modest contribution of atrial contraction to ventricular filling is lost in atrial fibrillation. Even patients with normal valves who experience atrial fibrillation often perceive a lack of well-being from the loss of ventricular filling as a result of atrial contraction. However, in patients with mitral stenosis, the afterload for *atrial* muscle and atrial pump function is increased. In this woman, atrial contraction had become more functionally important in overcoming the increased resistance to the flow of blood into the left ventricle. As a result, the sudden onset of atrial fibrillation forced the left ventricle to rely entirely upon passive filling. Moreover, the rapid ventricular rate did not allow adequate filling time. The result was a decrease in ventricular preload and a significant drop in CO.

It is often difficult to restore a coordinated *supraventricular rhythm*, and success is not guaranteed. In this case, the woman's physicians again placed her on digitalis and diuretics. In this case, however, the digitalis was prescribed because it prolongs the refractory period of the AV node. Thus, it helps to decrease the ventricular rate and allow more filling time. Finally, the patient was placed on an anticoagulant as a prophylactic measure against development of *thrombosis* in the left atrium resulting from blood stasis. She was referred to a surgeon to discuss correction of the valvular lesions.

REVIEW QUESTIONS

Directions: For each of the following questions, choose the **one best** answer.

1. The following equation involves heart rate (HR), stroke volume (SV), a resistance term (Res), and a pressure difference (or gradient, ΔP):

$$SV \times HR = \Delta P / Res$$

The term "ΔP" in this equation is

(A) an index of preload on the heart

(B) almost equal to central venous pressure *if* aortic blood pressure is 120/80 mm Hg

(C) identical to pulmonary capillary wedge pressure

(D) essentially equal to mean aortic blood pressure if right atrial pressure is about 0 mm Hg

(E) transmural pressure across the right atrium

2. The recordings in the figure below are most likely to be observed in a patient with

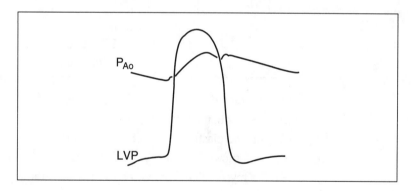

(A) a mitral valve that does not close completely during systole

(B) a mitral valve that does not open completely during diastole

(C) an aortic valve that is stenosed (abnormally narrow or obstructed)

(D) a left atrium that is fibrillating

(E) a left ventricular myocardium with low contractility

3. An increase in myocardial contractility has which of the following characteristics?

(A) It can be elicited by an increase in cardiac parasympathetic nervous activity

(B) It is induced by activation of a cardiac muscarinic receptor

(C) It tends to decrease end systolic volume

(D) It tends to decrease arterial systolic blood pressure

(E) It tends to decrease the amount of work performed by the myocardium

4. The following values are obtained from a patient: radial artery blood pressure, 132/88 mm Hg; heart rate (HR), 72 bpm; cardiac output (CO), 5.8 L/min; pulmonary arterial pressure, 26/15 mm Hg; pulmonary capillary wedge pressure, 8 mm Hg; Pa_{O_2}, 96 mm Hg; respiratory rate, 14/min. Which of the following statements is correct?

   (A) Left atrial pressure is dramatically elevated above normal

   (B) Stroke volume (SV) is ≈80 mL

   (C) Mean arterial blood pressure is 120 mm Hg

   (D) Oxygen exchange across this patient's lungs is extremely poor

   (E) The compliance of this patient's left ventricle is very low

5. Which of the following statements about the figure below is correct?

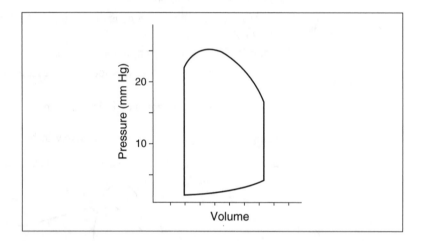

   (A) This recording is from the right ventricle

   (B) The ejection fraction is 20%

   (C) The end diastolic pressure is 25 mm Hg

   (D) The atrioventricular (AV) valve opened at a pressure of 25 mm Hg

   (E) The myocardium contracted isometrically throughout ejection

6. Which of the following statements concerning the right ventricular and the pulmonary circulation is correct?

   (A) Pulmonary systolic pressure is much higher than systemic arterial pressure

   (B) The volume of blood ejected by the right ventricle with each beat is significantly less than that ejected by the left ventricle

   (C) The volume of blood flowing through the pulmonary circulation over a given time equals that which flows through the systemic circulation

   (D) The pulmonary vascular resistance is identical to the total peripheral resistance

   (E) The work performed by the right ventricle for each beat equals that of the left ventricle

7. Stimulating the cardiac sympathetic nerves tends to

   (A) decrease the time required for isovolumic contraction and isovolumic relaxation

   (B) increase the duration of ejection

   (C) decrease the rate of rise and rate of fall of left ventricular pressure

   (D) increase the time between heartbeats (i.e., the interbeat interval)

   (E) increase the duration of the action potential recorded from a ventricular myocyte

8. The systolic arterial blood pressure (SBP) for the heartbeat below is

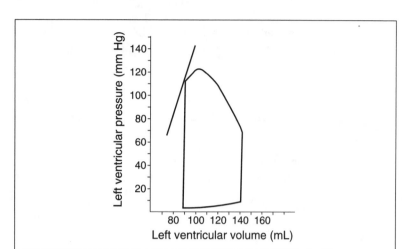

(A) 20 mm Hg

(B) 65 mm Hg

(C) 84 mm Hg

(D) 112 mm Hg

(E) 122 mm Hg

ANSWERS AND EXPLANATIONS

1. The answer is D. ΔP is the pressure gradient driving blood around the circulation, and it equals mean aortic pressure minus right atrial pressure. Right atrial pressure approaches 0 mm Hg, so its contribution to the overall gradient is often ignored.

2. The answer is C. A large pressure drop occurs across the abnormally small orifice of a stenosed valve. A significant component of the potential energy stored in the blood pressure would be lost as blood moved through the narrow valve opening. Consequently, aortic blood pressure would no longer be nearly identical to left ventricular pressure but would be significantly lower.

3. The answer is C. Since stroke volume tends to increase with an increase in myocardial contractility with no change in end diastolic volume, end systolic volume must decrease.

4. The answer is B. SV may be computed by dividing CO, 5800 mL/min, by HR to yield ≈ 80 mL/beat. The normal filling pressure coupled with a normal CO indicates that ventricular compliance is also normal.

5. The answer is A. The pressure–volume loop generally resembles that of Figure 9-4C for the left ventricle; however, the systolic pressure is within the normal range for the pulmonary circulation, not for the systemic circulation.

6. The answer is C. Even though systemic arterial pressure, stroke work, and vascular resistance are much higher than for the pulmonary circulation, on the average the same volume of blood flows through them in a given time since they are connected in series.

7. The answer is A. Activation of the cardiac sympathetic nerves increases the rate of development of tension. This decreases the time required for the events of the cardiac cycle, including the isovolumic contraction and relaxation and the duration of ventricular depolarization. Answer D is also wrong because the interbeat interval tends to *de*crease.

8. The answer is E. Do not confuse SBP with the pressure at which the aortic valve closes (≈ 112 mm Hg) or with mean arterial blood pressure [≈ 65 mm Hg + $\frac{1}{3}$ (122 − 65) = 84 mm Hg].

REFERENCES

1. Swan HJ, Ganz W, Forrester J, et al: Catheterization of the heart in man with use of a flow-directed balloon-tipped catheter. *N Engl J Med* 283:447–450, 1970.

10 CARDIAC PUMP FUNCTION

CHAPTER OUTLINE

INTRODUCTION OF CLINICAL CASE

A 31-year-old woman presented to the outpatient clinic because of shortness of breath on effort. She reported that she first noticed the dyspnea about 2 months ago and that it had progressively worsened to the extent that she was currently unable to perform routine physical tasks. She had previously been told during a routine physical examination that she was hypertensive. She was given medication to lower her blood pressure, but she did not continue to take it.

On examination, the woman's pulse was 100 beats/min, with a regular rhythm. Simultaneous palpation of the radial and femoral arteries revealed that the femoral pulse was weak and delayed on both sides. Blood pressure was 190/120 mm Hg from either arm but was only 90/70 mm Hg when measured from the lower limbs. A basal ejection systolic murmur could be detected by auscultation. Chest radiograph revealed an increased ratio of heart size to chest size (cardiothoracic ratio) and pulmonary vascular congestion. Echocardiography showed a localized aortic narrowing just distal to the origin of the left subclavian artery with an estimated pressure gradient of 75 mm Hg. The left ventricular wall was markedly thickened, and its cavity was moderately dilated. Left ventricular shortening dynamics were also noticeably depressed.

The woman was admitted to the hospital and was given antihypertensive medication under close supervision. After 2 days, her brachial blood pressure was 150/95 mm Hg, and her dyspnea improved markedly. She was then informed about the nature, congenital etiology, and probable consequences of her condition. A cardiac catheterization was strongly recommended to assure a more accurate diagnosis. She was also told that surgical correction would probably be required to deal effectively with her problem.

However, the patient was hesitant to undergo surgery. She was released from the hospital at her request. Her physician urged that she comply rigorously with the antihypertensive medication and that she return regularly for follow-up visits.

Two months later, the patient presented to the emergency room with a compound fracture of her left femur as a result of an automobile accident. The wound had bled profusely for about 10 minutes after the accident. The hemorrhage was controlled by the ambulance paramedics; they estimated the total blood loss at 1000–1200 mL. Her pulse was 132 beats/min; blood pressure taken at the arm was 80/60 mm Hg; respiratory rate was 44 breaths/min; central venous pressure was 2 cm H_2O. She was given a blood transfusion and additional intravenous fluids, but her hemodynamic status remained critical for several hours before improving. After 24 hours, her condition stabilized with a blood pressure of 130/80 mm Hg, pulse rate of 96 beats/min, and central venous pressure of 14 cm H_2O (normal value: < 12 cm H_2O).

EFFECTS OF CHANGES IN PRELOAD AND AFTERLOAD ON CARDIAC OUTPUT

Key Question
How does the heart increase or decrease CO to adjust to changing circulatory demands?

"The heart more deceitful than all else and is desperately sick; Who can understand it?" (Jeremiah 17:9, New American Standard)

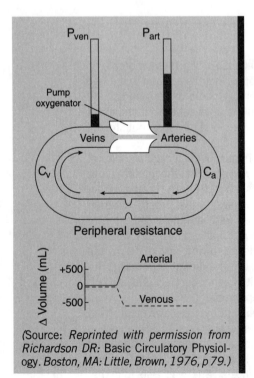

(Source: *Reprinted with permission from Richardson DR: Basic Circulatory Physiology. Boston, MA: Little, Brown, 1976, p 79.*)

The primary objective of this chapter is to examine the effects of changes in preload, afterload, and inotropic state upon the ability of the heart to eject blood and to interpret these effects in terms of the functional properties of heart muscle. The myocardium possesses marvelous adaptive mechanisms involving changes in preload and inotropic state that allow it to alter cardiac *pump* performance to meet increased demands by the tissues for delivery of oxygenated blood. Because of these extremely effective adaptive abilities, it is possible for cardiac output (CO) and blood pressure to be nearly normal, even though the myocardium is severely diseased. *The physician must somehow see through the "deceit" of the heart—as a pump—to recognize when the muscle constituting that pump is "desperately sick."*

Adaptations to Changing Preload

The amount of blood returned to the right atrium over a given time, the *venous return*, constitutes one of the primary demands placed upon the heart pump. The simple model of the circulation in Chapter 3, Figure 3-4 showed that with each beat the heart must transfer to the arterial system the same volume of blood it has just received from the venous system. This occurs in part because venous return helps determine the preload. Starling's law of the heart is a fundamental concept that relates the amount of blood returned to the heart to the amount of blood ejected by the heart.

STARLING'S LAW OF THE HEART

During the closing years of the nineteenth century, the German physiologist Otto Frank showed that increasing the stretch on the ventricle of the frog heart during diastole—*the preload*—increased the pressure developed during systole. He concluded that increasing the stretch on the myocardium allowed the frog heart to perform more work. During the second decade of the twentieth century, Ernest Starling and his colleagues used a canine *heart–lung preparation* to demonstrate a similar relationship in the mammalian heart. Figure 10-1A illustrates the heart–lung preparation.

Understanding the role of the venous reservoir is the key to grasping Starling's experiment and its ultimate physiologic impact. Starling replaced the normal venous inflow to the heart with a blood-filled reservoir. By varying the height of the reservoir with respect to the heart, he was able to control the volume of blood entering the ventricles prior to each heartbeat; that is, the pressure gradient driving blood to the heart was determined by the height of the column of blood above heart level. The *heavily shaded* cross section of the heart in Figure 10-1A shows the volume of the ventricles when the reservoir was at position 1. When the reservoir was raised to position 2, the filling pressure increased and the volume of blood entering the heart during the filling phase consequently increased. This new preload is indicated by the *lightly shaded* outline of the

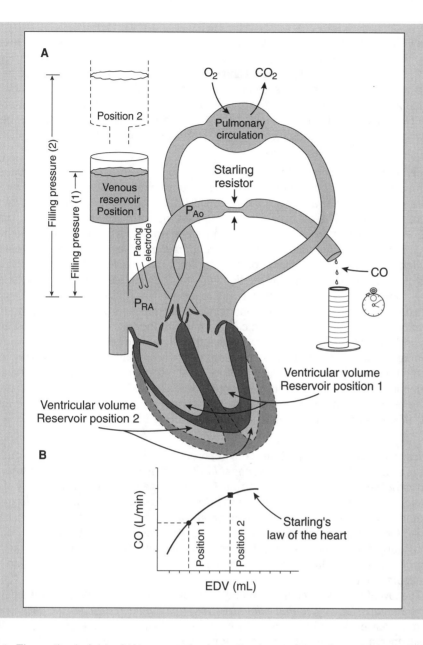

FIGURE 10-1
Starling's Heart–Lung Preparation. The purpose of the experiment is to determine the effects of changes in preload, the independent variable, on cardiac output (CO) [volume of blood pumped in a given time]. (A) This panel illustrates how raising the venous reservoir from position 1 to position 2 increases the filling of the ventricles, as shown. Therefore, position 1 produces a smaller ventricular preload than does position 2. A pacing electrode on the atrium maintains a constant heart rate. Appropriate adjustments of a physical clamp on the aorta, called a Starling resistor, keeps arterial blood pressure constant irrespective of changes in reservoir position. (B) This panel plots CO against left ventricular preload. CO measured when the reservoir is at position 1 is indicated by "●." Increasing the height of the reservoir above the heart to position 2 elevates CO, indicated by "■." Starling tested the effects of a large number of preloads to obtain the relationship now known as Starling's law of the heart. EDV = end diastolic volume; P_{RA} = right atrial pressure; P_{Ao} = aortic blood pressure.

heart. Thus, *the height of the reservoir above the heart determines the end diastolic volume (EDV) of the ventricle.* Using this technique, Starling controlled the preload (the independent variable) and observed the effects upon CO (or pump function, the dependent variable).

Pump function may be assessed directly by measuring stroke volume (SV). SV directly reflects CO if the heart rate (HR) is fixed at a constant rate by an electrical pacemaker (i.e., CO = HR × SV). Starling also maintained aortic pressure by using a hydraulic resistor. Keeping the aortic pressure constant was important for two reasons: First, it prevented the afterload from changing, which allowed Starling to investigate the effects of preload without worrying about changing afterload; second, it can be shown mathematically that if arterial pressure is constant, then changes in CO also indicate changes in the work performed by the heart. Therefore, Starling's heart–lung preparation allowed him to ask the following question: What are the effects of changing the amount of blood delivered to the heart upon CO and upon the amount of work performed by the heart?

The results of a typical heart–lung experiment are shown in Figure 10-1B. Setting the reservoir at position 1 results in a certain volume of blood entering the ventricles during the filling phase prior to each heartbeat. This important volume is called *left (or right) ventricular end diastolic volume* (LVEDV/RVEDV). As explained in Chapter 9, be-

The venous reservoir controls the input to the right ventricle, while the CO measurement is for the left ventricle. This is not a problem, since under the conditions of the experiment, RVSV must equal LVSV. It is easier to focus on the pumping action of the left ventricle; however, similar results could be obtained for the right ventricle.

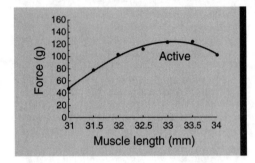

First Answer to Key Question
Starling's law of the heart.

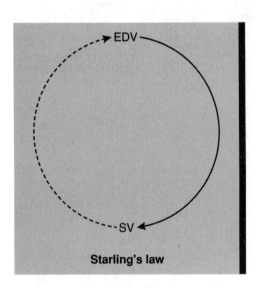

Starling's law

cause EDV constitutes the preload, it determines the stretch on the ventricular muscle fibers just prior to contraction. EDV at position 1 is indicated on the x-axis in Figure 10-1B; the CO at this initial preload is shown on the graph by "●." Increasing the height of the venous reservoir to the second level increases the EDV to the value shown at position 2, and CO to the value indicated by "■." The gently curved line passing through these two points would be obtained if the CO were measured for a large number of preloads. This is a graphic representation of Starling's law of the heart.

Intracellular Mechanisms of Starling's Law. The shape of the Frank–Starling relationship is immediately reminiscent of the active length–tension relationship for striated muscle (Figure 4-3). Laser diffraction experiments show that the lengths of the myocyte sarcomeres at normal EDVs are considerably less than the optimal overlap (i.e., L_{max}) value of 2.2 − 2.3 μ. Therefore, unlike skeletal muscle in which the in situ length is normally ≈L_{max}, *cardiac muscle functions on the ascending limb of its length–tension relationship.* Indeed, the classic explanation for Starling's law was formulated exclusively in terms of the active length–tension relationship: increasing preload increased the stretch on the myocytes closer to L_{max}, thereby increasing active tension. More recent experiments have revealed an additional phenomenon in heart muscle called *length-dependent activation* [1, 2]. This means that in cardiac muscle, the fraction of the total potential cross bridges that are activated at any given intracellular free calcium (Ca^{2+}) concentration increases with increased sarcomere length. This is probably a result of differences in troponin C in skeletal versus cardiac muscle. Whatever the precise cellular mechanism, the fundamental principles of muscle function described in Chapter 4 show that increasing the preload on the muscle increases the amount of shortening (ΔL). In the intact heart, this increase in ΔL translates into an increase in SV.

Implications of Starling's Law. One of the important messages of Starling's law is that the heart is a *demand pump: within practical limits, the heart pumps whatever amount of blood is delivered to it*! This implies that EDV is normally well below the peak of the Frank–Starling curve, closer to preload 1 than preload 2 in the previous example. Therefore, as implied above, *the heart normally functions on the ascending limb of the Frank–Starling relationship.* Consequently, the heart can increase its CO by becoming more engorged with blood as a result of an increased preload. Dilation of the heart as a result of increased preload is mechanistically different from the increase in heart size that occurs in elite athletes.

The law of the heart includes another profound truth: *The Frank–Starling relationship is a homeostatic cycle that minimizes variations in heart size.* An increase in EDV acts to increase SV; an increase in SV empties the heart more, thereby offsetting the original increase in EDV. This cycle operates independently of neurohumoral control systems external to the heart.

PRESSURE–VOLUME RELATIONSHIP FOR CONTROL AND ELEVATED PRELOAD

The effects of changes in preload upon cardiac pump function may be examined productively from the perspective of the pressure–volume loop. Figure 10-2 shows one heartbeat at a lower preload in a *solid line* (e.g., position 1, Figure 10-1) with a second beat at a higher preload in a *broken line* (e.g., position 2, Figure 10-1). The diastolic pressure–volume relationship is also shown with extensions above and below its EDV and end systolic volume (ESV), respectively. The conditions of the experiment also stipulate that the afterload (i.e., arterial diastolic pressure) and inotropic state are identical for the two heartbeats. Assume the first beat starts at point 1 and proceeds through the trajectory indicated by points 2–4. Filling for the second beat with increased preload starts with the opening of the atrioventricular (AV) valve at 5. However, because of the increased preload, filling does not cease at point 2; instead, the ventricle continues to increase in volume to point 6. The additional filling proceeds along the passive pressure–volume relationship, even though this portion of the curve could not have been determined during the control beat. Also, since afterload is constant, the aortic valve opens at the same pressure in both the beats (points 3 and 7). The following list summarizes the major lessons of Figure 10-2 and recapitulates the action of the law of the heart upon cardiac pump performance:

- The preload was increased, as shown in the greater EDV for beat 2 (EDV_2) as compared to beat 1 (EDV_1).
- The end of ejection was delineated by the end systolic pressure–volume relationship (ESPVR) for both beats; the resulting ESV was similar for the two beats.
- The SV (i.e., EDV − ESV) was significantly increased because of the elevated preload; the increased SV was due to the increase in EDV (point 6 > point 2) as opposed to a decrease in ESV.
- The amount of work performed by the heart (the area within each pressure–volume loop) was increased with the increase in preload.
- The increased SV increased arterial systolic pressure at a constant peripheral vascular resistance.

There is another way to look at the implications of Starling's law for cardiac homeostasis. The natural tendency is to regard SV as "the" regulated variable in this simple cycle. However, since this is a closed-loop cycle, each variable in the cycle is regulated! Therefore, it is entirely legitimate to view EDV as a regulated variable. From that perspective, the Starling relationship could be said to maintain constancy of EDV. In fact, a person might conclude that the heart is nothing more than a sump pump, removing blood from the venous system at a rate appropriate to maintain stable central venous blood volume.

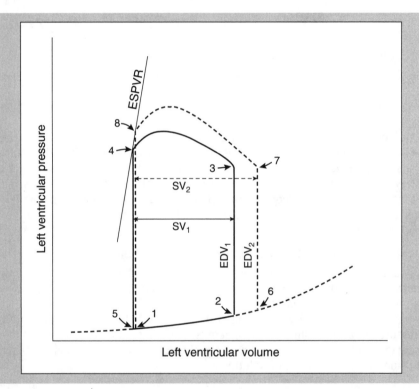

FIGURE 10-2
Left Ventricular Pressure–Volume Loops for Control Beat (solid line, EDV_1) and Second Beat with Increased Preload (broken line, EDV_2). Afterload (points 3 and 7) and inotropic state (reflected in the end systolic pressure–volume relationship, ESPVR) are identical for the two beats. Stroke volume (SV) increased with increased preload as a result of increased end diastolic volume (EDV).

Figure 10-3 illustrates a series of left ventricular pressure–volume loops from an experiment in which the canine autonomic nervous system (ANS) was blocked using appropriate drugs. This elimination of neural reflexes fulfills the stipulation of a constant inotropic state that was made in deriving Figure 10-2. The data shown in panel A were recorded while blood was drained away from the heart in a manner analogous to standing upright. The loops shown in this panel did not vary much from heartbeat to heartbeat. (The variations that do appear result from an interaction between the dog's respiration and heartbeat—another example of *cardiopulmonary* integration.) Panel B shows the changes that occurred when the blood was suddenly free to move from the peripheral veins toward the heart. Similar transformations would occur if a person were gently lowered from an upright to a supine position. EDV and SV progressively increased during the first five or six individual loops after the shift. Blood pressure also increased, at least in part because of the increased SV. Panel C shows a series of loops recorded after cardiac function had stabilized under the new conditions. Note that ESV is approximately the same in panels A and C; therefore, the increase in SV is attributable largely to the elevated EDV. Blocking the ANS eliminated any neurohumoral changes in myocardial inotropic state, and, under these conditions, the heart's response to the increased preload clearly followed Starling's law.

FIGURE 10-3 ▶

Left Ventricular Pressure–Volume Loop from a Healthy Dog with Blocked Autonomic Nervous System (ANS) Reflexes.
(A) Blood pooled in the lower body as a result of the gravitational field. (B) A series of loops during changes in the dog's position in the gravitational field allows some of the blood previously pooled in the lower body to shift into the chest. (C) This panel shows data after the blood shifted into the chest. Stroke volume (SV) increased primarily as a result of increased end diastolic volume (EDV). Similarly, increasing preload in contracting papillary muscle preparation increases muscle shortening. (Source: *Reprinted with permission from White GN, Knapp CF, Evans JM, et al: Control of left ventricular function during acceleration-induced blood volume shifts.* Aviat Space Environ Med *59:436, 1988.)*

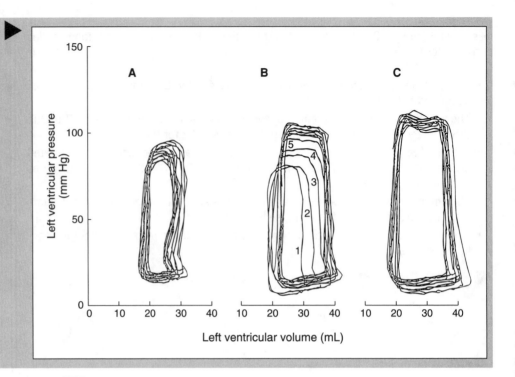

One could easily construct pressure–volume loops for control versus *decreased* preload and see that SV decreases. A decreased preload explains the brief feeling of faintness everyone occasionally experiences in going from the supine to standing position. Gravity causes blood to pool in the newly dependent legs and abdomen; this, in turn, decreases venous return, preload, SV, and blood pressure. Normally, the baroreflex (see Chapter 13) quickly adjusts cardiac and peripheral vascular function to counter the drop in blood pressure.

IMPLICATIONS OF LAPLACE'S LAW FOR CARDIAC PUMP FUNCTION

A physical principle known as Laplace's law dictates that the pressure produced within the ventricles depends not only on the tension developed by myocardial contraction but also on the size and shape of the heart. This relationship was formulated in the early nineteenth century by the French scientist the Marquis de Laplace. His law states that the pressure (P) within a thin-walled sphere is proportional to the wall tension (T) and inversely to the radius of the sphere (r). A simplified form of the relationship (that does not consider the contributions of wall thickness) is:

$$P = \frac{2T}{r}$$

To understand the implications of Laplace's law, suppose the heart needed to maintain a mean arterial pressure of 100 mm Hg to move blood around the circulation. If its radius were normally 1 unit, the tension required to develop the 100 mm Hg would be 50 units. If the heart were to dilate to a radius of 2 units, the wall tension required to develop the 100 mm Hg would rise to 100 units. *Laplace's law demonstrates that any increase in the size of the heart increases the load on the myocardium.* Clearly, it would be metabolically and mechanically advantageous if the heart were able to increase CO without physically dilating.

PHYSIOLOGIC APPLICATIONS OF THE LAW OF THE HEART

Chapter 20 examines the relative roles of the Starling mechanism and alterations in myocardial contractility in controlling CO in humans during exercise. In two other situations, the direct effects of preload on CO are worthy of special consideration:

1. *The law of the heart maintains the balance between right and left ventricular stroke volumes.* For example, suppose the right ventricle were to pump 0.1 mL more blood per heartbeat than the left ventricle. In 10 beats, 1 mL of blood would be trans-

ferred from the systemic circulation to the pulmonary circulation. If this were to continue indefinitely, the pulmonary circulation would become engorged with blood. However, any such shift of volume would quickly increase the preload on the left ventricle and increase its SV to equal that of the right ventricle. This restores the balance of right and left ventricular pump performance.

2. *Ventricular volume can become dangerously large during heart failure.* However, even in moderate failure, the heart may be able to maintain nearly normal values of arterial blood pressure (ABP) and CO (i.e., cardiac pump function) because of the adaptive power of the Frank–Starling relationship! The function of the failing heart is discussed in more detail later in this chapter.

Over the years, a spirited discussion has centered on whether there is a "descending limb" on the Frank–Starling relationship. Several factors must be considered. First, as noted in Chapter 4, the compliance of the myocardium at high preloads is much less than that for skeletal muscle; it would be difficult to stretch the heart muscle beyond the peak of the Starling relationship. Moreover, the pericardium limits the expansion of the heart. In any case, if the heart were to dilate beyond the peak in the Starling curve and enter the descending limb, any further increase in preload would *decrease*—not increase—SV. This would initiate a short-lived, downward spiral where further increases in preload would cause a further decrease in SV, and so forth. In effect, a positive-feedback cycle would become active and heart function would terminate in *asystole* (failure to contract) within a few heartbeats. (See Chapter 7, Figure 7-4C for further discussion.)

Adaptations to Changing Afterload

The ventricles must eject blood "against" ABP. This means that ejection, or myocardial shortening, cannot occur until ventricular pressure rises to meet ABP. Therefore, at least to a first approximation, arterial diastolic blood pressure constitutes the afterload on the ventricles. The present task is to apply the principles of muscle performance to understand how changes in afterload alter the pumping ability of the heart.

PRESSURE–VOLUME RELATIONSHIP FOR CONTROL AND ELEVATED AFTERLOAD

Figure 10-4 shows a control heartbeat (*solid line*) at a normal afterload and a second heartbeat (*broken line*) at an elevated ABP. In this example, the preload and inotropic state of the heart do not differ between the two beats. As in Figure 10-2, the control beat encompasses points 1–5; filling begins for the second beat at point 5. Points 2 and 6 are identical, since preload is the same in the two beats. A major difference between the two loops is that ejection does not begin until a much higher pressure is attained (point 7) for the beat with elevated afterload. Ejection ends at point 8, as demarcated by the ESPVR. Figure 10-4 illustrates two principal points:

1. *The increase in afterload decreases SV* in the absence of changes in preload or neurohumorally mediated changes in inotropic state.
2. The work performed by the left ventricle, as indicated by the relative areas enclosed by the two curves, is either relatively unchanged or perhaps modestly increased. Since the SV is smaller for the second beat, *the heart expends more energy to eject a unit volume of blood.*

The decrease in SV secondary to an increase in afterload follows directly from the principles inherent in the force–velocity relationship. In particular, increasing the afterload for any given preload decreases the shortening of the papillary muscle preparation. This translates directly into a decrease in SV in the intact heart. The increase in afterload also decreases the rate of muscle shortening. Similarly, an increase in ABP tends to decrease the rate of ejection of blood into the aorta in the absence of changes in preload and inotropic state.

CLINICAL IMPLICATIONS OF ELEVATED AFTERLOAD–HYPERTENSION

Many individuals have undiagnosed, chronically elevated ABP, a disease known as *hypertension*. Since oxygen (O_2) is required to produce adenosine triphosphate (ATP),

It is not easy to identify a variable equivalent to the afterload weight A in Chapter 4, Figure 4-4. The muscle plays no role in determining the value of weight A. Conversely, the left ventricle clearly helps determine the value of arterial pressure. Laplace's law clarifies the problem of identifying a realistic afterload. "Tension" may be expressed more accurately as wall thickness (w) times wall stress (σ, force per unit cross-sectional area of the wall; see Chapter 3). Laplace's equation would then be written $P = 2\sigma w/r$. Afterload (with a small contribution from preload) determines the stress developed by muscle during isotonic contraction. Therefore, wall stress faithfully reflects afterload. Rearranging the equation above shows that $\sigma = Pr/2w$. The afterload on the heart (σ) changes during ejection. In fact, the reduction in both P and r during late systole decreases afterload and facilitates late ejection. Although arterial diastolic pressure can be used to measure afterload, this approach has limitations.

FIGURE 10-4 ▶

Left Ventricular Pressure–Volume Loops for Control Beat (solid line) and Second Beat with Increased Afterload (broken line). Preload (points 2 and 6) and inotropic state (reflected in the end systolic pressure–volume relationship, ESPVR) are identical for the two beats. Stroke volume (SV) decreases with increased afterload as a result of increased end systolic volume. Similarly, increasing afterload in the papillary muscle experiment decreases shortening and velocity of shortening.

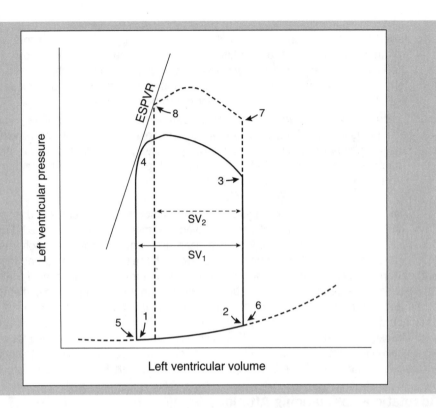

the energy expenditure of the myocardium (M) may be assessed by measuring the amount of O_2 it consumes over a given time. This variable is known as $M\dot{v}o_2$. (The dot over the V in this expression signifies the *rate* at which a volume of, in this case, O_2 is utilized.) Figure 10-5 compares $M\dot{v}o_2$ in an individual at rest, during infusion of a drug that activates alpha receptors to increase afterload (via increased peripheral resistance), and during moderate exercise. The latter two conditions are given as a percent of resting $M\dot{v}o_2$. The amount of energy expended by the heart with each beat at rest can be partitioned into that needed to (1) eject the SV, (2) impart the potential energy of pressure, and (3) produce a heartbeat. (A positive inotropism produces an additional energy cost that is discussed later under "Inotropic Response to Environmental and Behavioral Challenges.") The SVs for the resting state and for the increased afterload are roughly similar; conversely, the total energy expenditure is markedly greater with the increased afterload. Virtually all of this increase is attributable to the energy cost of developing a greater ABP. In the human, hypertension is likely to be associated with *coronary artery disease*. Narrowed coronary vessels are less capable of increasing the delivery of oxygenated blood to the myocardium than are normal vessels. Finally, chronically elevated blood pressure induces myocardial *hypertrophy*, a physical increase in the muscle mass. The increased metabolic demand that results from the hypertension itself and the increased muscle mass, coupled with a decreased ability to deliver O_2 to the muscle, is a potentially lethal combination and accounts for large numbers of *myocardial infarctions* (death of the myocardium). The data for exercise in Figure 10-5 are considered later in this chapter.

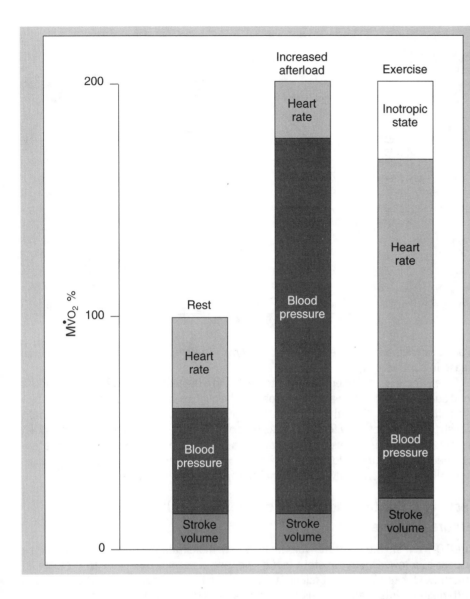

Increased
afterload

Exercise

Rest

FIGURE 10-5
Energy Expenditure, Measured by the Rate at which Myocardium Consumes Oxygen ($\dot{M}vo_2$). Left panel: individual at rest. Middle panel: after infusion of α-adrenergic agonist drug to produce arteriolar vasoconstriction (increasing peripheral resistance and thereby afterload). Right panel: during exercise. Energy utilization is apportioned between the costs of producing stroke volume, arterial pressure, heart rate, and inotropic state. Basal and activation oxygen consumption are not shown. Hypertension secondary to increased afterload dramatically increases the metabolic load on the heart, even though the heart pumps a similar volume of blood. Exercise increases $\dot{M}vo_2$, largely as a result of increased tachycardia and the "energy-wasting" effect of positive inotropism. (Source: Adapted with permission from Braunwald E, Ross J, Sonnenblick EH: Mechanisms of Contraction of the Normal and Failing Heart. Boston, MA: Little, Brown, 1976, p 184.)

EFFECTS OF CHANGES IN INOTROPIC STATE ON CARDIAC OUTPUT

A key question in this chapter is, "How does the heart control the amount of work it performs?" The first answer to this question, Starling's law of the heart, is intrinsic to the function of the heart because it does not depend upon neural or hormonal influences. However, other considerations, such as the implications of Laplace's law, prompt scientists to seek other answers to this question. An alternative mechanism, a change in the inotropic state of the myocardium, has potent effects upon cardiac pump function. It requires elevated ANS activity or circulating catecholamines.

Second Answer to Key Question
An increase in myocardial contractility.

Effects of a Positive Inotropism upon the Frank–Starling Relationship

Assume in Figure 10-1 that the reservoir is set at position 1 and the heart is ejecting a CO equal to the previously observed value; this is denoted by "●" in both Figure 10-1B and Figure 10-6. If epinephrine was added to the blood in the reservoir, CO would quickly increase to a higher value, denoted by the symbol "○" in Figure 10-6. *This increase in CO*

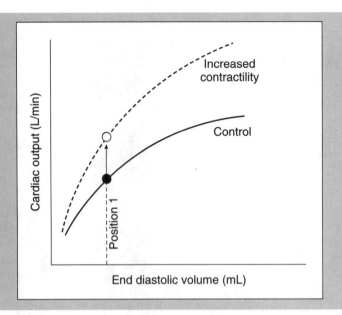

FIGURE 10-6 ▶

Starling Curves for Control State (solid line) and for Increase in Contractility (broken line). Position 1 refers to Figure 10-1A. Cardiac output (CO) in the control state is indicated by "●"; after an increase in contractility, CO increases to a value indicated by "○." The heart increases CO without an increase in preload. This is, by definition, an increase in contractility.

An increase in contractility occurs when the heart performs more work than before starting from the same, or smaller, EDV.

was achieved without an increase in preload; it results from a positive inotropism (i.e., an increase in contractility).

If the effects of adding epinephrine to the blood were tested at a series of preloads, a second curve would shift upward with respect to the control relationship; this is shown by a *broken line* in Figure 10-6. In fact, any number of these *ventricular function curves* could be constructed theoretically for varying degrees of hormonal or ANS activity. In the intact organism, a positive inotropism normally results from activation of β_1-adrenergic receptors by neurotransmitters released from the sympathetic nerve varicosities or by circulating catecholamines (primarily epinephrine) from the adrenal medulla.

Effects of a Positive Inotropism on the Ventricular Pressure–Volume Loop

Figure 10-7 enlists the pressure–volume loop to demonstrate the differences between a heartbeat at a lower inotropic state (*solid line*) and a second beat with an increase in contractility (*broken line*). The preload is the same for the two beats (points 2 and 6), as is the afterload (points 3 and 7). The following list describes the differences between the two loops (positive inotropism versus control):

- With the increase in inotropism, the trajectory of the second pressure–volume loop crosses the control ESPVR (E) to a new ESPVR (E'). As a result, *the SV increases significantly*. The slope of the ESPVR, in fact, is highly dependent upon the inotropic state of the heart [3].
- *The increase in SV is due to a decrease in ESV*. This differs qualitatively from the mechanism in the Frank–Starling phenomenon, where the SV increase is due to an increase in EDV.
- Arterial (and ventricular) systolic blood pressure are increased (given no change in vascular resistance) with the positive inotropism because a larger volume of blood is injected into the great arteries.
- *The total work performed is significantly greater with an increase in contractility*: the heart performs more work without becoming engorged with blood.
- Since ESV is decreased, the pressure at the opening of the AV valve (point 9) is lower than for the control beat (point 1). The value of the pressure at point 9 is determined by the diastolic pressure–volume relationship.

Alterations in inotropic state have now been viewed from three perspectives: the Wiggers diagram (Chapter 9, Figure 9-5), the ventricular function curve (Figure 10-6), and the ventricular pressure–volume loop (Figure 10-7). Although each viewpoint

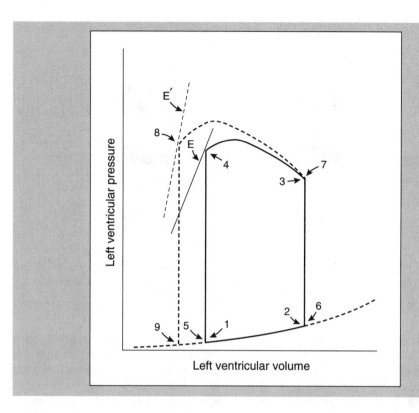

◀ **FIGURE 10-7**
Left Ventricular Pressure–Volume Loops for Control Beat (solid line) and Second Beat with Increased Contractility (broken line). Preload (points 2 and 6) and afterload (points 3 and 7) are identical for the two beats. The loop for the positive inotropic beat transgresses the original end systolic pressure–volume relationship (E) to abut a new ESPVR (E'), demonstrating the sensitivity of this relationship to changes in inotropic state. Stroke volume and stroke work increase with the increase in contractility that results from decreased end systolic volume. Similarly, increasing contractility in the papillary muscle experiment increases shortening and velocity of shortening.

reveals a somewhat different perspective, they all show how an increase in contractility allows the heart to perform more work, more rapidly, while minimizing the mechanical and metabolic costs of physical dilation.

Inotropic Response to Environmental and Behavioral Challenges

What role do changes in cardiac contractility play in adapting cardiac function in the intact subject to environmental and behavioral demands? Figure 10-8 shows the response of the heart in a healthy, awake monkey to a *sympathomimetic* drug (a β-agonist); the animal's heart's response is similar in many ways to what occurs as a result of activation of the SNS during challenges such as behavioral stress. The first two channels are recordings of left ventricular pressure and its rate of change (i.e., dP/dt). The *bottom* channel shows an isometric force recording from a strain gauge attached to the left ventricular wall; this recording is conceptually similar to the isometric papillary muscle recordings from Chapter 4. One cardiac cycle was recorded at a fast chart paper speed in both panels to show the waveform of each recording. The *left* panel was recorded while the animal was sitting quietly. The drug was injected intravenously at the *upward arrow* in the *right* panel. The increase in contractility caused both the isometric contractile force and the rate of rise of pressure (i.e., dP/dt) to increase. This shows how a positive inotropism increases the work the heart performs and its power output. This would result in a larger SV and a more rapid ejection. HR also increased, as would CO. (Blood pressure did not increase in this example because the β-agonist decreased peripheral resistance, thereby offsetting the tendency of increased CO to elevate pressure.)

The energy cost of changes such as those during exercise is shown in Figure 10-5. The increase in $M\dot{v}O_2$ compared to rest shows that there is an energy cost to increasing SV and HR during exercise. The energy cost attributable to generating blood pressure, however, is only modestly higher than during rest. Moreover, stimulating the α-adrenergic receptor increased the energy cost attributed to generating blood pressure much more than did exercise.

Effects of Myocardial Ischemia on Myocardial Contraction

Failure of the coronary circulation to deliver an adequate supply of oxygenated blood to the myocardium creates a condition known as *myocardial ischemia*. Prolonged ischemia

The rate of change in left ventricular pressure over time, dP/dt, shows how rapidly the ventricle is able to develop pressure. The peak (i.e., maximum) value of dP/dt is often used to index the inotropic state of the heart, though both preload and afterload can also alter dP/dt_{max}. See also Figure 9-6.

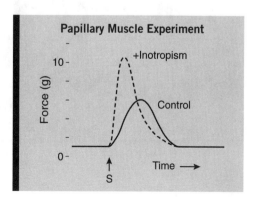

Papillary Muscle Experiment

FIGURE 10-8 ▶

Cardiac Response of an Awake Monkey to Intravenous Infusion of a β-Agonist Drug (Isoproterenol) at "Inject." Recordings are of left ventricular pressure, its first time derivative (dP/dt), and contractile force from an isometric strain gauge attached to the left ventricle. A single heartbeat is shown in detail both before and after drug infusion. The positive inotropism increases both the force and rate of pressure development, indicative of how the heart is able to perform more work, more quickly, with increased sympathetic nervous system drive. (Source: Reprinted with permission from Randall DC: Concurrent measurement of left ventricular dP/dt$_{max}$, isometric contractile force and cardiac loading in the intact monkey. Cardiology 59:309, 1974.)

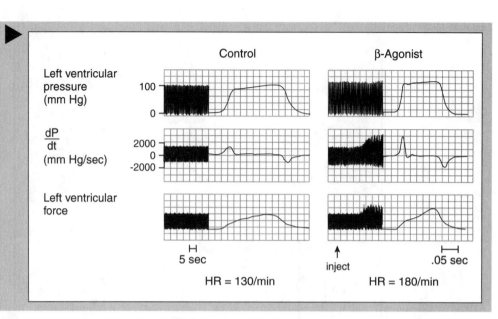

Stretching of Ischemic Muscle during Systole

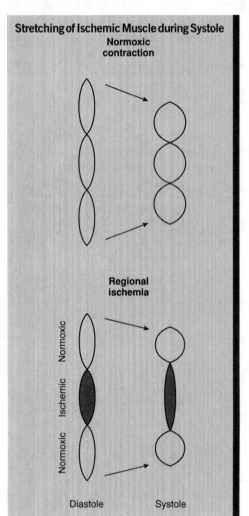

may result in the death of heart muscle—*myocardial infarction.* Figure 10-9 shows recordings from a healthy monkey before and at progressively later times after the anterior descending coronary artery was occluded at a point about halfway between the base and apex of the heart. The uppermost contractile force recording was made toward the base of the heart; this part of the heart was above the occlusion, so the muscle never experienced ischemia. The lowest tracing is from a force gauge placed near the apex of the heart; the blood supply to this muscle was cut off by the occluder. Both strain gauge recordings show robust force development during the control beats before onset of the occlusion. By 2 min after occlusion, the gauge below the occluder shows changes in the shape of the contraction including an early negative deflection and a decrease in the amplitude of developed force. These changes continued to develop at 5 minutes, and by 9 minutes the gauge on the ischemic muscle did not detect any active contraction at all. In fact, the force decreased during systole in this gauge because the ischemic muscle was being stretched by the contraction of the surviving muscle.

The dP/dt for ventricular pressure showed an increase during the ischemia, especially at 5 minutes. This increase was due to a reflex increase in cardiac SNS activity, which also explains the modest increase in ventricular systolic pressure. Despite the loss of contractile function in the ischemic muscle, compensatory mechanisms allowed the animal's heart to maintain adequate pump function. This example illustrates why it is important to consider both cardiac pump and muscle function and that it is essential to determine the underlying causes for the ischemia so that further myocardial infarction can be avoided.

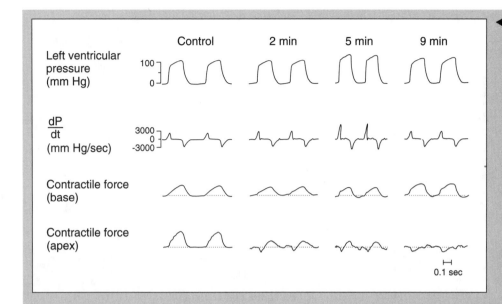

FIGURE 10-9

Impact of Myocardial Ischemia upon Myocardial and Cardiac Performance. *Two heartbeats are shown prior to (control), and at selected times after, occlusion of the distal portion of the anterior descending coronary artery in a monkey. Uppermost contractile force recording is from an isometric strain gauge arch attached to the myocardium at the base of the left ventricle above the occluder. The bottom recording is from a gauge attached to muscle at the apex of the heart below the occluder. Active contractile tension deteriorated rapidly in the apical segment after the occlusion. By 9 minutes, this recording showed a decrease in tension resulting from the ends of the gauge being pulled apart because noncontracting muscle under the arch was stretched during systole. Despite the loss of contracting muscle, ventricular pressure was maintained, partly as a result of reflexly elevated sympathetic drive. dP/dt = time rate of change of left ventricular pressure.*

THE FAILING HEART

The ventricles *must* transfer a volume of blood from the venous system to the arterial system equal to the volume delivered to them from the peripheral (or pulmonary) vessels. The healthy heart is able to accomplish this even during heavy, sustained exercise. Unfortunately, the ventricles may become less competent in a variety of pathologic conditions (e.g., myocardial infarction secondary to coronary artery disease, chronic pressure or volume overload, or infectious processes).

How does a failing heart respond to the demands of increased preload? Figure 10-10 illustrates an imaginary scenario to help answer this question. Figure 10-10A shows a ventricular function curve for a healthy human heart. The heart is functioning at the point on this curve indicated by "●" (beat 1), and this volume of blood must be pumped each minute to meet this person's bodily needs for oxygenated blood. Suddenly, the person's heart fails, so that the ventricular function curve becomes *depressed*, as indicated by the lower line, labeled "failing." The patient's CO suddenly drops in the space of one heartbeat to the value indicated by "□" (beat 2). The new CO is clearly below the minimal required value. For example, if the SV were 80 mL (i.e., 5 L/min ÷ 60 beats/min) in beat 1, it might be only 70 mL in beat 2. During this sudden cardiac event, the amount of blood that is in the process of returning to the heart could not have changed—it was already "committed" to returning to the heart. Therefore, essentially 80 mL of blood will be delivered to a heart that is now able to pump only 70 mL! What happens to the "extra" 10 mL of blood?

If the heart is not able to eject 10 mL of the 80 mL that had been delivered to it during the previous filling cycle, its preload for the next heartbeat must increase by 10 mL. As shown in Figure 10-10A, this will force the heart to dilate to point 3 on the depressed curve, as indicated by a smaller *open box*. As a result, the heart is now capable of ejecting a somewhat larger SV, perhaps 75 mL. Nevertheless, approximately 80 mL of blood will have arrived at the right atrium from the periphery during the third beat, leaving an additional 5 mL of extra blood in the heart. In effect, ventricular preload has now increased by almost 15 mL (10 + 5), so that beat 4 takes place from an even more elevated position on the depressed ventricular function curve. Over the course of a few beats, the heart would attain the required CO at the point indicated by a small, *solid square* (beat 7). The heart has no "choice"—it must either eject the volume of blood delivered to it or it must dilate until it can.

FIGURE 10-10 ▶

Simplified Scenario to Explain the Heart's Response to the Sudden Shift from a Normal Ventricular Function Curve (Healthy Heart) to a Depressed Function Curve (Failing Heart). (A) The individual's heart functioning at position 1 "falls" to position 2 as a result of sudden failure. At position 2, the amount of blood returning to the heart exceeds stroke volume (SV). Function progressively "migrates" through points 2–7 until SV again equals venous return. The heart is compensated at position 7. (B) This figure shows partial restoration of ventricular function (broken line) as a result of therapeutic intervention. The heart now functions at x, where cardiac output is normal, with only a modest increase in preload.

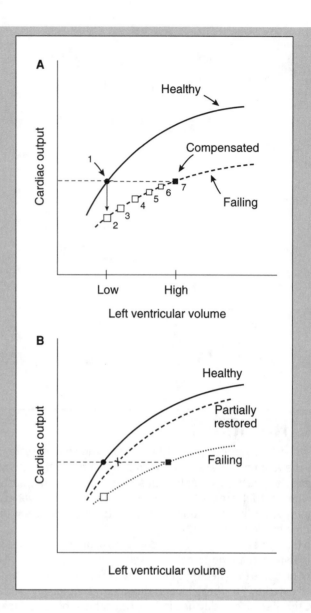

The heart has become *compensated* at its new operating point on the depressed ventricular function curve; CO is once again at the minimal required level and equals venous return. The heart is being "deceitful," however, since pump function has been sustained but only at the considerable cost of increasing preload from the normal value to a high value. The kidneys will retain fluid and increase total blood volume to maintain the elevated preload. The physician can "understand" this "deceit" only by assessing the state of the myocardium. For example, measuring pulmonary capillary wedge pressure would reveal that the preload on the muscle is abnormally high (Chapter 9, Figure 9-5). Eventually, the patient depicted in Figure 10-10 is likely to present to a physician because his CO cannot increase much further, severely limiting his daily activities. In addition, the *congestion*, or backup, of blood into the pulmonary circulation causes water to filter out of the pulmonary capillaries and accumulate around and within the alveoli ("wet lung"). This decreases the ability of the patient's lungs to exchange O_2, leading to dyspnea.

What can be done to reestablish acceptable levels of ventricular function? The classic therapeutic approach is threefold: (1) reduce the metabolic demand on the heart by reducing its work load, (2) reduce plasma volume, thereby countering the dilation of the heart, and (3) improve ventricular function. The most efficacious way to accomplish the first objective is to recommend that the patient rest as much as possible and to reduce ABP with drugs that cause vasodilation or block vasoconstriction. The second objective can be accomplished by prescribing a *diuretic* that causes the kidneys to increase water excretion. This offsets the mechanical disadvantage of Laplace's law. The physician may achieve the third objective by prescribing positive inotropes such as digitalis.

If this approach is successful, the patient's cardiac function may be somewhat restored to the point indicated by the *x* on the *broken line* (labeled "partially restored") in Figure 10-10B. Unfortunately, digitalis and related drugs have a narrow therapeutic range, so their usefulness is somewhat limited. Newer drugs that inhibit angiotensin-converting enzyme (ACE inhibitors) offer alternate approaches to the treatment of congestive heart failure (CHF). These drugs block the conversion of angiotensin I to angiotensin II, thereby also decreasing the production of mineralocorticoids from the adrenal cortex. This reaction restricts the kidney's reabsorption of sodium and water, limiting the expansion of blood volume normally seen in CHF. Because angiotensin II is a potent vasoconstrictor, the ACE inhibitors also decrease the afterload on the heart. In addition, because angiotensin II potentiates the action of the SNS at the effector junction, ACE inhibitors blunt this facilitatory interaction with the ANS. Finally, recent data have shown that angiotensin stimulates the myocytes to hypertrophy; this action would also be limited by the ACE inhibitors.

SUMMARY

The primary objective of this chapter has been to understand how changes in preload, afterload, and inotropic state influence the ability of the heart to eject blood. In each case, the effects upon CO have been seen to follow directly from fundamental properties of muscle function. The increased stretch that results from elevated preload increases SV, as described by Starling's law of the heart. Increased afterload decreases muscle shortening and, in the functioning heart, SV. A positive inotropism increases the degree and rate of muscle shortening; this yields an increase in stroke work and power without requiring an elevation in preload. However, Chapter 13 shows that these issues have not yet been resolved: a critical interaction between the heart and vasculature must still be considered.

RESOLUTION OF CLINICAL CASE

The woman presented at the beginning of the chapter has a congenital narrowing of her aorta known as a *coarctation*, which worsened over time. The narrowing is due to a shelf-like protrusion of the tunica media of the anterior, posterior, and superior aortic walls into the lumen of the vessel. This partial obstruction of aortic flow caused the systolic ejection murmur (see Chapter 9) and a large pressure gradient along that segment of the vessel. Whereas blood pressure proximal to the coarctation was high (i.e., to both arms, the neck, the head), pressure distal to the narrowing was relatively low. The coarctation also caused a noticeable delay in the pulse in the femoral as compared to radial arteries.

This high resistance produced a long-term, and gradually worsening, increase in left ventricular afterload. The woman's survival to adulthood is attributable to the interplay of a number of compensatory mechanisms. First, *the increased afterload caused her left ventricle to hypertrophy*, probably starting in childhood, as a result of a parallel replication of myofibrils, thickening of myocytes, and increased collagen deposition. This wall thickening prevented muscle stress (see Chapter 3) from rising, despite the increased afterload, but at the price of a significant increase in myocardial oxygen demand (i.e., $M\dot{v}O_2$). For approximately 30 years, this mechanism was able to maintain adequate CO without symptoms of pump failure. Eventually, however, the gradually increasing afterload could no longer be matched by hypertrophy; wall stress began to increase, shortening dynamics became depressed, and SV began to decrease.

What happened when this mechanism was no longer able to compensate adequately? *As the heart's ability to transfer blood from the venous side of the circulation to*

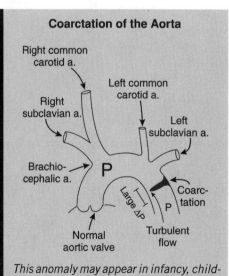

Coarctation of the Aorta

This anomaly may appear in infancy, childhood, or adulthood, depending on the site and severity of obstruction and the state of collateral circulation across the area of narrowing.

Ventricular hypertrophy is thought to be mediated by local growth factors that are normally dormant after birth but become activated upon abnormal rise in wall stress. Other neurohumoral factors such as growth hormone, cortisol, angiotensin, and increased sympathetic nervous system (SNS) stimulation are thought to contribute to the development of cardiac hypertrophy.

the arterial side began to decline—however imperceptibly—preload inevitably increased by the mechanisms described in Figure 10-10A. The woman's heart was able to continue to maintain pump function via the Frank–Starling mechanism. The cost of this adaptive mechanism was an increase in ventricular volume, which was detected by chest radiograph and echocardiography.

In this patient, *activation of the renin-angiotensin-aldosterone axis* was a third important adaptive mechanism in conjunction with the increase in preload. Presumably, this mechanism was activated by a tendency for renal blood flow to decrease, to which the kidney responded by retaining salt and water, driven largely by increased circulating levels of aldosterone. This increased the woman's effective blood volume and helped maintain high levels of ventricular preload. Again, there was a cost: venous and pulmonary congestion. The elevated pulmonary pressure interfered with respiratory function. The patient's dyspnea can be attributed to an increased diffusion barrier, thickening of the alveolar membrane as a result of plasma transudation, decreased lung compliance, and stimuli from overworked respiratory muscles.

The amount of blood the woman lost as a result of the automobile accident would normally be tolerated fairly well in a healthy subject. What accounted for the near fatal collapse in her cardiovascular status? At this advanced stage in her overall disease process, her heart had become dependent on the high preload to maintain CO. When the rapid contraction of blood volume deprived the left ventricle of the Frank–Starling compensation, CO fell precipitously. The patient's physicians were able to restore cardiac function only after sufficient fluid was replaced to return central venous pressure to unusually elevated levels.

REVIEW QUESTIONS

Directions: For each of the following questions, choose the **one best** answer.

1. If left ventricular preload, inotropic state, and heart rate were held constant, then an *increase* in arterial blood pressure would tend to *increase*

    (A) the rate of ejection of blood during systole

    (B) left ventricular end systolic volume (ESV)

    (C) the rate of rise in left ventricular pressure (dP/dt)

    (D) pulmonary capillary wedge pressure

    (E) the intensity of the first heart sound

2. Which of the following statements is consistent with the principles inherent in Starling's law of the heart?

    (A) Going from a supine to standing posture would tend to drop stroke volume (SV)

    (B) A patient with right ventricular failure would tend to have a pressure in the thoracic superior and inferior vena cavae lower than that in a healthy person

    (C) Pulmonary capillary wedge pressure in a patient with untreated left heart failure would be abnormally low

    (D) A patient experiencing an acute hemorrhage tends to have a large SV

    (E) Left ventricular SV routinely exceeds right ventricular SV

3. The pressure–volume loop drawn with a *broken line* shown below illustrates a heartbeat with

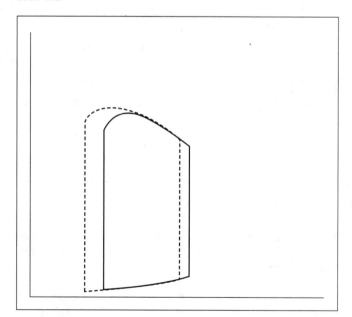

    (A) smaller end diastolic volume (EDV) and decreased afterload

    (B) a depressed contractility

    (C) a decreased preload and increased contractility

    (D) a decreased stroke volume (SV) and increased preload

    (E) an increased arterial diastolic pressure and an increased end systolic volume (ESV)

4. Which of the following statements regarding the work performed by the heart is correct?

   (A) Part of the energy expended by the contraction of the heart is used to eject physically (i.e., move) blood out of the ventricles

   (B) Very little of the energy expended by the heart appears as "potential" energy in the form of blood pressure

   (C) A positive inotropism allows the heart to eject a larger stroke volume (SV) without requiring any additional oxygen (O_2) consumption

   (D) The amount of energy the heart expends can be assessed by measuring the amount of O_2 in the coronary arterial blood

   (E) An increase in preload tends to decrease the rate at which the myocardium consumes oxygen ($M\dot{v}o_2$)

5. The active length–tension relationship for papillary muscle is most closely related to

   (A) changes in the pressure inside the ventricle as it is developing pressure isovolumically

   (B) the effect of changes in afterload upon the amount of blood ejected with each heartbeat

   (C) the rate of pressure generation during isovolumic contraction after a positive inotropic intervention

   (D) the relationship between intraventricular pressure and ventricular wall tension during diastole

   (E) the effect of changes in the amount of blood in the ventricle at the end of diastole upon force generation by the ventricular muscle

6. Which of the following statements concerning the function of the heart is true?

   (A) *Cardiac* muscle *active* tension increases with a positive inotropic stimulus from the parasympathetic nervous system (PNS)

   (B) Cardiac muscle inotropic state decreases with activation of its α-adrenergic receptors

   (C) *Passive* muscle tension measured before the beginning of isometric muscle contraction depends upon the length of the muscle

   (D) Ejection occurs during isovolumic relaxation

   (E) An increase in afterload increases the rate of ejection of blood into the aorta

ANSWERS AND EXPLANATIONS

1. **The answer is B.** The increased afterload will decrease the emptying of the heart by increasing ESV, which in turn decreases stroke volume and the rate of ejection of blood from the heart.

2. **The answer is A.** Gravity pools blood in the periphery, transiently decreasing the preload on the heart. SV must decrease until neural reflexes compensate for the decreased preload. Right heart failure causes fluid to congest in the venous system, increasing central venous pressure. The decrease in blood volume from hemorrhage tends to decrease preload and ventricular SV.

3. **The answer is C.** The preload (i.e., EDV) is decreased, and inotropic state is increased (i.e., second loop crosses original end systolic pressure–volume relationship [ESPVR]).

4. **The answer is A.** The heart works to: (1) develop pressure; (2) physically eject blood; (3) perform certain "chores," including producing a heartbeat and producing the "energy-wasting" effect of a positive inotropism. The physician can assess $M\dot{v}o_2$ by knowing the value of the coronary blood flow and the difference in O_2 content between the arterial and coronary venous blood.

5. **The answer is E.** The studies of muscle function in Chapter 4 have corollaries in the area of heart function. The isometric phase of muscle contraction corresponds to isovolumic contraction. Changing afterload on the papillary muscle changes muscle shortening, just as changing aortic pressure (or vascular resistance) alters stroke volume. Positive inotropic effects on muscle tension and rate of tension development are reflected in the rate of change in pressure within the ventricles. The passive length–tension relationship in muscle is closely related to the diastolic pressure–volume relationship.

6. **The answer is C.** Stretching the muscle increases preload, passive tension, and the potential for the muscle to perform work. The PNS has little direct influence on ventricular inotropic state. Finally, increases in afterload decrease the rate of ejection of blood into the aorta, all other things being constant.

REFERENCES

1. te Keurs HEDJ, Noble MIM: *Starling's Law of the Heart Revisited*. Dordrecht, Germany: Kluwer Academic, 1988.
2. Allen DG, Kentish JC: The cellular basis of the length–tension relation in cardiac muscle. *J Mol Cell Cardiol* 17:821–840, 1985.
3. Suga H: Ventricular energetics. *Physiol Rev* 70:247–277, 1990.

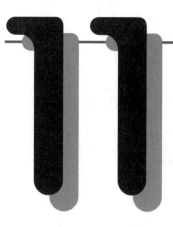

REGULATION OF TISSUE BLOOD FLOW

INTRODUCTION OF CLINICAL CASE

The clinical case presented in Chapter 3 is used here with added information. As described in Chapter 3, the patient's left leg felt "tight" and cramped after walking for several minutes. Physical examination showed weak or absent pulsations in the major arteries of his legs. More recently, the patient stated that he sometimes wakes up during the night with cramps and pain in his left leg, but the pain subsides if he stands up and walks to the bathroom. Further examination of the patient showed some ankle edema in the left leg and *dependent rubor* in the left foot. The patient has a 50-year history of cigarette smoking and a 20-year history of diabetes mellitus.

> **Dependent rubor** is redness of the skin when the foot is placed below the heart.

STRUCTURE OF THE MICROCIRCULATION

Some of the salient features of the microcirculation are described in Chapter 5. This section expands this description to define the structural framework of the microcirculation upon which the regulation of tissue blood flow is based.

Terminology

The generic term *microcirculation* is defined as the microscopic subdivisions of the vascular system that lie within the tissue and are exposed to the medium of the interstitial fluid. The juxtapositioning of microvessels with the tissue medium allows blood flow and blood–tissue exchange to be coupled to metabolic needs. The range and size of microvessels varies somewhat from tissue to tissue but in general encompasses all vessels less than about 0.1 mm in diameter. These vessels include the smallest of the arteries, the arterioles, the capillaries, the venules, and the smallest of the veins.

The arterioles offer the most resistance to the flow of blood (see Chapter 5, Figure 5-1); therefore, they are collectively termed "resistance vessels." The regulation of blood flow is achieved primarily by adjustments in the *tone* of vascular smooth muscle surrounding arterioles. For these reasons, the structure of the arterioles is emphasized in this chapter.

In keeping with current terminology, an arteriole is the vascular branch from a small artery that marks the entrance into the microcirculation [1]. The arterioles are invested in one or more tightly packed layers of smooth muscle, and their diameters are regulated primarily by the sympathetic division of the autonomic nervous system (ANS). Arterioles give rise to the next order of branching, the terminal arterioles. These vessels serve as the parent vessels of capillaries, and as their name implies, they terminate in a capillary network. Terminal arterioles are invested proximally in vascular smooth muscle. The final smooth muscle wrapping at the entrance to a capillary is termed a *precapillary sphincter*. Not all capillaries are invested at their entry points by vascular smooth muscle. Accordingly, this chapter uses only the terms "arteriole" and "terminal arteriole" to describe blood flow regulation.

The specific topographic structure of the microcirculation is geared toward serving the functional needs of the tissue being perfused. Nonetheless, most microcirculatory networks have common features that have an impact on the regulation of tissue blood flow. Figure 11-1 illustrates the microcirculation as found in the intestinal mesentery. Two arterioles supply blood to the region: one in the lower left and one in the upper right. Each of these arterioles can be traced back to a *different* intestinal artery. This redundancy of arterial input is a safety feature that assures capillary perfusion in the event that one of the supply arteries becomes dysfunctional (e.g., because of an embolism). This ability of the capillary network to derive blood from several sources is critical in tissues, such as the heart, that rely heavily on aerobic metabolism.

Note that the arterioles follow a serpentine pattern. Such tortuosity provides a certain amount of *geometric hindrance* (i.e., resistance) to the blood flow. An increase in the tortuosity of arterioles is a typical feature of hypertension. Figure 11-2 illustrates geometric hindrance. Note that the two capillaries branch from the terminal arteriole at very sharp angles, are narrow at their points of origin, and initially follow a tortuous path. All these geometric factors contribute to resistance to blood flow. Geometric hindrance is one of the factors that determines tissue blood flow; however, it does not regulate flow on a moment-to-moment basis. On a long-term basis, however, changes in geometric hindrance contribute to chronic adjustments in vascular resistance. For example, geometric hindrance increases in hypertension.

Finally, note that in Figure 11-1, large plasma gaps can be seen in several of the capillaries. These indicate regions in which capillary flow is stagnant or extremely slow. This reflects the fact that at any moment in time the number of perfused capillaries (those through which blood is flowing) is less than the total number of capillaries in a tissue. However, as a result of vasomotion of arterioles (discussed in this chapter in the section entitled "Local Regulation") the population of perfused capillaries is constantly shifting; over a given period of time, most, if not all, capillaries within a tissue participate

Intestinal mesentery is a thin, highly vascularized connective tissue surrounding the intestines. Because the mesentery of an anesthetized laboratory animal can easily be draped over the stage of a light microscope, it has been used extensively in investigations of microcirculatory structure and function.

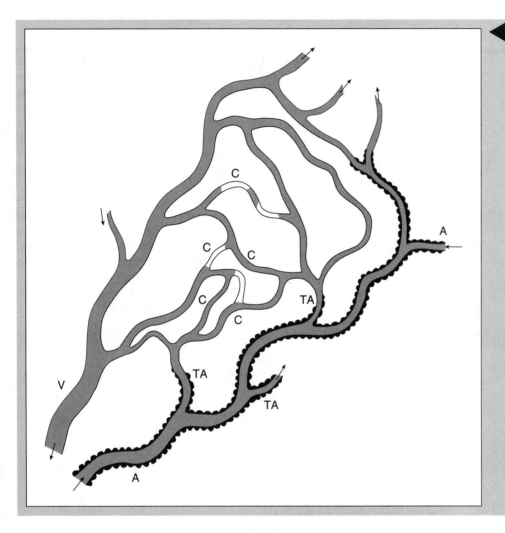

FIGURE 11-1
Structure of the Microcirculation as Exemplified in the Mesentery. *There are two arteriole inputs, each of which can be traced to a separate supply artery. Multiple inputs of this nature provide a safety factor to assure adequate blood flow to the capillary network. A = arteriole; TA = terminal arteriole; C = capillary; V = venule.*

in active circulation. The situation is analogous to a basketball game in which there are ten players on the floor; however, at any one moment, only one of them has the ball. Analogously, the passing of blood from capillary to capillary assures that all tissue cells have a chance to exchange substances with the blood.

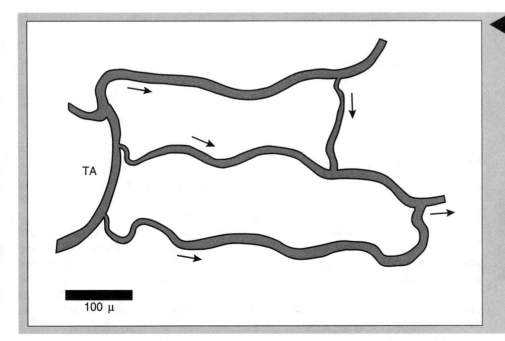

FIGURE 11-2
Capillaries Branch from a Terminal Arteriole in a Tortuous and Narrow Fashion. *These structures provide geometric hindrance to blood flow. TA = terminal arteriole. (Source: Adapted with permission from Zweifach BW, Lipowsky HH: Handbook of Physiology, Bethesda, MD: American Physiological Society, 1984, p 257.)*

100 μ

DETERMINANTS OF VASCULAR TONE

Blood flow regulation is achieved primarily by adjustments in the tone of arteriolar smooth muscle. The term "tone" as applied to muscle refers to the existing level of contractile force. In skeletal muscle, tone is maintained by asynchronous activity of motor units, and the level of tone is determined by the number of participating units and their frequency of contraction. Thus, a muscle group, such as the biceps, can maintain a steady level of contractile force even though individual muscle fibers are contracting and relaxing in a cyclic manner.

In contrast to skeletal muscle fibers, individual vascular smooth muscle cells have the ability to maintain a continuous level of force and are always contracted to a certain extent. The level of this contractile force at any particular time is synonymous with the term "tone." Vascular smooth muscle contraction elicits vasoconstriction; therefore, "vascular smooth muscle tone" refers to the existing level of *net* vasoconstrictor activity, as determined by the interaction of vasoconstrictor and vasodilator influences. Figure 11-3 gives an overview of the major extracellular mechanisms that initiate vasoconstriction (*dashed lines*) or vasodilation (*solid lines*) and, hence, regulate vascular tone.

FIGURE 11-3 ▶
Overview of Factors That Determine the Diameter of Blood Vessels. Dashed lines *indicate factors that reduce vessel diameter by increasing* the constrictor *tone of vascular smooth muscle.* Solid lines *indicate factors that increase vessel diameter by reducing smooth muscle tone. EDRF = endothelial-derived relaxation factors (nitric oxide is thought to be a major EDRF); EDCF = endothelial-derived constrictor factor (endothelin is thought to be a major EDCF).*

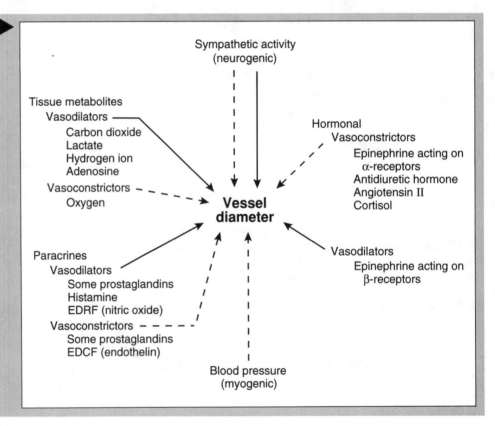

Neural Regulation

The *top* of Figure 11-3 shows the neurogenic contributions to vascular tone. Vascular smooth muscle is innervated primarily by the sympathetic nervous system (SNS); "neurogenic tone" refers to the collective effect of sympathetic neural activity on vascular diameter.

As illustrated, sympathetic activity can elicit either vasoconstriction or vasodilation. This differentiation depends upon the type and concentration of receptors on vascular smooth muscle. The dominant receptors in the circulatory system are α-adrenergic receptors, which mediate vasoconstriction in response to catecholamines. In fact, most tissue circulations contain only the alpha type of sympathetic receptors. This being the case, the *systemic* effect of a general increase in sympathetic activity is vasoconstriction (i.e., an increase in vascular tone).

There is some evidence for parasympathetic innervation of blood vessels in a few vascular beds, such as the salivary glands and sex organs; however, the physiologic significance of the parasympathetic system in regulating blood flow is unclear.

Although there are far fewer dilatory receptors on vascular smooth muscle compared to constrictor (alpha) receptors, dilatory receptors are found in a variety of types. The best known, and most understood, of these are the β_2-adrenergic receptors, which respond primarily to circulating epinephrine and which fall under the category of hormonal regulation. However, evidence shows that some sympathetic neural junctions release transmitters that interact with dilatory receptors on blood vessels [2]. It is not entirely clear what these transmitters or their associated receptors are; therefore, they are called simply *nonadrenergic–noncholinergic (NANC)*.

In contrast to α-adrenergic receptors, which are found throughout the circulatory system, vasodilatory innervation and receptors are located only in specific tissues. For example, β_2-adrenergic receptors exist within the skeletal muscle circulation, where (it is hypothesized) they play a role in mediating the increase in blood flow associated with exercise. At present, the extent and roles of the NANC neural innervation in humans are not known [2].

Hormonal Regulation

Moving clockwise in Figure 11-3, some of the hormones involved in circulatory control are listed. This list is by no means inclusive, but these particular hormones are thought to play major roles in determining, if not regulating, vascular resistance and tissue blood flow. Epinephrine is clearly the most versatile of these hormones; it can elicit either vasoconstriction or vasodilation, depending upon whether it binds with α- or β_2-adrenergic receptors, respectively.

Epinephrine is the major hormone released from the adrenal medulla in response to an increase in sympathetic neural activity to that tissue. Because alpha receptors are the dominant adrenergic receptors in the circulatory system, the net effect of epinephrine secretion in the resting individual is vasoconstriction and an increase in total peripheral resistance.

Antidiuretic hormone (ADH) is also known as vasopressin because of its ability to raise blood pressure by direct constrictor action on vascular smooth muscle. It is likely that normal plasma levels of ADH contribute to basal vascular tone, but the degree to which this may be important quantitatively is not known.

Angiotensin II has a direct constrictor effect on vascular smooth muscle, and, possibly more important, it potentiates the constrictor effects of sympathetic activity by inhibiting the reuptake of norepinephrine into the postganglionic sympathetic nerve terminals. Sympathetic activity to the kidneys releases renin, the enzyme that initiates the series of chemical events leading to angiotensin II; consequently, conditions characterized by a high sympathetic drive (e.g., exercise) are usually attended by an increase in the level of circulating angiotensin II.

The maintenance of basal vascular tone, and hence blood pressure, is dependent on a normal level of circulating cortisol. However, it is thought that cortisol does not act directly on blood vessels but rather acts by *supporting* the SNS as a permissive hormone. The lack of cortisol is one reason patients with adrenal insufficiency have a tendency to develop hypotension.

Myogenic Regulation

Blood pressure exerts a distorting force on the walls of blood vessels, and the resultant stretch of the vessels elicits a vasoconstrictor response. This property was first thought to be inherent in vascular smooth muscle; therefore, it is referred to as a "myogenic" response. Chapter 1 described how myogenic vasoconstriction contributes to hypertension in a positive feedback manner. However, in the normotensive state, the myogenic mechanism is one of the factors that maintains a steady-state level of basal tone in vascular smooth muscle.

Paracrine Regulation

Paracrines are humoral substances that are secreted by one type of cell and affect neighboring cells. Histamine, secreted from local cells, is a potent vasodilator and is one of the first paracrines known to affect vascular tone. However, it is thought that histamine may also be a neural transmitter released from dilatory neurons (e.g., the NANC neurons of the SNS).

The vascular endothelial cells are interposed between the circulating blood and vascular smooth muscle. Because of their strategic location, endothelial cells play an extremely important role in the regulation of blood flow by secreting a variety of constrictor and dilator paracrines. Among these are the prostaglandins, which are derived from arachidonic acid in the endothelium, as well as from platelets. These substances elicit either vasoconstriction or vasodilation, depending upon their exact chemical nature. For example, prostacyclin is a vasodilator, and thromboxane is a vasoconstrictor.

The more recently discovered endothelial cell factors may be the most important of the local paracrines in the regulation of blood flow. The best known of these are the endothelial-derived relaxation factors (EDRF). Nitric oxide (NO), a highly lipid-soluble vasodilator substance derived from the amino acid tyrosine, is considered the major EDRF. Conversely, endothelin, a potent vasoconstrictor, is considered the major endothelial-derived constrictor factor (EDCF).

Although paracrines elicit significant effects on vascular tone, the mechanisms responsible for their synthesis and release, as well as the way in which they fit into the overall scheme of circulatory regulation are not presently known.

Metabolic Regulation

Several by-products of tissue metabolism collectively elicit vasodilation. Since parenchymal cells produce these by-products in direct proportion to tissue metabolic activity, they serve to couple tissue blood flow to ongoing local metabolic demands.

These metabolic products adjust blood flow to steady-state levels commensurate with tissue activity.

Laboratory studies have shown oxygen to be a vasoconstrictor; however, it is not clear if oxygen itself has a direct constrictor effect or if it acts through a local paracrine. Furthermore, arterial oxygen tension remains stable in healthy individuals, even under extreme metabolic demands; therefore, it is not certain that oxygen plays a role as a physiologic regulator of tissue blood flow.

Summary

In any given situation, vessel diameter (i.e., vascular tone) is determined by a balance of constrictor and dilator influences. Some of these (e.g., sympathetic activity, circulating hormones) play a systemic role in maintaining homeostasis of arterial blood pressure so that cardiac output (CO) may be distributed according to the needs of the body. Other substances (e.g., paracrines, tissue metabolites) serve the local needs of specific tissues to maintain blood flow commensurate with tissue activity.

SYMPATHETIC INNERVATION AND NEURAL CONTROL

Pattern of Innervation

One of the salient structural features in relation to blood flow regulation is the pattern of sympathetic innervation. Figure 11-4 shows the general pattern of sympathetic innervation to the circulation within a tissue. The distributing arteries have the richest sympathetic innervation in terms of neurons traversing the adventitia. However, only when the small arteries and arterioles are reached do the neuron varicosities, from which transmitters are released, begin to appear in sizable numbers. Varicosities are sparse, or nonexistent, in the region of the terminal arterioles. From a functional point of view, this distribution pattern indicates that the small arteries and arterioles are the major sites of sympathetic activity and, as such, serve systemic needs; the terminal arterioles are more responsive to local paracrines and metabolites and are thus positioned to serve the needs of individual tissues.

In comparison to innervation on the arterial side, venous innervation is quite sparse. Furthermore, the effect of vasoconstrictor activity on venous vessels is to reduce vascular compliance rather than increase vascular resistance.

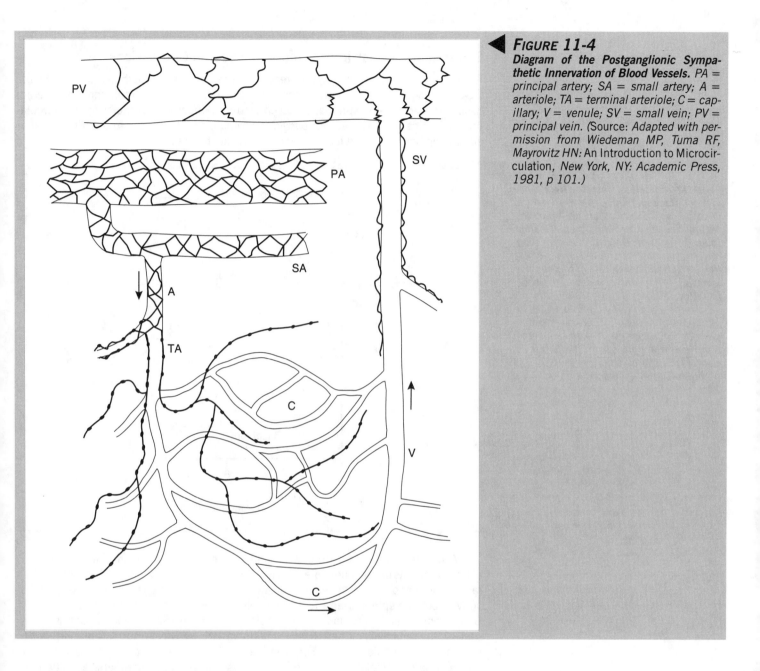

FIGURE 11-4
Diagram of the Postganglionic Sympathetic Innervation of Blood Vessels. PA = *principal artery; SA = small artery; A = arteriole; TA = terminal arteriole; C = capillary; V = venule; SV = small vein; PV = principal vein.* (Source: *Adapted with permission from Wiedeman MP, Tuma RF, Mayrovitz HN:* An Introduction to Microcirculation, *New York, NY: Academic Press, 1981, p 101.*)

Sympathetic Transmitters

It was once thought that a given neuron secretes only one transmitter; it is now known that this is the exception rather than the rule. Most neurons—postsynaptic sympathetic neurons included—secrete more than one transmitter at their terminals [3]. Postganglionic sympathetic adrenergic neurons secrete at least two transmitters: norepinephrine and the more recently discovered neuropeptide Y (NPY). Norepinephrine is a vasoconstrictor when it interacts with α-adrenergic receptors and a vasodilator when it interacts with beta receptors; the former interaction is much more common than the latter. In contrast, NPY is only a vasoconstrictor, and the nature of its receptor on vascular smooth muscle is not entirely known. With regard to the differential effects of norepinephrine and NPY, present evidence suggests that NPY is the more potent vasoconstrictor [4].

Evidence suggests that certain postganglionic sympathetic neurons, primarily those to the skin, secrete vasodilators. At present the transmitter substances are not known, but a long list of candidates has been proposed [2]. Where particular transmitters are located, what their functional significance is, and how their release is regulated are all questions that have yet to be answered.

Sympathetic Constrictor Effects in Specific Circulations

Individual circulations, in general, respond differently to sympathetic activity. Figure 11-5 is a logarithmic graph that compares the effects of the circulations in different tissues to sympathetic stimulation. Even with no sympathetic stimulation, the circulation maintains a certain level of *basal tone*, which is probably due to the interaction of circulating hormones and local autoregulatory mechanisms.

FIGURE 11-5 ▶

Logarithmic Scale of Vascular Resistance in the Cutaneous, Muscle, and Renal Circulations as a Function of the Action Potential Frequency of Sympathetic Neurons Innervating These Organs. *With no sympathetic stimulation, there is a baseline tone, which for the purpose of this comparison was set at unity. However, the baseline tone differs from one circulation to another as a result of variations in the interactions of circulating hormones and local autoregulatory mechanisms.* (Source: Reprinted with permission from Smith JJ, Kampine JP: Circulatory Physiology, Baltimore, MD: Williams & Wilkins, 1984, p 149.)

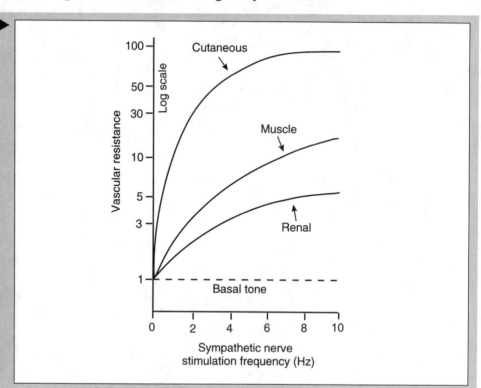

A sizable portion of day-to-day sympathetic activity occurs within the range of 2–6 action potentials per second, noted in Figure 11-5 as frequency in Hertz (Hz). Within this range, norepinephrine is the major transmitter released; at higher levels of sympathetic activity, both norepinephrine and NPY are released. However, even within the range of 2–6 Hz, considerable variation in the sensitivity of the particular circulations is represented. The sensitivity of these tissues to sympathetic activity is inversely proportional to their basal metabolic activity. For example, in Figure 11-5, cutaneous tissue has the lowest basal metabolic rate and the highest sensitivity to sympathetic activity. Conversely, the kidneys have a high basal metabolic rate and a relatively weak response to sympathetic stimulation. The muscle circulation resides somewhere between those of cutaneous and renal tissues.

LOCAL REGULATION

Autoregulation of Blood Flow

Autoregulation refers to the tendency for tissue blood flow to remain constant amid changes in local perfusion pressure [5]. However, this definition does not imply that blood flow is the only variable being regulated. Autoregulation maintains homeostasis of blood–tissue exchange, one of the focal concepts in the study of the cardiovascular system, by influencing tissue blood flow, capillary pressure, and capillary permeability.

Variations in local perfusion pressure trigger autoregulatory mechanisms. This section describes situations in which local perfusion pressure tends to vary independently of systemic arterial pressure. The most common example relates to the effects of posture.

Figure 11-6 illustrates that in the upright posture, tissues below the heart, the approximate reference level for systemic arterial pressure, undergo elevated arterial pressure; those above the heart, such as the head, the brain, and the forearms (when extended over the head), experience a decrease in arterial pressure. Autoregulatory adjustments tend to prevent these regions from becoming over- and underperfused, respectively. Although venous pressure (not shown in the figure) is also affected by gravity, it usually does not vary to the degree that arterial pressure does, because venous return mechanisms (discussed in Chapter 10) oppose gravitational effects on the venous side of the circulation.

Atherosclerotic vascular disease presents a chronic situation in which local arterial pressure can be affected. If a sclerotic lesion on a supply artery (e.g., one of the coronary arteries) becomes more than about 70% occluded, then downstream perfusion pressure begins to be compromised. However, autoregulatory vasodilation in the downstream arterioles and terminal arterioles tends to maintain blood flow and capillary pressure within a normal range. Conversely, autoregulatory adjustments to chronic hypertension prevent tissues from being overperfused. However, as pointed out in Chapter 1, these adjustments can generate a positive feedback cycle that contributes to the hypertensive state.

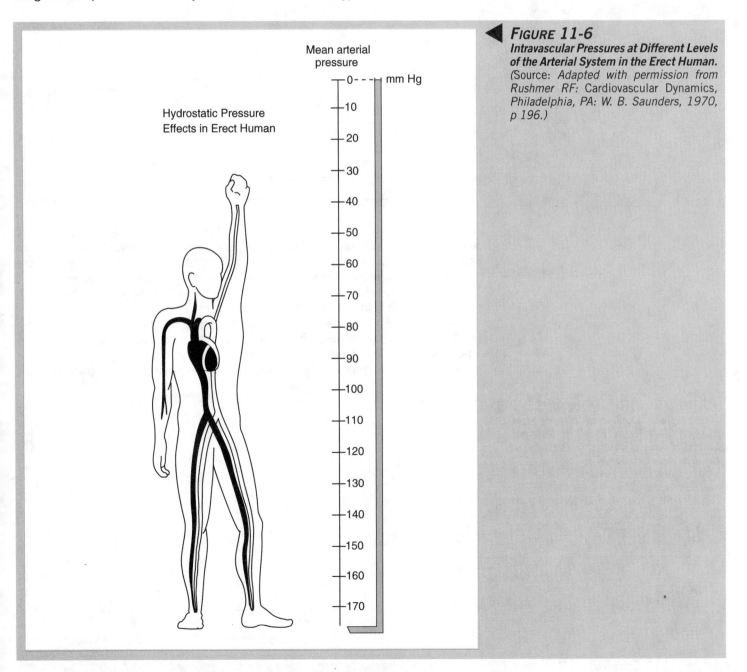

FIGURE 11-6
Intravascular Pressures at Different Levels of the Arterial System in the Erect Human.
(Source: *Adapted with permission from Rushmer RF:* Cardiovascular Dynamics, *Philadelphia, PA: W. B. Saunders, 1970, p 196.*)

Figure 11-7 shows the temporal changes in local perfusion (arterial) pressure and blood flow that are characteristic of autoregulation. When perfusion pressure increases (point A), blood flow initially increases in proportion. Within less than a minute following the pressure change, autoregulatory adjustments constrict local arterioles and return blood flow toward its control level. When perfusion pressure returns (point B), blood flow initially drops below control, because arterioles remain constricted; shortly thereafter, however, the arterioles relax, and blood flow returns to its control level. A reduction in arterial pressure (point C) causes temporal adjustments in flow that are the mirror image of those that occur when pressure increases.

FIGURE 11-7
Temporal Effects of Changes in Arterial Perfusion Pressure on Local Blood Flow. *The adjustments in blood flow following each pressure change are indicative of autoregulation.*

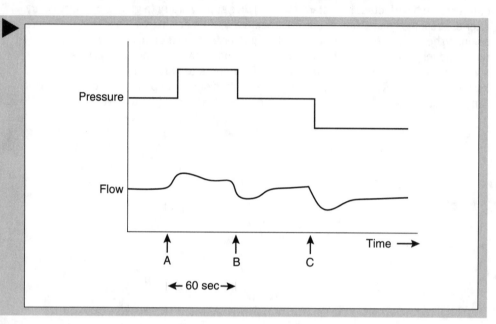

Figure 11-8 is a graph of initial (*dashed line*) and steady-state (*solid line*) values of blood flow to the kidneys as a function of local arterial pressure. These lines were obtained from initial and steady-state blood flow data similar to those shown in Figure 11-7. This figure also shows that the operative range of autoregulation is between 60 and 180 mm Hg perfusion pressure. Like all compensatory adjustments of the body, autoregulation is limited in its ability to maintain homeostasis.

Two fundamental mechanisms have been proposed for autoregulation of blood flow. From a historical perspective, the first of these is the myogenic mechanism by which arterioles respond to increases and decreases in transmural pressure (intravascular pressure–interstitial pressure) by vasoconstriction and vasodilation, respectively. This

FIGURE 11-8
Initial (solid line) and Steady-State (dashed line) Tissue Blood at Different Levels of Arterial Perfusion Pressure in the Renal Circulation. *The relatively flat area on the solid line between 60 and 180 mm Hg is indicative of autoregulation. (Source: Reprinted with permission from Smith JJ, Kampine JP:* Circulatory Physiology, *Baltimore, MD: Williams & Wilkins, 1984, p 155.)*

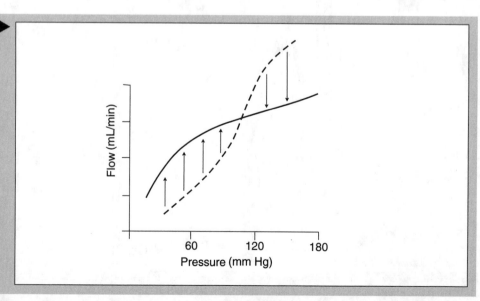

mechanism was first proposed in 1902 by W. M. Bayliss; consequently, it is also called the Bayliss response. Despite almost 95 years of investigation, the mechanism of the myogenic, or Bayliss, response is not entirely known. Johnson has proposed a tension-sensing element in vascular smooth muscle [5], and more recent investigations have pointed to the release of an endothelial factor [6, 7]. These mechanisms are not mutually exclusive; it is possible that both are operative.

The second fundamental mechanism proposed for autoregulation is the metabolic theory [3]. According to this hypothesis, if a decrease in blood flow occurs without a corresponding decrease in metabolic rate (e.g., by a decrease in perfusion pressure), then a net accumulation of metabolic by-products will occur. The accumulated metabolites then elicit vasodilation (i.e., a reduction in vascular tone) and a return of tissue blood flow toward control. Conversely, an increase in arterial pressure elicits an overperfusion of tissues, resulting in a washout of metabolic by-products. This shifts the balance of vascular tone toward constrictor influences and a return of blood flow toward control levels. Although the metabolic theory is reasonably straightforward, attempts to identify which specific metabolite (or metabolites) mediates autoregulation have thus far been unsuccessful. With our more recent understanding of vascular actions of local paracrines, it now seems possible that metabolic autoregulation may not be directly mediated by metabolites but rather by dilatory paracrines (e.g., EDRF) released by metabolites. Accordingly, the term "metabolite" in reference to blood flow regulation is generic in nature and includes metabolic by-products as well as local paracrines that may be released by metabolites.

The myogenic and metabolic hypotheses of autoregulation are not mutually exclusive; both mechanisms may play a role. The possible interactive nature of these roles is depicted in Figure 11-9. An increase in local arterial pressure increases tissue blood flow and simultaneously stretches the arterioles. An increase in tissue blood flow reduces the accumulation of local metabolites, which shifts the regulatory balance toward vasoconstrictor influences. Thus, arteriole diameter decreases, and tissue blood flow returns toward control levels. In the meantime, the increased stretch on the arterioles elicits myogenic vasoconstriction and a reduction in arteriole diameter, which lessens the degree of stretch on these vessels. In accordance with this scheme, the degree of arteriolar adjustment is the collective effect of metabolic and myogenic mechanisms. As a result of these adjustments, both tissue blood flow and local capillary pressure tend to be maintained.

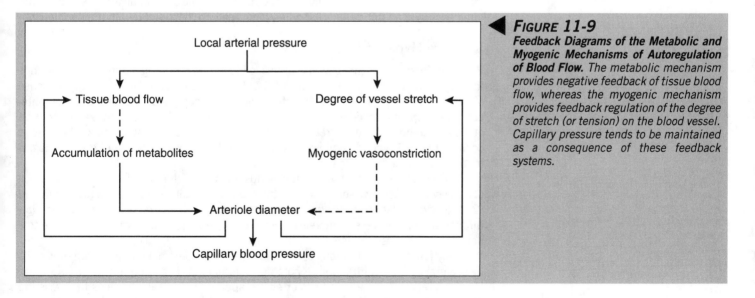

FIGURE 11-9
Feedback Diagrams of the Metabolic and Myogenic Mechanisms of Autoregulation of Blood Flow. *The metabolic mechanism provides negative feedback of tissue blood flow, whereas the myogenic mechanism provides feedback regulation of the degree of stretch (or tension) on the blood vessel. Capillary pressure tends to be maintained as a consequence of these feedback systems.*

Figure 11-9 shows that in autoregulation tissue blood flow is maintained as part of a feedback loop, whereas the maintenance of capillary pressure occurs as a consequence of the feedback system. In the more global scheme of homeostasis, this figure illustrates how feedback regulatory systems can affect variables that are coupled to, but outside, the feedback loop.

Active hyperemia refers to the vasodilation and increase in local blood flow associated with an increase in tissue function.

Flow-Dependent Vasodilation

As discussed in Chapter 6, blood flows through vessels in laminar fashion. As shown in Figure 11-10, the laminar flow sets up a shear stress that tends to distort the endothelial cells. The shear stress forces are hypothesized to release dilatory factors (e.g., EDRF), which then elicit relaxation of the adjacent vascular smooth muscle [8]. This phenomenon, now known as flow-dependent vasodilation, is thought to occur in the small arteries and may be a mechanism contributing to *active hyperemia*.

FIGURE 11-10 ▶
The Hypothesized Mechanism of Flow-Dependent Vasodilation. *The arrows represent the velocities of individual lamina within the blood as it flows through a blood vessel. The resultant shear stress distorts the endothelial cell, resulting in the secretion of an endothelial relaxation factor (e.g., nitric oxide). The endothelial-derived relaxation factor (EDRF) then enters the smooth muscle cell, eliciting vasodilation. As blood flow increases, flow velocity increases, resulting in a greater shear stress, an increase in the secretion of EDRF, and, hence, an increase in flow-dependent vasodilation.* (Source: Adapted with permission from Davies PF: How do vascular endothelial cells respond to flow? News Physiol Sci *4:24, 1989.*)

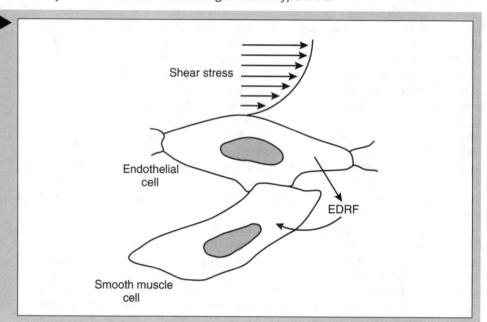

Flow-dependent vasodilation in active hyperemia follows a sequence of events: an increase in tissue activity elicits vasodilation of the terminal arterioles. The resultant increase in blood flow increases flow velocity in the associated arterioles and small arteries. The resultant increase in shear stress on the endothelial cells of the small arteries elicits the release of dilator factors, which then mediate vasodilation and a reduction of resistance to the flow of blood. In this manner, the small arteries that are not directly subjected to tissue metabolites participate in local regulation of blood flow.

Reactive Hyperemia

Reactive hyperemia is the response of tissue blood flow following a brief period (seconds to minutes) of local ischemia. Figure 11-11 shows a typical reactive hyperemic response in the human forearm. At the 2-minute mark, flow is occluded by inflating a pneumatic cuff on the upper arm for 30 seconds. When occlusion is released, there is a brief period of flow overshoot, termed "reactive hyperemia." At the 8-minute mark, the flow is occluded for 60 seconds, followed by a reactive hyperemic response of greater magnitude and duration, as indicated by the *solid line.*

It is hypothesized that during the occlusion period arteriole dilation is mediated by (1) a myogenic response secondary to a decrease in arterial pressure distal to the cuff and (2) the accumulation of tissue metabolites. Upon release of occlusion, blood flow through the dilated vessels increases markedly. The increased flow may contribute to a flow-dependent vasodilation.

Very few natural situations can induce reactive hyperemia (compression of vessels by skeletal muscle contraction, a notable exception, is discussed in the next section). However, reactive hyperemia tests often are applied in clinical situations to assess the ability of the peripheral circulation to respond to vasodilator stimuli. The *dashed line* following the 1-minute occlusion in Figure 11-11 represents the hyperemic response that would occur in a patient with arterial obstructive disease (e.g., sclerosis) in the limb being tested. The peak response is markedly reduced, and the whole response pattern is delayed. This response is typical of a tissue in which the arterioles either have lost most of

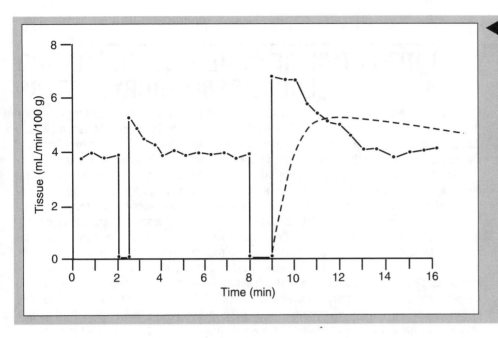

FIGURE 11-11
Reactive Hyperemia in the Human Forearm. Solid lines *denote the healthy subject;* dashed line *represents a reactive hyperemic response from an individual with atherosclerotic disease of the limb being tested.* (Source: *Adapted with permission from Smith JJ, Kampine JP: Circulatory Physiology, Baltimore, MD: Williams & Wilkins, 1984, p 154.)*

their ability to vasodilate or are already vasodilated as a compensatory mechanism in response to a chronic reduction in perfusion pressure.

Vasomotion

Steady-state blood flow does not necessarily mean that blood flow remains invariant. Quite often, flow oscillates as a result of alternate dominance of constrictor and dilator influences on vascular smooth muscle. Such oscillations are called *vasomotion*, which is considered a local phenomenon because it occurs in tissues from which the neural innervation has been removed. An example of vasomotion is given in Figure 11-12, which presents arterial perfusion pressure and blood flow in a capillary within a denervated intestinal circulation of a laboratory animal. The oscillatory behavior of flow between 0 and 40 seconds represents vasomotion. As blood pressure is reduced to about 80 mm Hg, mean blood flow remains approximately the same as a result of autoregulatory adjustments; however, vasomotion disappears and does not reappear until after the reactive hyperemia response following the restoration of blood pressure at 210 seconds. The vasomotion appears when the blood pressure is relatively high; consequently, it is hypothesized that this phenomenon is due to alternate dominance of myogenic vasoconstriction and metabolic vasodilation.

The reader should be able to construct feedback diagrams to show how myogenic vasoconstriction and metabolic vasodilation could interact to produce vasomotion.

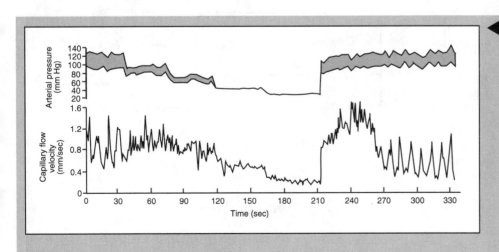

FIGURE 11-12
Blood Flow in a Capillary within the Intestinal Circulation of a Laboratory Animal at Different Levels of Arterial Perfusion Pressure. *The oscillatory behavior of flow from 0–40 seconds and after 270 seconds is indicative of vasomotion. Vasomotion is due to intermittent dominance of constrictor and dilator influences. During the periods of low perfusion pressure and the period of reactive hyperemia following the restoration of pressure (at 210 seconds), vasodilatory influences dominate and vasomotion does not occur.* (Source: *Adapted with permission from Johnson PC: Peripheral Circulation, New York, NY: John Wiley, 1978, p 120.)*

INTERACTION OF SYSTEMIC (NEURAL) AND LOCAL REGULATORY FACTORS

Physical exercise is a good example of the interaction of the various factors that regulate the circulatory system because this activity affects blood flow in a variety of tissues. Figure 11-13 gives the general scheme of blood flow regulation associated with exercise, and Figure 11-14 presents the distribution of CO at increasing levels of exercise intensity.

As indicated in Figure 11-13, the initial event in the exercise sequence is a central nervous system (CNS) *command* that increases muscle activity through somatomotor neurons. The muscle contractions tend to compress blood vessels, thereby reducing blood flow. However, the transmural pressure across the arterioles (blood pressure–interstitial pressure) simultaneously decreases as a result of an increase in the interstitial pressure caused by the contracting muscle. The reduction in transmural pressure elicits a myogenic-induced vasodilation. Figure 11-15 shows the blood flow response of the human calf muscle to a 2-minute static (sustained) muscle contraction at 15% of the subject's maximum voluntary contractile force (MVC). There is an approximate doubling of the blood flow during contraction. According to Sparks [4], about one-third of this response is due to the aforementioned myogenic mechanism; it is likely that the remainder is primarily due to metabolic-induced vasodilation. When the sustained contraction is released at the end of 2 minutes, there is a dramatic rise in blood flow similar to that seen in reactive hyperemia (Figure 11-11). This rise indicates that during the sustained contraction, the muscle is underperfused relative to metabolic needs, and metabolites accumulate, much the same as when flow to a limb is occluded in a reactive hyperemia test.

The information provided in Figure 11-15 makes it possible to predict that during rhythmic exercise the majority of the blood flow will occur during the relaxation phase of the contraction cycle, much the same as coronary blood flow is most prominent during

FIGURE 11-13 ▶

General Scheme of Blood Flow Regulation Associated with Physical Exercise. The upper portion of the figure summarizes the factors responsible for blood flow distribution during exercise. A complete explanation is in the text. The lower portion of the figure illustrates the sequence of events by which the blood flow response of a tissue is augmented by the flow-dependent vasodilation of small arteries. The asterisk (*) indicates identical vasodilatory mechanisms in the upper and lower portions of the figure. Dashed lines indicate inverse relationships, and solid lines indicate direct relationships. + = to increase; − = to decrease. CNS = central nervous system; SNS = sympathetic nervous system.

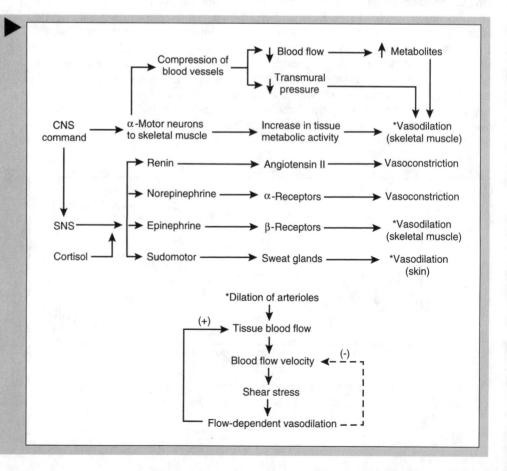

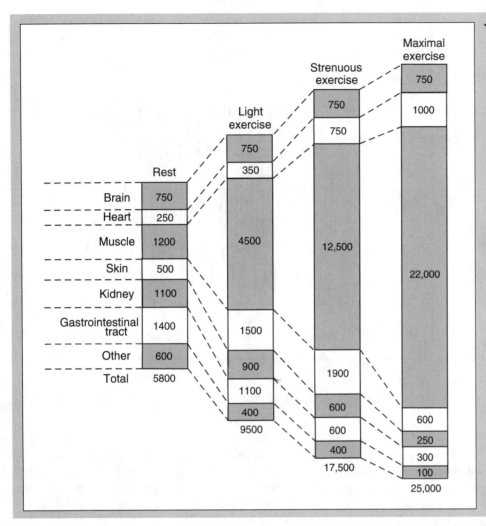

FIGURE 11-14
Distribution of Cardiac Output during Exercise. (Source: Adapted with permission from Chapman CB, Mitchell JH: The physiology of exercise. Sci Am 212:91, 1965.)

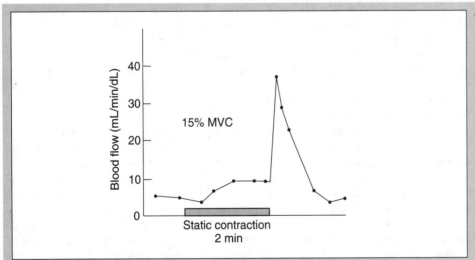

FIGURE 11-15
Blood Flow Responses of the Human Calf Muscle during and after a Static (Isometric) Contraction at 15% of the Subject's Maximal Voluntary Contractile Force (MVC). (Source: Adapted with permission from Richardson D: Blood flow response of human calf muscles to static contractions at various percentages of MVC. J Appl Physiol 51:931, 1981.)

diastole. Figure 11-16 shows this to be the case. During the contraction phases of the rhythmic cycle, blood flow is somewhat higher compared to controls, as with a sustained contraction. However, the flow during contraction is nowhere near the peak flows that occur during relaxation. An explanation for this phenomenon is that during the high metabolic state of exercise, muscle contraction tends to compress arterioles, causing a net accumulation of metabolites and possibly some myogenic relaxation of the blood vessels such that during muscle relaxation the resultant reactive hyperemia supplies most of the blood flow.

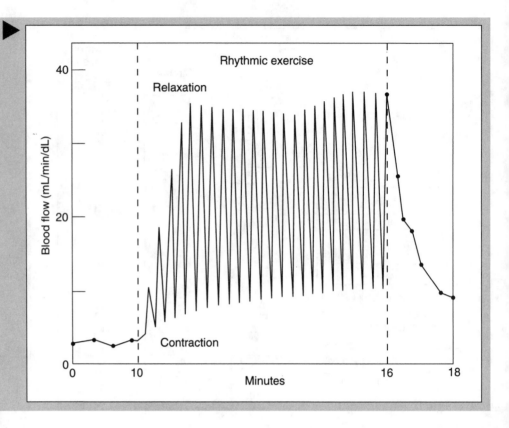

FIGURE 11-16

Pattern of Human Calf Muscle Blood Flow during Rhythmic Contractions of the Legs. *During the contraction phase, blood flow is low as a result of compression of the blood vessels in the legs. The majority of the blood flow is obtained during the relaxation phase when the compression is removed. (Source: Reprinted with permission from Austrand PO, Rodahl K: Textbook of Work Physiology, New York, NY: McGraw-Hill, 1977, p 179.)*

> ***Flow-dependent vasodilation*** *appears to elicit a positive feedback effect on tissue blood flow. However, as Chapter 6 explains, vasodilation tends to reduce flow velocity because blood flow through a vessel is equal to the product of cross-sectional area, which is determined by diameter times the velocity of blood flow. Because a reduction in flow velocity tends to reduce shear stress, the positive feedback nature of flow-dependent vasodilation is limited.*

This fundamental balance of compression and dilation is modified by other regulatory influences. Paralleling the increase in somatic motor activity is a proportionate increase in sympathetic activity to the entire cardiovascular system. Furthermore, because exercise is a physiologic stress, sympathetic effects are bolstered by an increase in circulating cortisol. The work of Honig suggests that the initial sympathetic activity at the onset of exercise may involve vasodilatory influences to skeletal muscle [10]. Although this could explain the rapid increase in muscle blood flow that occurs at the onset of exercise, there is, as yet, no solid evidence of NANC receptors in human skeletal muscle [2].

Once skeletal muscle contractions begin, the associated increase in metabolic activity leads to local dilation of skeletal muscle arterioles. As illustrated in the *bottom* portion of Figure 11-13, the associated increase in blood flow and shear stress elicits flow-dependent vasodilation of the small arteries, which contributes in a limited positive feedback manner to tissue blood flow.

In the case of autoregulation (see Figure 11-9), metabolic activity and tissue blood flow interact in a negative feedback manner. During exercise, this negative feedback relationship achieves a higher steady-state level of blood flow in keeping with the increased metabolic needs of the tissue. As pointed out in the earlier discussion of autoregulation, metabolic-linked vasodilation may involve the local release of paracrines as well as the direct action of metabolites on vascular smooth muscle.

Metabolic-elicited vasodilation is also thought to be the major mechanism by which coronary blood flow to the heart is increased during exercise. However, the active hyperemia in both skeletal and cardiac muscle during exercise is inversely dependent upon the degree of preexisting vasodilation; that is, if the arterioles are already vasodilated, then metabolic activity may add very little to the established blood flow. This scenario is illustrated in Figure 11-17, which depicts a major supply artery (a coronary artery) and the downstream arterioles. In the normal control situation, metabolic activity causes normal dilation of the arterioles (20–40 μ) and an increase in blood flow. However, as the artery becomes progressively narrowed by a sclerotic plaque (a 70% occlusion, in this example), autoregulatory adjustments in the downstream arterioles compensate to maintain normal resting tissue blood flow. These adjustments impair the ability of the arterioles to vasodilate further in response to an increase in metabolic demands during exercise. In this example, the dilatory reserve of the arterioles is decreased by one-half; that is, the arteriole can

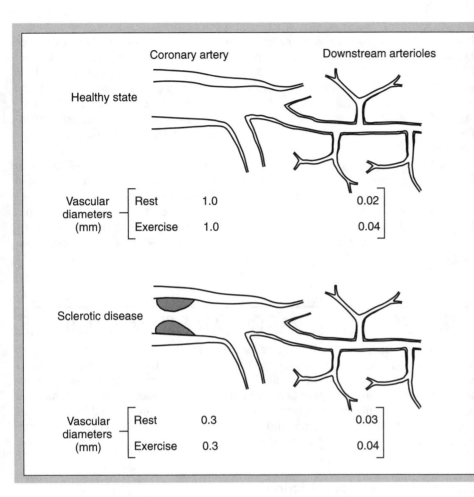

Coronary artery

Downstream arterioles

Healthy state

| Vascular diameters (mm) | Rest | 1.0 | 0.02 |
| | Exercise | 1.0 | 0.04 |

Sclerotic disease

| Vascular diameters (mm) | Rest | 0.3 | 0.03 |
| | Exercise | 0.3 | 0.04 |

FIGURE 11-17
Process by Which Autoregulatory Adjustments of Arterioles Downstream from a 70% Sclerotic Lesion of a Coronary Artery Compromise the Ability of the Arterioles to Dilate in Response to an Exercise Demand. In the normal state, shown in the upper half, exercise elicits a doubling of arteriole diameter. A narrowing of the artery by a sclerotic lesion, shown in the lower half, elicits autoregulatory adjustments of the arteriole, which then compromise the ability of the arteriole to increase diameter during a period of exercise.

dilate only by 10 μ (from 30 to 40) instead of 20 μ. As a result of a reduced dilatory ability, atherosclerotic patients typically have reduced exercise tolerance.

The sympathetic activity attending exercise elicits an α-adrenergic–mediated vasoconstrictor activity throughout the circulatory system. Theoretically, this effect is more potent during exercise because of the higher levels of cortisol (mentioned previously), and as a result of a renin-mediated increase in circulating angiotensin II. However, the effects of circulating hormones in modifying sympathetic activity during exercise have not been quantified.

In tissues where the balance of constrictor effects outweigh dilatory influences, a net decrease in blood flow occurs. As shown in Figure 11-14, this net constrictor effect occurs in the renal and gastrointestinal (GI) circulations at all levels of exercise. However, the degree of vasoconstriction is tempered by autoregulation and active hyperemia. In some cases, this sets up a "conflict-of-interest" scenario. For example, the vasoconstrictor influences of an increase in sympathetic activity juxtaposed to vasodilation related to local metabolic needs could be the source of GI discomfort when a person attempts to exercise after eating a large meal.

Sympathetic neurons innervate blood vessels within skeletal muscle; consequently, it is correct to assume that during exercise, muscle blood flow is determined by a balance between the constrictor effects of α-adrenergic activity and dilatory influences. The dilatory influences come from at least two sources: the metabolic activity mentioned previously and circulating epinephrine acting on β_2-adrenergic receptors located on skeletal muscle arterioles. The blood flow distribution chart, shown in Figure 11-14, indicates that even at light levels of exercise there is a net vasodilatory influence on skeletal muscle. This influence reflects the dominance of active skeletal muscle. In skeletal muscle that does not participate in the exercise, blood flow either decreases or changes very little from its rest state.

The cutaneous circulation is an example of the balance of constrictor and dilator influences. At levels of submaximal exercise, dilator influences derived from sweat gland activity (the sudomotor system), and possibly from NANC neurons, dominate, and skin

Evidence suggests that the balance between constrictor and dilator influences may involve more than a simple opposition of forces. It is thought that local metabolites and paracrines may decrease the effectiveness of α-adrenergic receptors on vascular smooth muscle [11].

*The **sudomotor system** is the branch of the SNS that innervates sweat glands. The postsynaptic transmitter is acetylcholine (ACh), rather than norepinephrine. ACh stimulates the production of sweat. By-products from the production of sweat elicit a local dilatory effect on cutaneous arterioles.*

blood flow rises in proportion to the exercise level. However, at a maximal exercise level, the larger constrictor influences of sympathetic activity, which are perhaps a result of NPY, almost completely balance out dilator influences, and skin blood flow differs very little from that of pre-exercise levels. The thermoregulatory role of skin blood flow is compromised under these conditions; however, because the duration of maximal exercise is, at best, only about a minute (e.g., an all-out sprint), constrictor influences at maximal exercise do not adversely affect the overall regulation of body temperature.

Finally, blood flow to the brain remains essentially unchanged at all levels of exercise. It was once thought that blood flow to brain tissue in general remained invariant through autoregulatory mechanisms [12]. However, more recent techniques for detecting the distribution of flow among specific areas of the brain indicate that while total CNS blood flow may remain invariant, blood flow is redistributed continually such that the most active areas in the brain receive higher flow compared to less active areas [13].

SIGNAL TRANSDUCTION IN VASCULAR SMOOTH MUSCLE

In the case of vascular smooth muscle, signal transduction refers to the series of biochemical and physiologic events initiated by a regulatory molecule, such as a neurotransmitter or a hormone, and culminating in either vasoconstriction or vasodilation. Structural features that may play a role in signal transduction are small, sac-like inpocketings on the plasma membrane called *caveoli*. These are thought to exist in all cells; however, their function is not entirely known. In some cells, particularly smooth muscle, caveoli may contain the plasma membrane receptors that bind signal molecules.

Mechanisms of Vasoconstriction

Fundamentally, any factor that causes an increase in intracellular calcium (Ca^{2+}) within vascular smooth muscle also causes vasoconstriction. Chapter 4 provides information on the coupling between an increase in intracellular Ca^{2+} and muscle contraction in smooth muscle.

Figure 11-18 summarizes the mechanisms by which intracellular Ca^{2+} is increased in smooth muscle. On the *top left* of the plasma membrane are two types of channels by which Ca^{2+} gains entry into smooth muscle from the extracellular environment, a voltage-gated and a ligand-gated channel. The former can be opened by an action potential (e.g., propagated from an adjacent coupled cell) or by membrane depolarization caused by Ca^{2+} entering from a ligand-gated channel. The Ca^{2+} entering vascular smooth muscle via plasma membrane channels can either (1) directly participate in the contractile process by binding to calmodulin or (2) serve as *trigger Ca^{2+}* by opening Ca^{2+} channels (probably voltage-gated) on the sarcoplasmic reticulum, thus mediating a further increase in intracellular Ca^{2+}.

To the *right* of the ligand-gated channel shown in Figure 11-18 is a different type of plasma membrane receptor that, when interacting with a ligand, activates a membrane-bound G protein. The activated G protein in turn activates phospholipase C, another membrane-bound protein. The active portion of phospholipase C is an enzyme that converts intracellular phosphatidylinositol bisphosphate (PIP_2) to inositol triphosphate (IP_3) plus diacylglycerol (DAG). IP_3 then attaches to the ligand-gated Ca^{2+} channel on the sarcoplasmic reticulum, thereby eliciting an increase in cytosolic Ca^{2+}. By this pathway, contraction can occur without a change in membrane potential; consequently, this mechanism is known as *pharmacomechanical coupling*.

With regard to specific ligand–receptor interactions, it is thought that norepinephrine and epinephrine may open ligand-gated Ca^{2+} channels as well as generate IP_3. This suggests that the pharmacomechanical and ligand-gated Ca^{2+} channel receptors are α-adrenergic receptors or components of an alpha receptor. However, a wide variety of nonadrenergic vasoconstrictors also elicit their direct vasoconstrictor action by

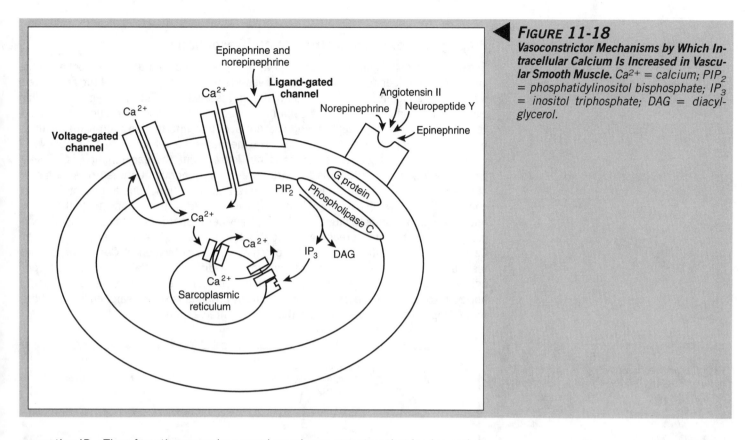

◀ FIGURE 11-18
Vasoconstrictor Mechanisms by Which Intracellular Calcium Is Increased in Vascular Smooth Muscle. Ca^{2+} = calcium; PIP_2 = phosphatidylinositol bisphosphate; IP_3 = inositol triphosphate; DAG = diacylglycerol.

generating IP_3. Therefore, there may be several membrane receptors that lead to activation of phospholipase C, the α-adrenergic receptor among them.

Mechanisms of Vasodilation

Any mechanism that reduces the Ca^{2+} level within vascular smooth muscle cells also causes vasodilation. However, intracellular Ca^{2+} is reduced in smooth muscle primarily by activation of a cyclic guanosine monophosphate (cGMP)–dependent protein kinase. This particular protein kinase then triggers a sequence of events, leading to an increase in the activity of Ca^{2+} pumps on the plasma membrane of the cell and on the membrane of the sarcoplasmic reticulum within the cell. This activity, in turn, elicits a net transport of Ca^{2+} to the extracellular environment and a resequestering of Ca^{2+} within the sarcoplasmic reticulum.

Cyclic adenosine monophosphate (cAMP), the intracellular messenger of β-adrenergic receptors, elicits vasodilation. Lincoln and his colleagues [14] have shown that the cAMP elicits its vasodilatory effect by activating cGMP-dependent protein kinase. Figure 11-19 presents the general scheme of this model. β-Adrenergic and nonadrenergic dilatory receptors elicit, respectively, through G proteins, the activation of membrane-bound adenosine and guanosine cyclase enzymes. These enzymes, in turn, generate cAMP and cGMP, both of which activate the cGMP-dependent protein kinase, which then triggers a series of steps leading to activation of Ca^{2+} pumps. In addition, vascular smooth muscle contains a soluble guanosine cyclase within the interior of the cell. This enzyme may be activated by lipid-soluble vasodilators such as NO. The ability to bypass a membrane receptor may be why NO is such a powerful vasodilator.

Again, some vasodilators, such as catecholamines, operate by attaching to plasma membrane receptors on vascular smooth muscle, while others, such as ACh, exert their dilatory effects by attaching to endothelial receptors, which in turn elicit the secretion of NO. An understanding of the different functions of specific vasodilators will aid physicians in combating cardiovascular diseases such as hypertension.

The nitrogen-containing compounds used to elicit rapid vasodilation in patients with heart disease are lipid-soluble and function by activating soluble guanosine cyclase.

Propagation of Vasoconstriction and Vasodilation

Segal and his colleagues [15] have shown that the application of both vasoconstrictor and vasodilator ligands directly on a blood vessel results in propagation of the associated response to adjacent upstream and downstream vessels. This observation fits with earlier evidence that only certain "key" cells in a smooth muscle complex, such as a blood vessel, contain ligand receptors and that intracellular information is in some manner passed to adjacent "coupled" cells [16]. The mechanism by which propagation between vascular smooth muscle cells occurs is not known, but the gap junction is a likely candidate. Figure 11-20 shows the structure of gap junctions between plasma membranes of adjacent smooth muscle cells. Note that these junctions form protein-lined channels that allow the passage of ions. With this in mind, one could speculate that Ca^{2+} released from one smooth muscle cell (e.g., a key cell) can diffuse into adjacent cells via gap junctions, thereby spreading the contractile influence. The reverse could occur if Ca^{2+} were removed from the cytosol of a key cell by activation of Ca^{2+} pumps. The resultant reduction in cytosolic Ca^{2+} would elicit diffusion of Ca^{2+} into the cell from adjacent cells, and hence a spread of vasodilation. Admittedly, these are speculations; however, speculation of possible mechanisms by physicians and researchers is one of the initial steps in the discovery of new therapeutic interventions.

FIGURE 11-19 ▶

Vasodilator Mechanisms by Which Intracellular Calcium Is Decreased in Vascular Smooth Muscle. ATP = adenosine triphosphate; Ca^{2+} = calcium; cAMP = cyclic adenosine monophosphate; cGMP = cyclic guanosine monophosphate; GTP = guanosine triphosphate; NO = nitric oxide.

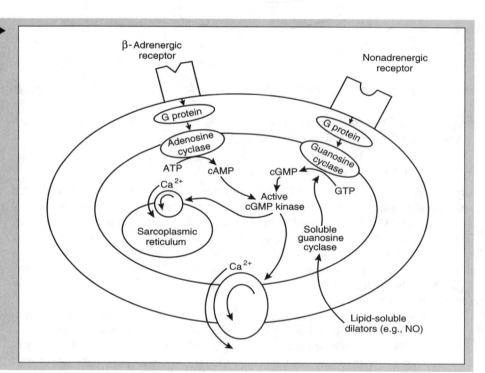

RESOLUTION OF CLINICAL CASE

As mentioned in Chapter 3, the patient described at the beginning of the chapter has peripheral vascular disease. The particular disease in this case is known as *claudication*, a term derived from Latin, meaning "to limp." Claudication is a severe sclerotic disease within the major arteries of the legs. In this patient, the lesions were primarily in the arteries of the left leg, as indicated by his symptomatology and by the total lack of pulsations in the left popliteal, dorsal pedis, and posterior tibialis arteries. The reduced blood flow and drop in perfusion pressure downstream from the lesions elicit compensatory vasodilation (autoregulation) of the downstream arterioles. The compensatory vasodilation reduces vasodilatory reserve such that blood flow cannot be adequately adjusted

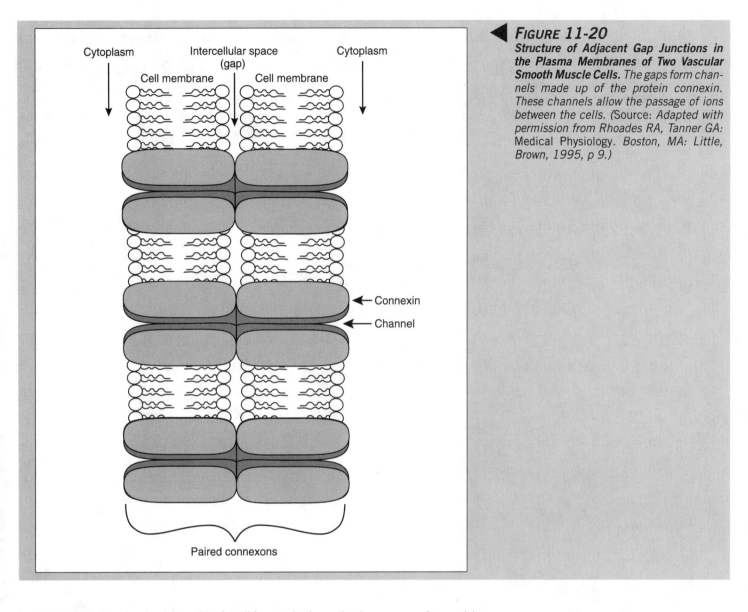

FIGURE 11-20
Structure of Adjacent Gap Junctions in the Plasma Membranes of Two Vascular Smooth Muscle Cells. *The gaps form channels made up of the protein connexin. These channels allow the passage of ions between the cells. (Source: Adapted with permission from Rhoades RA, Tanner GA:* Medical Physiology. *Boston, MA: Little, Brown, 1995, p 9.)*

to meet even the simple demands of walking and, thus, the leg cramps (caused by ischemia) when the patient walks even a short distance.

With a severe arterial lesion and compensatory downstream arteriole dilation, this patient's leg can receive adequate perfusion only when it is in the dependent position (below the heart) where gravity can move the blood. At night, when the patient is lying down, the leg becomes underperfused, sometimes causing ischemic pain that wakes the patient. Standing up and moving the leg (e.g., walking to the bathroom) establishes some perfusion, and the ischemic pain subsides.

The dependent rubor and ankle edema suggest that the disease has progressed to the extent that it has affected the arterioles. Normally, when a person places a foot below the heart (the dependent position), the increased intravascular pressure in the arterioles (see Figure 11-6) causes myogenic vasoconstriction. If this constriction does not occur, then the subepidermal vessels of the skin become overperfused, rendering the skin a reddish color (dependent rubor). Furthermore, without myogenic vasoconstriction in the arterioles of the legs, capillary pressure increases and the tissues become edematous. Thus, this patient's dependent rubor and ankle edema suggest that his arterioles are incapable of vasoconstriction. They are also incapable of vasodilation, which may be a result of either the disease or the possibility that the arterioles are maximally dilated as an autoregulatory compensation.

Ischemic tissues tend to heal quite slowly, hence the patient's foot ulcer. Skin ulcers are also prevalent in diabetics; consequently, the patient's history of diabetes is undoubt-

From the information in Chapter 6, the reader should be able to describe how inhibition of RBC aggregation results in a decrease in whole blood viscosity.

edly a factor in this case. However, since claudication is prominent among smokers, the most likely causal agent is the patient's 50-year history of tobacco smoking.

There are two major arms of therapy for patients with claudication. The most conservative arm is the administration of drugs that inhibit red blood cell (RBC) aggregation. This improves perfusion by reducing blood viscosity. Patients who do not respond to drug therapy may then undergo surgery (the second therapeutic arm) in which the surgeon places a vascular graft around the localized obstructions.

REVIEW QUESTIONS

Directions: For each of the following questions, choose the **one best** answer.

1. A variety of medications used in the treatment of hypertension elicit a reduction in vascular smooth muscle tone. These medications relieve hypertension by reducing

    (A) cardiac output (CO)

    (B) blood viscosity

    (C) geometric hindrance

    (D) peripheral vascular resistance

    (E) intracellular levels of cyclic guanosine monophosphate (cGMP)

2. A depressed reactive hyperemia response is indicative of

    (A) atherosclerotic vascular disease

    (B) hypertension

    (C) congestive heart failure

    (D) a low level of tissue metabolic activity

3. Consider the curve below, which depicts the relationship between sympathetic nerve activity and vascular resistance for skeletal muscle. Assuming that the curve shown is for resting skeletal muscle, the curve shifts in which direction during exercise?

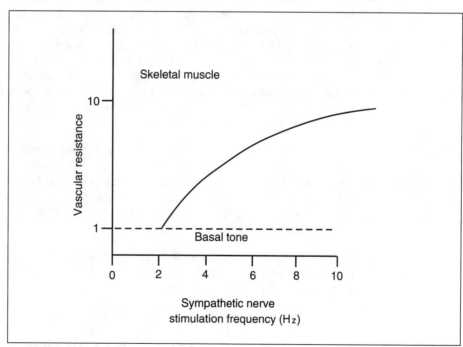

    (A) Up and to the left

    (B) Up and to the right

    (C) Down and to the left

    (D) Down and to the right

4. Which of the following treatments could be used to reduce vascular smooth muscle tone?

    (A) Medications that inhibit nitric oxide (NO) synthase, the enzyme that converts tyrosine to NO

    (B) Medications that promote endothelin synthesis

    (C) Medications that inhibit β-adrenergic receptors

    (D) Medications that inhibit renin synthesis

ANSWERS AND EXPLANATIONS

1. The answer is D. A variety of medications used in the treatment of hypertension elicit a reduction in vascular smooth muscle tone. These medications relieve hypertension by reducing peripheral vascular resistance. A reduction in vascular smooth muscle tone elicits vasodilation, which reduces vascular resistance. If the reduction in vascular smooth muscle tone is limited to the venous side, then CO might be reduced if cardiac filling pressure is reduced, but this would occur only under limited circumstances. Vasodilation might reduce blood viscosity if tissue blood flow is increased, but this would be unlikely to lower resistance sufficient to affect blood pressure. Geometric hindrance often increases in hypertension, but this is not altered by vasodilatory therapy. Reducing intracellular levels of GMP causes vasoconstriction, not vasodilation.

2. The answer is A. A depressed reactive hyperemia response is indicative of atherosclerotic vascular disease. Atherosclerotic lesions reduce local blood flow. This, in turn, elicits downstream vasodilation of arterioles by metabolic autoregulation. Because arterioles are in a state of vasodilation, the reactive hyperemia curve would be depressed. In hypertension, the reactive hyperemia response would be either unchanged or increased if arterioles have a higher than normal constrictor tone. A reactive hyperemia response would be unaffected by congestive heart failure; a low level of tissue metabolic activity would be expected to increase a reactive hyperemia response because the local circulation would be in a state of higher initial vasoconstriction.

3. The answer is D. The curve shown in the question represents resting skeletal muscle. During exercise, the curve would shift down and to the right because the vasodilator influences of exercise would reduce the constrictor effects of sympathetic activity, which would shift the curve down, and reduce the level of basal vascular tone, which would shift the curve to the right (i.e., it would take some sympathetic activity simply to bring vascular tone up to the resting basal level).

4. The answer is D. Inhibition of renin would reduce the production of angiotensin. Angiotensin is a vasoconstrictor. Removal of this vasoconstrictor will result in net vasodilation. All of the other choices listed in the question will promote vasoconstriction.

REFERENCES

1. Wiedeman MP: Architecture. In *Handbook of Physiology. Section 2: The Cardiovascular System IV. Microcirculation Part 1*. Bethesda, MD: American Physiological Society, 1984, pp 11–40.
2. Rowell LB: *Human Circulation: Regulation during Physical Stress*. New York, NY: Oxford University Press, 1986, pp 107–108.
3. Milhorn DE, Hokfelt T: Chemical messengers and their coexistence in individual neurons. *News Physiol Sci* 3:1–5, 1988.

4. Lundberg JM, Tatemoto K: Pancreatic polypeptide family (ATP, BPP, NPY and PYY) in relation to sympathetic vasoconstriction resistant to alpha-adrenoceptor blockade. *Acta Physiol Scand* 116:393–402, 1982.

5. Johnson PC: Principles of peripheral circulatory control. In *Peripheral Circulation*. Edited by Johnson PC. New York, NY: John Wiley, 1978, pp 111–139.

6. Harder DR: Pressure induced myogenic activation of cat cerebral arteries is dependent on intact endothelium. *Circ Res* 60:102–107, 1987.

7. Katusic ZS, Shepherd JT, Vanhoutte PM: Endothelium dependent contraction to stretch in canine basilar arteries. *Am J Physiol* 255:H783–H788, 1987.

8. Davies PF: How do vascular endothelial cells respond to flow? *News Physiol Sci* 4:22–25, 1989.

9. Sparks HV: Skin and muscle. In *Peripheral Circulation*. Edited by Johnson PC. New York, NY: John Wiley, 1978, pp 193–230.

10. Honig CR: *Modern Cardiovascular Physiology*. Boston, MA: Little, Brown, 1981, pp 251–262.

11. Burcher E, Garlick D: Effects of exercise metabolites on adrenergic vasoconstriction in the gracilis muscle of the dog. *J Pharm Exp Ther* 192:149, 1975.

12. Lassen NA: Brain. In *Peripheral Circulation*. Edited by Johnson PC. New York, NY: John Wiley, 1978, pp 337–358.

13. Pantano P, Baron JC, Lebrun-Grandie P, et al: Regional cerebral blood flow and oxygen consumption in human aging. *Stroke* 15:635–641, 1984.

14. Lincoln TM, Cornwell TL, Taylor A: cGMP-dependent protein kinase mediates the reduction of Ca^{2+} by cAMP in vascular smooth muscle cells. *Am J Physiol* 259:C399–C407, 1990.

15. Segal SS, Damon DN, Buling BR: Propagation of vasomotor responses coordinates arteriolar resistance. *Am J Physiol* 256:H832–H837, 1989.

16. Bulbring E, Brading AF, Jones AW, et al: *Smooth Muscle*. Baltimore, MD: Williams & Wilkins, 1970.

12

BLOOD-TISSUE EXCHANGE

INTRODUCTION OF CLINICAL CASE

A Xosha mother brought her 2-year-old son to a clinic in the Transkei region of South Africa. The child was lethargic, and his skin was cold to the touch. His face was puffy, and his arms and legs were so severely edematous that the skin was cracked. He had a low pulse rate and low blood pressure.

Echocardiography showed reduced myocardial mass and stroke volume, which, when combined with heart rate and blood pressure data, indicated a reduced cardiac output (CO) and elevated total peripheral vascular resistance (TPR). A plasma sample showed elevated antidiuretic hormone (ADH) and a markedly reduced plasma albumin concentration.

OVERVIEW OF EXCHANGE MECHANISMS

Exchange vessels are those that allow a bidirectional transport of substances between blood and the interstitial space. This process occurs primarily across those microvessels, or portions of microvessels, in which blood is separated from the interstitium by only the vascular endothelial cells. These include portions of the terminal arterioles, the capillaries, and portions of the venules. However, the bulk of exchange occurs across the capillaries for the following reasons: (1) There are far more capillaries than any other microvessels; therefore, the area available for exchange is greatest in the capillary networks; (2) compared to other microvessels, the capillaries have the greatest surface-to-volume ratio so that proportionately more of the blood is exposed to the exchange surface; (3) the velocity of flow is slowest in the capillaries; therefore, more time is available for exchange to occur; and (4) plasma is mixed continuously as blood traverses the capillaries.

The exchange of substances across vascular endothelium takes place by one of three processes that are summarized in Figure 12-1. One process involves simple *diffusion* of lipid-soluble and water-soluble substances from regions of high concentration to regions of low concentration (i.e., from a state of low entropy to a state of high entropy). Another process is *ultrafiltration*, whereby plasma water, interstitial fluid, and their dissolved crystalloids move through *functional pores* in response to pressure gradients. The third process is *vesicular transport*, whereby molecules move from one side of the vascular endothelium to the other in one or a series of small membrane-bound packets called vesicles.

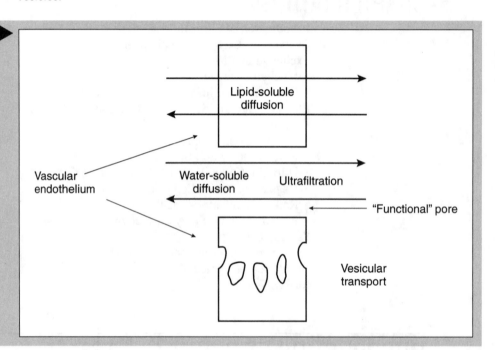

FIGURE 12-1 ▶

Blood–Tissue Exchange Mechanisms. Lipid-soluble substances can diffuse across the lipid-rich plasma membranes of the vascular endothelial cells; the diffusion of water-soluble substances is restricted to the same "functional" pores used for ultrafiltration. Finally, vesicular transport is a means by which large molecules can be transported across vascular endothelial cells in plasma membrane–surrounded spherical vesicles. (Source: Reprinted with permission from Richardson DR: Basic Circulatory Physiology. Boston, MA: Little, Brown, 1976, p 134.)

EXCHANGE BY DIFFUSION

Mechanics of Diffusion

The majority of substances that pass between blood and the interstitium do so by simple diffusion. The rate at which a substance diffuses across the vascular endothelium ($\dot{Q}x$) is equal to the permeability coefficient of the substance (Px), times the area available for exchange (A), times the difference between the concentration of the substance in the plasma (Cp_x) and in the interstitial fluid (Cif_x). In equation form:

$$\dot{Q}x = Px \cdot A(Cp_x - Cif_x)$$

A positive value means that a substance is moving from the blood into the interstitial fluid; a negative value indicates passage in the opposite direction.

For most substances, the plasma concentration remains within fairly narrow limits. This is in part due to mechanisms (discussed in Chapter 11) that enable tissue blood flow

This equation is another example of the application of Ohm's law. $\dot{Q}x$ is analogous to flow; Px is a measure of conductance (the inverse of resistance); and the concentration difference is the energy force driving the process.

to keep pace with metabolic needs. Thus, the rate of diffusion for a given substance is determined primarily by its interstitial fluid concentration, which is a function of the rate at which the substance is used or produced by cellular activity. For example, during exercise, the rate at which muscle cells produce carbon dioxide (CO_2) increases, thereby increasing the interstitial CO_2 concentration. This, in turn, results in an increase in the rate at which CO_2 diffuses into venous blood. If pulmonary mechanisms are functioning properly, then CO_2 elimination increases in proportion to production, resulting in a stable arterial CO_2.

The permeability coefficient of a diffusing substance (Px) is a measure of the ease with which vascular endothelium permits passage of the substance. This parameter is often difficult to separate from the area available for exchange (A), since for many substances they are interrelated. For example, as indicated in Figure 12-1, substances that are highly lipid-soluble, such as oxygen (O_2) and CO_2, have essentially the total endothelial surface available for diffusion; however, diffusion of substances that are water-soluble is restricted to aqueous pores. However, for both lipid- and water-soluble substances, the surface area for exchange is controlled by adjusting the number of capillaries through which blood is flowing. For example, in resting skeletal muscle, the ongoing vascular tone shuts off flow to most capillaries. However, during the vasodilation that accompanies an increase in metabolic activity, the number of capillaries being perfused increases in proportion to the degree of vasodilation.

The magnitude of Px is an interactive effect of the capillary endothelium and the diffusing substance. As shown in Figure 12-2, the structure of capillaries varies considerably from tissue to tissue. Muscle capillaries (A) have thick endothelial cells, a discernible basement membrane, and narrow intracellular junctions or gaps (labeled IC in the figure); however, liver (B) and intestinal (C) capillaries have relatively thin endothelial cells, have little or no basement membrane, and are perforated with *fenestrations*. These are window-like areas where the endothelium is reduced to an extremely thin membrane. Therefore, the permeability of most substances is much greater in liver and intestinal capillaries than in skeletal muscle capillaries.

> When there is no flow through a capillary, concentrations between blood and interstitium rapidly equilibrate, and the driving force for diffusion is lost. Therefore, unperfused microvessels do not contribute to exchange.

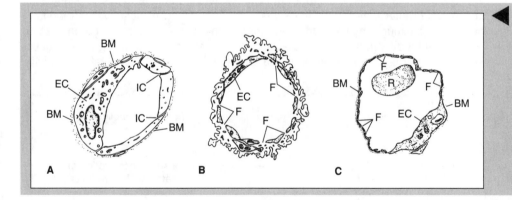

◄ **FIGURE 12-2**
Capillaries from Three Different Tissues.
(A) Muscle capillary. (B) Liver capillary. (C) Intestinal capillary. BM = basement membrane; EC = endothelial cell; P = perictye; IC = intercellular cleft; L = lumen; V = vesicle; S = extravascular space; F = fenestrations; R = red blood cell. (Source: Reprinted with permission from Selkurt EE: Physiology, 5th ed. Boston, MA: Little, Brown, 1984, p 212.)

Capillary permeability (Px) is determined not only by the endothelial structure but also by the molecular nature of the diffusing substance. Solutes that are highly lipid soluble penetrate the lipid endothelium quite easily and, therefore, have a high permeability factor. At the other extreme, water-soluble substances, such as sodium (Na^+), potassium (K^+), and chloride (Cl^-), have extremely low permeabilities because their diffusion is restricted to the aqueous medium of the pores.

Over the past half century, experiments with molecules of known size and water permeability have shown that capillaries behave as though they contain a population of *functional pores* of varying size. Despite considerable effort to identify these pores, their exact location is still not known. One hypothesis is that they are made up of the junctions between endothelial cells. These junctions are known as "small pores," "intercellular junctions," "tight junctions," and "intercellular clefts." Figure 12-3 diagrams the mosaic arrangement of endothelial cells that constitute a capillary with a cross-sectional view of one of the intercellular clefts. Toward the center of the cleft, the endothelial cells appear to touch. This is the region referred to as the tight junction. These junctions are

> The tight junctions referred to here are different in structure and function from the gap junctions described in Chapter 11 in conjunction with the spread of vasoconstrictor and vasodilator influences.

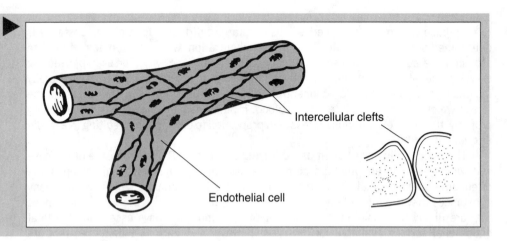

FIGURE 12-3 ▶
Mosaic of Endothelial Cells That Compose the Blood Capillaries. The intercellular clefts, also known as tight junctions, are probably the functional pores that allow for ultrafiltration and diffusion of water-soluble substances. (Source: Reprinted with permission from Vander AJ, Sherman JH, Luciano DS: Human Physiology, 6th ed. New York, NY: McGraw-Hill, 1994, p 439.)

examined in more detail in the following section, which discusses blood–tissue fluid exchange.

Even if all the intercellular cleft regions served as functional pores, the capillary surface area available for diffusion of water-soluble substances would still be far less than the surface area available for diffusion of lipid-soluble substances. This is because lipid-soluble molecules can easily cross the plasma membrane that occupies the surface of cells.

Coupling of Diffusion to Tissue Activity

Changes in the metabolic demand of a tissue are accompanied by corresponding changes in the rates at which metabolic substrates and by-products exchange with the perfused blood. Figure 12-4 illustrates the manner in which this coupling occurs with regard to the removal of metabolic products generated by tissue activity. A similar diagram could be drawn for the delivery of metabolic substrates. As indicated in the figure, metabolic-driven vasodilation increases both the number of perfused capillaries and capillary blood flow. The former increases the surface area for exchange; the latter provides a large sink for the rapid removal of metabolic by-products. As a result, plasma concentrations of metabolites are much smaller than concentrations in the interstitium, thereby increasing the gradient for diffusion. The increased surface area and concentration gradient collectively increase the rate of diffusion to match the increase in tissue metabolic activity.

FIGURE 12-4 ▶
Interaction of Factors That Couple an Increase in Tissue Metabolic Activity to a Corresponding Increase in the Rate of Blood–Tissue Exchange by Diffusion.

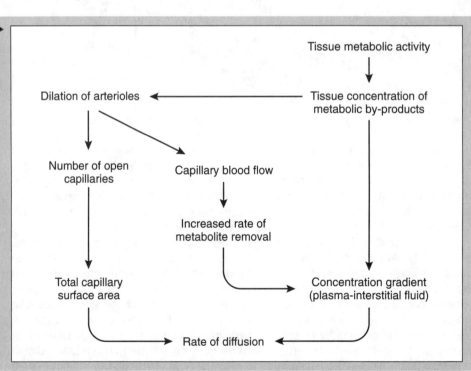

BLOOD-TISSUE FLUID EXCHANGE (ULTRAFILTRATION)

Overview

The capillary endothelial cell matrix behaves as a filter that allows the flow of plasma water and all dissolved solutes, such as electrolytes and glucose, but considerably inhibits the passage of suspended colloids, such as the large-molecular-weight proteins. Plasma so separated from its colloids is termed an *ultrafiltrate*. Tight junctions are considered to be the "pores" through which the ultrafiltrate moves. Figure 12-5 is a proposed model of a tight junction. The major features of this model are the narrow center region, known as the "neck," and the fiber-matrix protein aggregate that fills the junction. It is thought that the neck region imposes resistance to hydraulic conductivity and that the fiber matrix determines the selectivity of the junction to macromolecules. Thus, the tight junction behaves like a tube full of cotton: water can flow through the tube, but any large particles suspended in the solution will be trapped by the cotton.

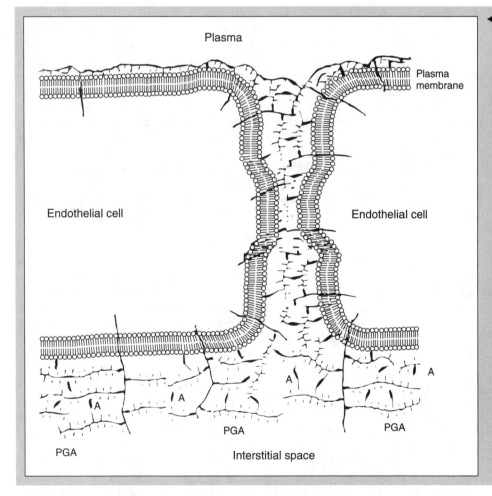

FIGURE 12-5
Structure of the Tight Junctions Between Endothelial Cells. *The characteristic features of tight junctions are a narrow center neck region, which gives hydraulic resistance to the junction, and a protein matrix, continuous with the interstitial space and plasma, which is responsible for molecular selectivity. PGA = protoglycan aggregate; A = albumin.*

Ultrafiltration is a bidirectional process in which fluid is constantly shifted back and forth between blood and interstitial fluid. In this context, the term "filtration" refers to a net movement of fluid *from blood to interstitium*; conversely, "absorption" refers to a movement *from interstitium into the blood*. Although there is a continuous bidirectional flow of ultrafiltrate across the capillaries, the volume filtered and the volume absorbed per unit time are rarely equal. The existence of lymph flow indicates that under normal conditions, filtration exceeds absorption on a total-body basis. However, if an individual becomes dehydrated, as could occur with severe sweating, a net absorption of interstitial fluid into the plasma occurs. Conversely, if an individual overhydrates by drinking too much, filtration increases and the extra fluid is transported to the interstitial space. Furthermore, the interstitium has an extremely high compliance and a large volume compared to the circulatory system; thus, it can take up and release large amounts of fluid with little change in interstitial pressure. For these reasons, the interstitium can serve as a fluid reservoir to buffer changes in plasma volume. In fact, *a major function of ultrafiltration is to maintain homeostasis of plasma volume.*

Ultrafiltration Forces

Given that ultrafiltration is the flow of a fluid, a hydrostatic pressure gradient would be the energy force that drives the process. More specifically, given that ultrafiltration is the flow of fluid across the capillaries, the hydrostatic pressures producing the gradient would be those in the blood capillaries and in the interstitial fluid. Blood pressure within the systemic capillaries ranges from about 20 to 40 mm Hg. This force drives outward filtration. Interstitial fluid hydrostatic pressure, the force opposing filtration, ranges from near 0 mm Hg during dehydration to less than 10 mm Hg in conditions of edema. If hydrostatic pressures alone were involved, there would always be considerable outward filtration, probably enough to cause severe edema. This fact indicates that forces other than hydrostatic pressure are involved in governing ultrafiltration.

Ernest Starling, the scientist who contributed Starling's law of the heart, is credited for recognizing a different type of ultrafiltration force called *colloid osmotic pressure* (COP) [1]. COP is the osmotic force created by the presence of proteins. The permeability of vascular endothelium to the large-molecular-weight proteins is small; thus, these molecules are essentially retained within either the plasma or the interstitium. Blood plasma has a protein concentration of 7%, as opposed to only 1% in the interstitium; this difference creates a net *colloid* osmotic force that favors the "pulling" of fluid from the interstitium into plasma. The higher protein concentration in the plasma and the resultant net pulling force provide the major opposition to outward filtration.

The direction and rate of ultrafiltration are determined by a balance between hydrostatic and colloid osmotic forces. However, in order to compare ultrafiltration forces quantitatively, COP must be expressed in the same units as hydrostatic pressure. This can be done by application of van't Hoff's law, given in the following expression:

$$\text{Osmotic pressure} = CRT$$

In the above equation, C is the concentration of the osmotic constituent, R is the gas constant, and T is the absolute temperature. This equation allows the concentration of an osmotically active substance to be expressed in terms of an equivalent hydrostatic pressure. From this equation, it is found that 1% of a protein concentration yields a hydrostatic pressure of 4 mm Hg. Plasma has a protein concentration of about 7%; therefore, normal plasma COP is approximately 28 mm Hg (7 × 4), whereas the interstitial COP is only about 4 mm Hg.

Figure 12-6 uses this information to insert numbers into the ultrafiltration process and compare the relative magnitudes of the hydrostatic and colloid osmotic forces involved. The figure illustrates a capillary with *arrows* showing the direction of ultrafiltration forces; the sizes of the arrows indicate their relative magnitudes. The *left portion* of the figure shows that blood pressure within the capillary (Pc) is the major filtration force serving to push fluid into the interstitium. This pushing force is aided by a slight pulling force resulting from the COP generated by the 1% protein concentration in the interstitial fluid (COPif). These outward-moving filtration forces are opposed by the two inward-moving absorption forces depicted on the *right* of the figure. The major absorptive force is the COP created by plasma proteins (COPp). This pulling force is aided by a slight hydrostatic pushing force in the interstitial fluid (Pif).

The mathematic relationship of the forces determining the rate of ultrafiltration is given in the equation below the capillary in Figure 12-6, where Jv is the rate of filtration and K is the capillary permeability coefficient; the remainder of the equation gives the hydrostatic and COP forces discussed previously. In this equation, the sum of the inward-moving forces is subtracted from the sum of the outward forces. By this convention, a positive value of Jv indicates outward filtration, and a negative value indicates inward absorption.

Plasma COP is the osmotic pressure that results from the presence of proteins, not the total osmotic pressure of the plasma. Total osmotic pressure takes into account not only the proteins but also all dissolved crystalloids, such as ions and sugars. The magnitude of the total osmotic force in plasma is about 6000 mm Hg, or about 60 times the mean arterial blood pressure. However, osmotic pressure gradients of this magnitude do not occur in living organisms, because crystalloids tend to have equal concentrations in the interstitium and plasma.

The equation for ultrafiltration given in Figure 12-6 is yet another example of Ohm's law applied to physiology. Jv is the rate of flow, and K is the inverse of resistance. The sum of the hydrostatic pressure and COP provides the energy force that drives the system.

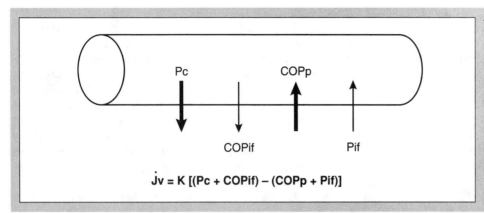

FIGURE 12-6
Relative Balance of Hydrostatic and Colloid Osmotic Pressure (COP) Forces in Ultrafiltration. As indicated by the relative size of the arrows, capillary hydrostatic pressure (Pc) is the major filtration force; colloid osmotic pressure of the plasma (COPp) is the major absorptive force. The equation below the figure represents the interaction of all factors determining the rate of ultrafiltration (Jv). K = capillary permeability coefficient; COPif = colloid osmotic pressure of the interstitial fluid; Pif = interstitial fluid hydrostatic pressure.

$$\dot{J}v = K[(Pc + COPif) - (COPp + Pif)]$$

Role of the Lymph System

In addition to returning excess filtrate to the circulatory system, the lymph system transports proteins that have "leaked" from the plasma, cellular debris from immune reactions, and ingested foods from the gastrointestinal tract, such as the fat-rich chylomicrons, to the circulatory system. Lymph flow takes place essentially in an uphill manner because interstitial hydrostatic pressure is normally much less than pressure within the subclavian veins where the systemic lymph system enters the circulation. These considerations raise two questions: how does lymph fluid flow uphill and how do large molecules, such as proteins, gain entry into the lymph system?

Figure 12-7 addresses the first question, presenting a sketch of a lymphatic tree beginning with a lymphatic capillary and ending with the main collecting channel. The

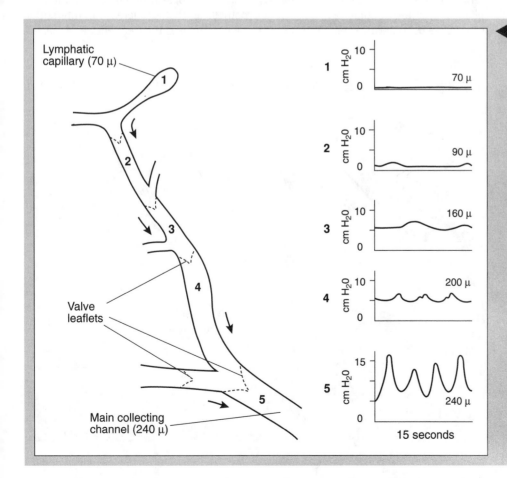

FIGURE 12-7
Micropressure Recordings in Successive Portions of Lymphatic Vessels in the Cat Mesentery. The lymphatic vascular tree, with a series of one-way valves, is shown on the left. On the right, there are tracings of pressure recordings within the five successive segments indicated in the drawing. Note that mean pressures rise from about 0.5 cm H_2O at the capillary level to about 10 cm H_2O at the collecting channel. (Source: Reprinted with permission from Crone C: Exchange of molecules between plasma, interstitial tissue and lymph. Pflugers Arch 336(Suppl):S68, 1972.)

lymph capillary is close-ended and much larger than a capillary in the blood circulatory system. Lymph passes through a series of one-way valves; on the distal side of each valve, pressure becomes higher and more pulsatile in nature. The pulsations are due to rhythmic contractions of smooth muscle, which surrounds the lymph vessels. The increase in lymphatic pressure resulting from the contraction of a muscle segment closes the upstream valve and opens the downstream valve. As indicated by the time scale on the pressure tracings, the contractions between valves occur asynchronously. The end result of the smooth muscle action along the lymph tree is that the valves are progressively closed and opened between a lymph capillary and the main channel. This action, in conjunction with the associated pressures, moves the lymph against a progressive pressure gradient in a manner analogous to a lock and dam system on a river.

The manner in which interstitial fluid and large substances enter the lymph system is shown in Figure 12-8. This figure illustrates the cross section of a lymph capillary, showing the anatomic positioning of three endothelial cells. Unlike those found in systemic capillaries, endothelial cells in lymphatic capillaries are not coupled by tight junctions. Instead, they are held in position by anchoring filaments, and there is considerable overlap of adjacent endothelial cells. Part A of the figure indicates the process during lymphatic muscle contraction in which pressure inside the lymph capillary exceeds interstitial pressure, thereby compressing the overlapping areas of endothelial cells. The compression of the endothelial cells against each other seals the interstitial-lymph pathways and forces fluid to move in the direction of the main channel. Parts B and C show the relaxation phase of lymph vessel smooth muscle. During these periods, interstitial pressure exceeds lymph capillary pressure. The higher interstitial pressure pushes the unsupported portions of the endothelial cells into the vessel lumen, thereby creating a large opening for the movement of interstitial fluid and any large substances, such as proteins and cellular debris, into the lymph capillary. When the lymph smooth muscle once again contracts, the system recycles back to the situation depicted in A.

The rhythmic contraction and relaxation of lymphatic vessels in conjunction with overlapping endothelial cells and one-way lymph valves moves lymph fluid from interstitial space into the circulatory system. It is hypothesized that an increase in interstitial pressure, as occurs with a net increase in filtration, increases the frequency and magni-

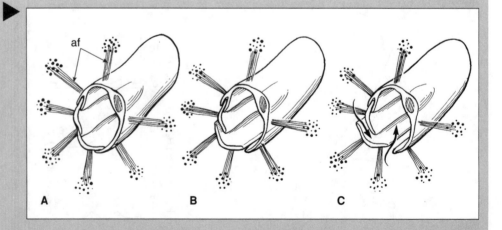

FIGURE 12-8
Lymphatic Capillary Interstitial Fluid Interface. *The anchoring filaments (af), the lack of adhesive connections between apposing endothelial cells, and the overlapping of endothelial cells collectively provide a mechanism to allow for the movement of interstitial fluid and large particles, such as proteins, into the lymphatic system and for the unidirectional flow of lymph toward the main collecting ducts. When interstitial pressure exceeds pressure in the lymphatic lumen, the portions of endothelial cells unsupported by anchoring filaments swing into the lymph capillary, thereby providing a wide channel between interstitium and lymph (B and C). When lymphatic smooth muscle contracts, pressure inside the vessel increases, closing the channels and forcing fluid in the direction of the one-way valves (A) [depicted in Figure 12-7]. (Source: Reprinted with permission from Hammersen F: Ultrastructure and functions of capillaries and lymphatics. Pflugers Arch 336 (Suppl):S52, 1972.)*

tude of lymph vessel contractions, resulting in an increase in lymph flow in proportion to an increase in filtration.

Ultrafiltration in Various Physiologic States

Table 12-1 lists hypothetical hydrostatic and colloid osmotic pressures that would occur in different physiologic states. In the normal state, shown in the first row of the table, the sum of the outward forces (Pc and COPif) is 30 mm Hg. This is opposed by inward-moving forces (COPp and Pif) totaling 29 mm Hg, for a net force of 1 mm Hg favoring filtration. The resultant filtrate enters the lymphatic system.

◄ **TABLE 12-1**
Ultrafiltration Pressure Forces (mm Hg)

| | Outward Forces | | | Inward Forces | | | |
	Pc	COPif	Sum of Outward	COPp	Pif	Sum of Inward	Net (Out–In)
Normal	26	4	30	28	1	29	+1
Vasoconstriction	20	5	25	28	0	28	−3
Vasodilation	30	3	33	28	2	30	+3
Dehydration	26	5	31	34	0	34	−3
Protein loss	26	3	29	24	2	26	+3

Note. Pc = blood pressure within the capillary; COPif = colloid osmotic pressure in the interstitial fluid; COPp = colloid osmotic pressure created by plasma proteins; Pif = pushing force in the interstitial fluid.

The second row depicts the situation during arteriolar vasoconstriction, which would cause a reduction in downstream capillary pressure. This reduction would result in a net absorption of fluid into the circulatory system, as indicated by the net ultrafiltration force of −3 mm Hg. The net shift of fluid from interstitium into plasma would concentrate interstitial proteins, resulting in an increase in COPif. A net loss of interstitial fluid would also cause interstitial pressure to fall somewhat, from 1 to 0 mm Hg in Table 12-1. A value of 0 mm Hg for interstitial pressure is not unreasonable; there is evidence that under some conditions interstitial pressure may even be subatmospheric [2].

The third row illustrates the opposite situation, that of arteriolar vasodilation. Under this condition, capillary pressure would increase, thereby increasing the rate of outward filtration. This increase would dilute the interstitial proteins and increase interstitial volume. As a result, COPif would decrease, and Pif would increase. The increase in Pif acts as a stimulant to increase the pumping action of the lymph vessels. This increases the rate of return of interstitial fluid to the general circulation and minimizes tissue edema.

The fourth row depicts the common condition of dehydration. A loss of water from the circulatory system results in a concentration of plasma proteins and an increase in COPp. The rise in COPp leads to a net absorption of interstitial fluid into the circulatory system, thereby buffering the loss of plasma volume. Absorption of interstitial fluid secondary to a rise in plasma COP is a major mechanism that protects circulatory volume in states of dehydration. The inward absorption elicits a rise in COPif and a decrease in Pif, just as with inward absorption in response to vasoconstriction.

The fifth row presents the pathologic state of hypoproteinemia. Conditions that cause this state include protein deficiency, malnutrition, and renal disease in which protein is excreted in the urine. When a loss of plasma protein occurs, the major colloid osmotic force that opposes outward filtration is diminished. This results in a net increase in filtration, which often leads to peripheral edema.

Regulatory Interaction of Ultrafiltration Forces

When an increase in net filtration occurs, interstitial volume tends to increase, causing edema. However, even in the most severe cases of edema, its progression subsides, and the system reaches a new steady state. Similarly, in dehydration states, interstitial volume is reduced only so far before a new steady state is established. Figure 12-9 diagrams the interaction of factors responsible for controlling ultrafiltration and, hence, interstitial volume. The *left* portion of the figure shows how changes in ultrafiltration are normally elicited by changes in COPp and Pc, the former retarding and the latter promoting outward filtration. The resultant changes in the rate of ultrafiltration elicit corresponding changes in interstitial volume. Because the filtrate is relatively protein-free, net filtration dilutes interstitial proteins, thereby reducing COPif and simultaneously increasing Pif. These changes "feedback" to inhibit further changes in ultrafiltration. Furthermore, an increase in Pif serves to stimulate lymph flow, which then stabilizes interstitial volume. In most situations, this system serves to prevent tissue edema or severe tissue dehydration. A notable exception is the inflammatory process, which involves changes in capillary permeability.

FIGURE 12-9 ▶
Interaction of Factors Determining the Rate of Ultrafiltration. Capillary pressure (Pc) and plasma colloid osmotic pressure (COPp) initiate changes in ultrafiltration. The interstitial forces provide feedback that brings these changes into a new steady state. COPif = interstitial fluid colloid osmotic pressure; Pif = interstitial fluid hydrostatic pressure.

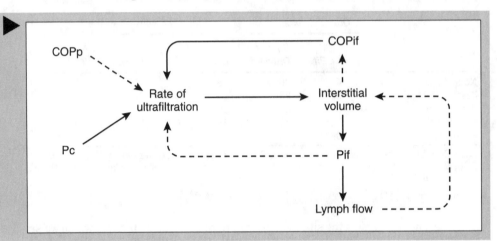

Role of Capillary Permeability

Not only does capillary permeability vary from one tissue to another, but within a given tissue, permeability can change from one situation to another. For example, the local inflammatory response that follows a bee sting is basically due to an increase in capillary permeability [3].

It is not entirely clear how capillary permeability increases in response to conditions such as a bee sting, but it is likely that inflammatory agents, such as histamine, which are released by foreign toxins, interact with receptors on endothelial cells. This interaction, through some signal transduction mechanism, may then lead to the activation of contractile proteins. This activation, in turn, opens up the neck region of tight junctions, thereby increasing hydraulic conductivity. Furthermore, since inflammation is usually attended by an increase in protein leakage into the interstitium, the fiber matrix complex may also be altered to allow an easier passage of proteins. It is probably the leakage of proteins into the interstitium that elicits inflammation by increasing the COP of the interstitial fluid, thereby drawing fluid from plasma into the interstitium.

It is thought that anti-inflammatory agents, such as cortisol, elicit the opposite action on capillary endothelial cells; that is, following a constriction of tight junctions, the lymph system clears the edema. Regardless of what the exact mechanisms might be, changes in capillary permeability play an important role in the ultrafiltration process.

Role of Total Capillary Surface Area

Finally, the overall rate of filtration in a given tissue is governed by the number of open capillaries through which blood is flowing, in addition to the rate of filtration across a single capillary. Figure 11-3 showed how metabolic activity can increase the number of open capillaries. This, in turn, increases the surface area available for filtration. Therefore, an increase in interstitial volume often accompanies an increase in tissue blood flow.

VESICULAR TRANSPORT

One of the most longstanding questions in circulatory physiology is how large molecules, such as whole proteins, are transported across the capillary endothelium. Most of the data on this point indicate that *plasmalemma vesicles*, also termed pinocytotic vesicles, are involved in this process. In the circulatory system, vesicles are small fluid-containing sacks within vascular endothelium, and the plasmalemma vesicles are those that are formed from invaginations of the plasma membrane. Figure 12-10 shows an electron micrograph cross section of a capillary. The *arrows* point to plasmalemma vesicles, which seem to be forming from the plasma membrane of the endothelial cell.

Plasmalemma vesicles are not the same as caveoli, mentioned in Chapter 11. Caveoli are, in general, smaller than vesicles and probably serve in signal transduction rather than in molecular transport.

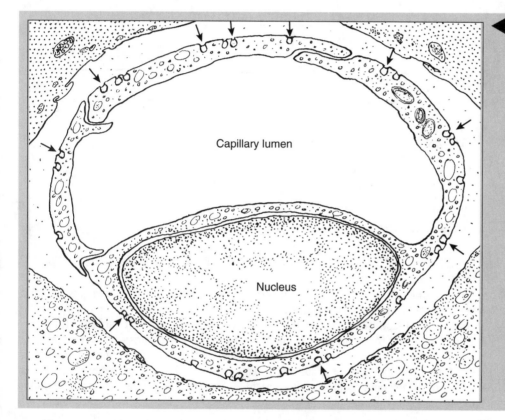

◀ **FIGURE 12-10**
Electron Micrograph Cross Section of a Capillary from the Heart, Showing Numerous Endothelial Vesicles at the Arrows. (Source: *Reprinted with permission from Fox SI:* Human Physiology, *5th ed. Dubuque, IA: Wm. C. Brown, 1996, p 370.)*

Capillary lumen

Nucleus

The process of vesicular transport is not entirely known. Figure 12-11 illustrates three models (A, B, and C) that have been proposed [4, 5]. In model A, a macromolecule first interacts with the plasma membrane of an endothelial cell; this interaction may be receptor-mediated. The macromolecule–plasma membrane interaction triggers an invagination of the plasma membrane into a vesicle that surrounds the macromolecule, a process called *endocytosis*. The vesicle breaks away from the plasma membrane and drifts to the opposite side of the endothelial cell, where the vesicle merges with the plasma membrane. This vesicle–plasma membrane interaction results in an emptying of the vesicular contents to the outside of the endothelial cell, a process termed *exocytosis*.

One of the criticisms of model A is that it is not certain that vesicles can drift through cytoplasm from one side of a cell to the other. Model B takes this criticism into account. According to this model, vesicular formation (termed *endocytosis*) occurs, as with model A; however, once inside the cytoplasm, vesicles merge with one another and exchange their contents, much like runners passing the baton in a relay race. The transported molecules eventually arrive at the opposite side of the cell, where they are discharged by the process of exocytosis.

Model C is much different from the other two in that it does not involve transport of macromolecules by a coupling of endocytosis and exocytosis. According to this model, intracellular vesicles are constantly in the process of merging, then dispersing. This merging of vesicles occasionally results in the formation of transcytotic channels that are

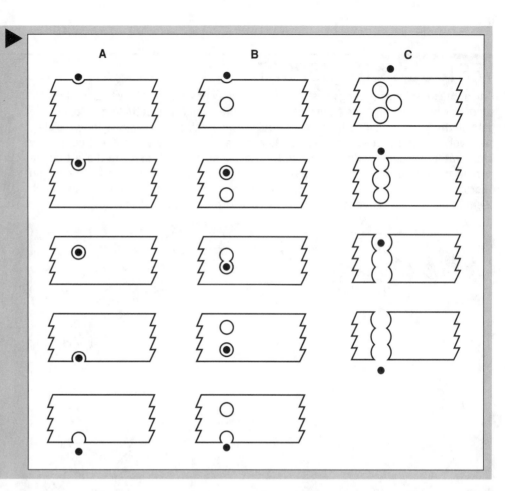

FIGURE 12-11 ▶

Models of Vesicular Transport. In model A, macromolecules interacting with the endothelial plasma membrane trigger the formation of a vesicle (endocytosis), which then breaks off and migrates to the opposite side where the process reverses (exocytosis), thereby discharging the macromolecule. In model B, the endocytotic vesicle transfers the macromolecule to other vesicles until it is ultimately discharged by exocytosis. In model C, the macromolecule diffuses through a transcytotic channel formed by the fusion of several vesicles.

wide enough to allow the passage of macromolecules by simple diffusion. Transcytotic channels are very short lived; consequently, they went undetected in early morphologic studies. When these channels were first found, they tended to be disregarded as artifacts. It is now believed that transcytotic channels are real, albeit transient, components of capillary endothelial cells. Furthermore, it is thought that they not only allow the transport of macromolecules but also participate in blood–tissue fluid exchange; in this context, they may be a major source of residual protein leak across the capillary endothelium.

EXCHANGE IN THE PULMONARY CIRCULATION

The pulmonary circulation has a unique role: it must extract, from the alveoli, all the O_2 used by the body and give off, to the alveoli, all the CO_2 produced by the body. Furthermore, the pulmonary circulation must do this by utilizing a total capillary surface area considerably smaller than the total surface area of the systemic capillaries. Figure 12-12 illustrates how this is achieved. Part A of the figure depicts the net-like fashion in which the pulmonary capillaries encase the alveoli. This provides a near maximal alveoli–capillary exchange surface. Part B of the figure is a cross section of a pulmonary capillary surrounded on both sides by alveolar space. The numbers 1, 2, and 3 indicate the pathway for O_2 diffusion from the alveolar space into an erythrocyte (EC). Note that the capillary endothelium (EN), the alveolus epithelium (EP), and the interstitial fluid layer between the two are extremely thin, particularly in the midregion where exposure to the alveolar air is maximal. The reduced blood–gas barrier and large alveoli–capillary surface area markedly enhance the rate of blood–gas exchange.

A major inhibitor to blood–gas exchange in the lungs is expansion of the interstitial space resulting from pulmonary edema. Under normal conditions, pulmonary edema is prevented by the fact that mean pulmonary capillary pressure, of about 10 mm Hg, is considerably lower than plasma COP. Thus, unlike systemic capillaries, pulmonary capillaries are pitched toward inward absorption, thereby keeping the lungs "dry." However, this situation can be easily reversed in pathophysiologic situations, such as congestive heart failure, where pulmonary pressures can be quite high. Thus, owing to the unique structure and low intravascular pressures of the pulmonary capillary system, the pulmonary circulation provides adequate blood–gas exchange even under conditions of extreme metabolic demand (e.g., maximal exercise).

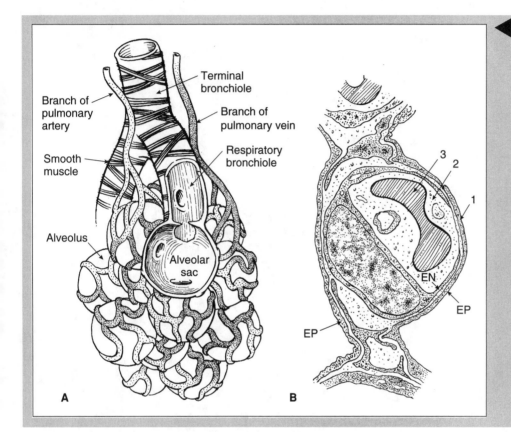

FIGURE 12-12

(A) The net-like manner in which pulmonary capillaries wrap around alveoli is illustrated. (B) An electron micrograph shows the coupling between pulmonary capillary endothelial cells (EN) and alveoli epithelial cells (EP). Note the thin interstitial space between the EN and EP membranes. The numbers 1, 2, and 3 indicate the relatively short path length for oxygen diffusion from the alveolar space into an erythrocyte. (Source: A, Reprinted with permission from Vander AJ, Sherman JH, Luciano DS: Human Physiology, 6th ed. New York, NY: McGraw-Hill, 1994, p 477. B, Reprinted with permission from West JB: Respiratory Physiology, 5th ed. Baltimore, MD: Williams & Wilkins, 1995, p 3.)

RESOLUTION OF CLINICAL CASE

The native African boy presented at the beginning of the chapter is suffering from the kwashiorkor form of protein energy malnutrition. This is considered a multifaceted disease triggered by malnutrition resulting from low protein intake. The classic features of kwashiorkor are lethargy, irritability, and severe peripheral edema. Low plasma albumin is a major cause of the peripheral edema; without sufficient albumin, the major force opposing outward filtration, plasma COP, is inadequate. Furthermore, an albumin deficiency would be expected to disrupt the tight junction matrix, thereby increasing the capillary permeability to an ultrafiltrate. However, edema in kwashiorkor may be more than just the result of low plasma albumin. Disrupted electrolyte metabolism, particularly K^+, may be related to the etiology of edema associated with kwashiorkor.

Severe edema also disrupts blood–tissue exchange of nutrients by increasing the path length for diffusion. Furthermore, low blood pressure and elevated TPR contribute to the deficiency of blood–tissue exchange by reducing the number of patent capillaries (i.e., reducing the surface area available for exchange).

The low blood pressure in this patient, and in most kwashiorkor patients, is due to low CO, which is secondary to reduced myocardial mass (i.e., decreased contractility) and reduced blood volume (i.e., decreased cardiac preload). The elevated TPR vis-à-vis a low heart rate suggests that the resistance adjustment is *not* secondary to a baroreflex response to the low blood pressure. Otherwise heart rate would be increased, not decreased. The most likely cause of the increased TPR is an elevated level of vaso-constrictor hormones, such as ADH.

Regardless of specific cause, the patient's cold skin is indicative of elevated TPR and is also, in part, reflective of reduced body metabolism. (Hypothermia is a common complication of kwashiorkor.)

In summary, kwashiorkor is a multifaceted disease that affects many aspects of the cardiovascular system, including blood–tissue exchange. A good overview of this disease is provided by Jelliffe and Jelliffe [6].

REVIEW QUESTIONS

Directions: For each of the following questions, choose the **one best** answer.

1. Which of the following is a mechanism by which the rate of blood–tissue exchange by diffusion is increased in response to an increase in tissue metabolic activity?

    (A) An increase in capillary blood pressure

    (B) An increase in the number of capillaries through which blood is flowing

    (C) An increase in pumping action of lymph vessels

    (D) Down-regulation of hormone receptors on vascular smooth muscle

2. In response to constriction of arterioles, fluid will be

    (A) filtered as a result of an increase in capillary blood pressure

    (B) filtered as a result of a decrease in plasma colloid osmotic pressure (COP)

    (C) filtered as a result of an increase in interstitial fluid COP

    (D) absorbed as a result of a decrease in capillary blood pressure

    (E) absorbed as a result of an increase in plasma COP

3. In response to dehydration (loss of water) that does *not* decrease either central venous pressure or mean arterial blood pressure, fluid will be

    (A) filtered as a result of an increase in capillary blood pressure

    (B) filtered as a result of a decrease in plasma colloid osmotic pressure (COP)

    (C) filtered as a result of an increase in interstitial fluid COP

    (D) absorbed as a result of a decrease in capillary blood pressure

    (E) absorbed as a result of an increase in plasma COP

4. In response to a decrease in protein content of the blood, fluid will be

    (A) filtered as a result of an increase in capillary blood pressure

    (B) filtered as a result of a decrease in plasma colloid osmotic pressure (COP)

    (C) filtered as a result of an increase in interstitial fluid COP

    (D) absorbed as a result of a decrease in capillary blood pressure

    (E) absorbed as a result of an increase in plasma COP

5. In response to an increase in the permeability of capillaries to proteins, fluid will be

    (A) filtered as a result of an increase in capillary blood pressure

    (B) filtered as a result of a decrease in plasma colloid osmotic pressure (COP)

    (C) filtered as a result of an increase in interstitial fluid COP

    (D) absorbed as a result of a decrease in capillary blood pressure

    (E) absorbed as a result of an increase in plasma COP

6. In response to dilation of arterioles, fluid will be

    (A) filtered as a result of an increase in capillary blood pressure

    (B) filtered as a result of a decrease in plasma colloid osmotic pressure (COP)

    (C) filtered as a result of an increase in interstitial fluid COP

    (D) absorbed as a result of a decrease in capillary blood pressure

    (E) absorbed as a result of an increase in plasma COP

ANSWERS AND EXPLANATIONS

1. The answer is B. An increase in the number of capillaries through which blood is flowing is a mechanism by which the rate of blood–tissue exchange by diffusion is increased in response to an increase in tissue metabolic activity. Tissue metabolites dilate terminal arterioles, which increases the number of capillaries with active flow. This increases the total surface area available for diffusion. An increase in capillary blood pressure would promote outward filtration but would have little effect on exchange by diffusion. An increase in the pumping action of lymph vessels would clear excess interstitial fluid but would not affect solute concentrations in the interstitium; therefore, concentration gradients, hence diffusion rates, would not be affected. Down-regulation of hormone receptors on vascular smooth muscle would probably elicit net vasodilation because there are more circulating constrictor hormones than dilator hormones. This might increase capillary pressure, but it would not have an effect on diffusion.

2. The answer is D. In response to constriction of arterioles, fluid will be absorbed due to a decrease in capillary blood pressure. Vasoconstriction decreases downstream pressure in the capillaries. Plasma COP would not be affected. Interstitial fluid COP would be increased as a result of fluid being absorbed.

3. The answer is E. In response to dehydration (loss of water) that does *not* decrease either central venous pressure or mean arterial blood pressure, fluid will be absorbed due to an increase in plasma COP. Dehydration concentrates plasma proteins, which increases plasma COP, the major force favoring absorption. If mean arterial pressure is not decreased, then capillary pressure would not be affected. Interstitial fluid COP would be increased, but again this would be as a result of fluid being absorbed.

4. The answer is B. In response to a decrease in protein content of the blood, fluid will be filtered due to a decrease in plasma COP. Plasma proteins create plasma COP, the major force opposing filtration. Capillary pressure would not be affected, and interstitial fluid COP would be decreased, not increased.

5. The answer is C. In response to an increase in the permeability of capillaries to proteins, fluid will be filtered due to an increase in interstitial fluid COP. An increase in permeability would cause proteins to leak into the interstitium. This would elevate interstitial fluid COP, a filtration force. None of the other choices apply in this case.

6. The answer is A. In response to dilation of arterioles, fluid will be filtered due to an increase in capillary blood pressure. This question is the reverse of question 2.

REFERENCES

1. Michel CC: One hundred years of Starling's hypothesis. *News Physiol Sci* 11:229–237, 1997.
2. Guyton AC: *Textbook of Medical Physiology*, 8th ed. Philadelphia, PA: W. B. Saunders, 1991, pp 175–177.
3. Curry FE: Determinants of capillary permeability: a review of mechanisms based on single capillary studies in the frog. *Circ Res* 59:376–380, 1986.
4. Rippe B, Haraldsson B: How are macromolecules transported across the capillary wall? *News Physiol Sci* 2:135–138, 1987.
5. Simionescu M, Ghitescu L, Fixman A, et al: How plasma macromolecules cross the endothelium. *News Physiol Sci* 2:97–100, 1987.
6. Jelliffe DB, Jelliffe EFP: Causation of kwashiorkor: toward a multifactorial consensus. *Pediatrics* 90:110–113, 1992.

13

CONTROL OF THE CARDIOVASCULAR SYSTEM

INTRODUCTION OF CLINICAL CASE

A 72-year-old woman was admitted to the hospital because of dizziness on assuming the upright posture with occasional *syncopal attacks* (fainting). Her arterial blood pressure when supine was 100/60 mm Hg; when she was seated, her blood pressure dropped to 80/50 mm Hg. Her heart rate (HR) was 75 beats per minute (bpm) in both the supine and sitting positions. Her hematocrit was 28 (normal: 37–48). Her jugular veins were distended to approximately 8 cm above the level of the right atrium (normal: 0–2 cm). Her white cell count, platelet count, and other hematologic tests were normal. Routine blood chemistry tests were also normal. She had ++ (moderate) peripheral edema and +++ (moderately severe) protein in her urine (*proteinuria*). Tests for prior *myocardial infarction* ("heart attack" or death of heart muscle) were negative, but an echocardiogram showed mild-to-moderate *ventricular hypertrophy*.

OVERVIEW OF THE REGULATION OF CARDIOVASCULAR FUNCTION

The prefix "baro" means pressure, as in the word barometer, a device that measures atmospheric pressure. Therefore, the baroreflex is a pressure reflex, and a baroreceptor is a sensor that detects changes in blood pressure.

*One of the most familiar examples of a **feedback system** is the cruise control in an automobile. This device maintains the speed of the car at a value determined by the driver (the set point) regardless of the driving conditions. If the road starts to climb, the slight decrease in the car's speed is sensed by an on-board computer that then increases the fuel delivered to the engine to maintain the desired speed. The driver can reset the operating point at any time so that the car's speed is maintained at a higher or lower value. Note that the cruise control contains all five of the required components for a functioning feedback system (see Figure 1-1).*

The arterial baroreflex has served as the primary example of a cardiovascular reflex since the description of the carotid sinus nerve by Hering [1] and the classical studies of the reflex by Heymans [2] and Koch [3]. *The neurally mediated baroreflexes with afferent information coming from the arch of the aorta and carotid sinus are responsible for minimizing fluctuations in arterial blood pressure that would otherwise result from changes in posture or other acute challenges.* This aspect of pressure regulation can be explained in terms of the classic biofeedback theory. Although this is a useful starting point for analyzing blood pressure regulation, the situation quickly becomes more complicated. For example, the value around which pressure is regulated—the *set point* (sometimes called the operating point)—appears to change to a new value (or *reset*), probably under direction of "higher" nervous centers, in response to internal motivational states or certain external challenges. Moreover, if an elevation in arterial pressure is sustained, the firing rate recorded from the afferent fibers gradually decreases or adapts. In fact, most physiologists agree that mechanisms other than the baroreflex dominate in the long-term regulation of blood pressure. These additional regulatory pathways probably involve receptors in the atria and perhaps other locations within the cardiopulmonary system, as well as nonneural intrinsic control mechanisms (see Chapter 7). These latter pathways and mechanisms are thought to regulate arterial pressure for days, weeks, and longer intervals largely by means of increases and decreases in total blood volume. Because the ability to maintain blood pressure is highly dependent on blood volume, it is not surprising that regulation of both variables involves common pathways and effector organs. This, of course, directly involves the kidney in the regulation of blood pressure. Finally, the possibility that a network of neurons residing within the heart helps regulate circulatory function is just beginning to be explored [4].

ARTERIAL BAROREFLEX

A helpful starting point for understanding the control of arterial blood pressure (BP) is the simple and familiar equation:

$$BP = CO \times TPR \tag{1}$$

where CO is cardiac output and TPR is total peripheral resistance. An even more useful formulation takes advantage of the fact that CO equals stroke volume (SV) times HR:

$$BP = (SV \times HR) \times TPR \tag{2}$$

Although these equations eventually prove to be overly simplified, they clearly show that *the nervous system can change (or regulate) arterial pressure by controlling the volume of blood that the heart pumps per minute and the resistance of the vasculature.* Figure 13-1 shows the first step in the construction of a feedback cycle built around this foundation. The convergence of the arrows from TPR and CO on "arterial pressure" is a standard visual representation of the mathematical rule that BP equals CO multiplied by TPR (i.e., BP = CO × TPR). The use of *solid arrows* indicates, as always, that an increase in CO (or TPR) tends to increase BP (or that a decrease in CO or TPR tends to decrease BP). The *dotted line* connecting TPR and CO is a useful, if unnecessary, tool to indicate that this is an explicit, quantitative (i.e., algebraic) relationship (likewise for SV and HR).

This chapter now proceeds step-by-step to develop a comprehensive cycle diagram of the arterial baroreflex (see Figure 13-6).

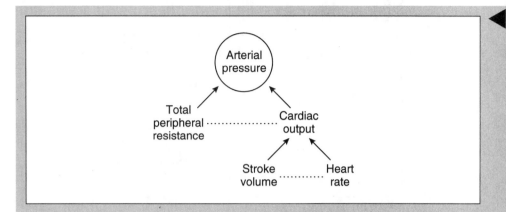

FIGURE 13-1
Foundation for a Cycle Diagram of the Baroreflex. This figure is a schematic representation of equation 2 on the previous page: blood pressure (BP) = total peripheral resistance (TPR) × stroke volume (SV) × heart rate (HR). Two variables converging on a third variable is a standard notation indicating that variable 1 times variable 2 equals variable 3. The dotted lines connecting TPR and CO, as well as SV and HR, are reminders that these are algebraic relationships. Solid arrows represent a direct relationship between two variables.

Baroreceptors in the Carotid Sinus and Aortic Arch

The walls of the left and right *carotid sinus* and the *arch of the aorta* contain sensory fibers that increase their firing rate as the respective intraluminal pressures increase. In effect, these are mechanical stretch receptors: increasing blood pressure inside the aorta or carotid sinus increases the stretch on the vessel wall and thereby on the stretch receptors within the wall. Bronk and Stella [5] isolated single afferent nerve fibers from the carotid sinus and showed that their firing frequency increased as the pressure inside the vessel increased. A sensory receptor that signals the prevailing value of the regulated variable is the first requirement for any feedback control system (see Chapter 1, Figure 1-1).

Figure 13-2A schematically illustrates the relationship between blood pressure within the carotid sinus and a recording from a single afferent baroreceptor fiber from within the wall of the carotid sinus. The overall firing frequency progressively decreases when blood pressure drops from a high to a normal value to a low value. Figure 13-2B shows the relationship that Franz and colleagues [6] described between carotid sinus pressure and the steady state frequency of firing for two single baroreceptor fibers from the rabbit carotid sinus. They found that increasing the pressure in the carotid sinus increased the baroreceptor's firing frequency; likewise, when carotid sinus pressure dropped, the firing frequency decreased. Normally, of course, carotid sinus pressure equals arterial pressure. Figure 13-2C depicts the direct relationship (i.e., *solid arrow*) between blood pressure and baroreceptor firing frequency that can now be added to the cycle diagram in Figure 13-1.

The afferent signals from the carotid sinus are carried via the carotid sinus nerve (also known as the nerve of Hering), which joins the glossopharyngeal nerve and projects to the nucleus of the solitary tract within the brainstem. Likewise, afferent fibers from the aortic arch project via the vagus nerve to the same destination (see Central Nervous System Pathways Mediating the Arterial Baroreflex for details of the brain's role in the baroreflex). This completes the first step in constructing the overall cycle diagram.

Effect of Arterial Pressure on Efferent Sympathetic Nerve Activity

Neuronal circuits within the brainstem compare the actual value of arterial pressure, as provided by the baroreceptors, with the optimal (or set point) value. If the actual arterial pressure is too high, the reflex causes efferent sympathetic nerve activity (SNA) to decrease; if the blood pressure is too low, the reflex increases SNA. *The inversion inherent in this relationship is ultimately expressed by a* dashed arrow *in the cycle diagram we are developing.*

Figure 13-3 is a simultaneous recording of arterial blood pressure and SNA. Blood pressure was initially at normotensive levels. However, it decreased starting at approximately 4 seconds because a drug was administered that caused vascular smooth muscle to relax and vascular resistance to fall. The overall activity in the sympathetic nerve

The use of the word "receptor" in physiology can be confusing. The mechanical stretch receptors in the carotid sinus are fine nerve endings in the vessel's wall. Stretching the nerve membrane by the pressure pulse results in action potentials, which have a frequency proportional to intraluminal pressure. Receptors on cell membranes, such as the α- or β-adrenergic receptors, are proteins that respond to the presence of a particular chemical agent (e.g., norepinephrine in the case of the sympathetic nervous system). Binding of norepinephrine to the receptor initiates a series of chemical events that alters the way the cell functions.

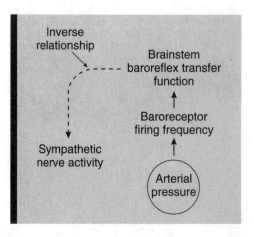

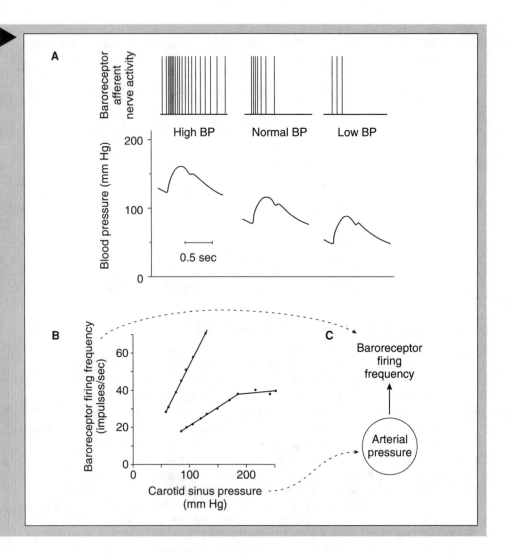

*In any feedback cycle, one can predict only what effect a change in one variable **tends** to have on a second variable. The effects of the one variable that is being deliberately manipulated may be swamped by other adjustments within the total cycle. When physicians treat a hypertensive patient with a drug that blocks a component of the baroreflex, for example, they generally know from experience what effect they will see on blood pressure, but there are no guarantees.*

increased as the blood pressure decreased. This is a direct demonstration of a compensatory change in SNA produced by the baroreflex. It is worth emphasizing again that the key inverse relationship that makes the baroreflex contribute to blood pressure stability is contained in this component of the cycle diagram.

Effect of SNA on Smooth Muscle Contraction and TPR

Chapter 4 explains that increases in SNA promote contraction of vascular smooth muscle. The classic neurotransmitter released from the varicosities of the sympathetic nerves is norepinephrine, which exerts its effects on the smooth muscle via an α-adrenergic receptor. The smooth muscle contraction tends to decrease the radius of the arteriolar resistance vessels and, by the principles of Poiseuille's law, increases peripheral resistance. Recall, however, that "peripheral resistance" is one of the terms in equations 1 and 2 and, in fact, appears as an "input" to arterial pressure in Figure 13-1. Therefore, *this step completes—or "closes"—one constituent loop of the baroreflex* (Figure 13-4).

The message inherent in Figure 13-4 is critically important to understanding how biofeedback systems work in general and how the baroreflex works in particular. To understand this important concept, start at arterial pressure in the figure and imagine that, for whatever reason, arterial blood pressure started to *decrease*. Following the arrows around the loop, note that the rate of action potential generation by the sensory fibers originating within the carotid sinus *decreases* because of the decreased stretch on the walls of this vessel due to the falling intraluminal pressure. The reflex response, mediated by neuronal networks within the brain (primarily within the medulla), *increases* SNA, thus promoting *contraction* of vascular smooth muscle in the peripheral circulation

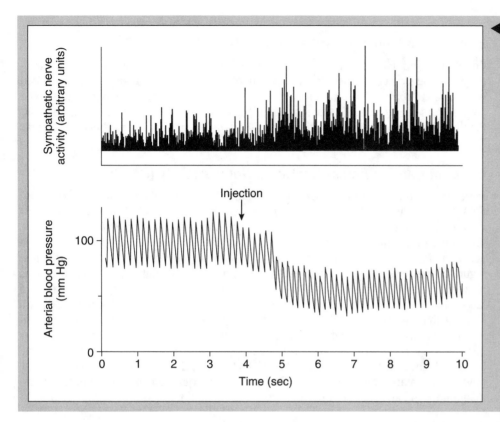

FIGURE 13-3
Changes in Sympathetic Nerve Activity (SNA) in Response to a Decrease in Arterial Pressure. *SNA was recorded from fine gold electrodes implanted around the renal nerve in a rat. This multifiber recording is the electrical signal produced by the combined action potentials from many individual sympathetic nerve axons. Nitroprusside was administered at the arrow to relax vascular smooth muscle. The resulting decrease in total peripheral resistance caused arterial blood pressure to fall. This drop in pressure increased SNA via the baroreflex. Nitroprusside, or similar drugs such as nitroglycerin, are used clinically to decrease myocardial metabolic oxygen demand by decreasing the afterload on the heart. (Source: These data were provided courtesy of Dr. David Brown, Center for Biomedical Engineering, University of Kentucky College of Medicine, Lexington, Kentucky.)*

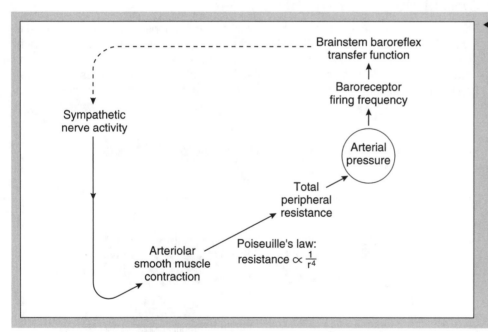

FIGURE 13-4
Loop of the Baroreflex That Helps Stabilize Arterial Blood Pressure by Changing Total Peripheral Resistance (TPR). *Increased levels of sympathetic nerve activity cause arteriolar smooth muscle to contract, thereby increasing TPR. TPR, however, is an element in Figure 13-1; therefore, the feedback loop is "closed" because the effects of changes in arterial pressure ultimately influence elements in the cycle that alter arterial pressure. The presence of an odd number of inverse relationships (in this case 1), represented by the dashed arrow, shows that this is a negative feedback cycle that promotes stability. Each arrow in the cycle represents a relationship between two variables. For example, the arrow between smooth muscle contraction and TPR embodies Poiseuille's law (see Chapter 3).*

with a consequent *rise* in TPR. *Because the effect of a rise in TPR is to promote an increase in arterial blood pressure, this sequence of physiologic changes offsets the incipient fall in blood pressure that started the whole cascade of events.* The reflex yields a decrease in TPR to drop blood pressure if the original challenge (or *perturbation*) acted to increase arterial pressure. Reduced to the simplest possible statement, the baroreflex counters any tendency for blood pressure to increase by decreasing SNA, and vice versa. Thus, the baroreflex minimizes transient pressor or depressor events, effectually stabilizing blood pressure around an optimal value: it produces moment-to-moment pressure homeostasis.

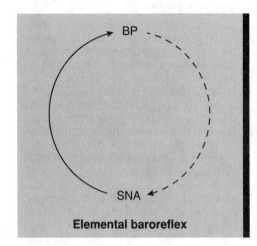

Elemental baroreflex

The most obvious effect of increased parasympathetic nerve activity is to decrease HR. Increased cardiac parasympathetic tone also depresses atrial contractility and AV-nodal conduction, and indirectly depresses ventricular contractility. For the sake of simplicity, these effects are ignored in many situations, including the diagram in Figure 13-6.

Effect of SNA on Myocardial Contractility, SV, and HR

Chapters 9 and 10 explain that increased cardiac SNA increases myocardial contractility; the classic neurotransmitter is norepinephrine acting on a β_1-adrenergic receptor. A positive inotropism, in turn, tends to increase SV. This completes another limb of the baroreflex (see Figure 13-6) because SV is one of the original variables in Figure 13-1. Finally, a third loop is closed by simply recalling the direct relationship between cardiac SNA and HR: $\uparrow$SNA → $\uparrow$HR or $\downarrow$SNA → $\downarrow$HR.

Effect of Cardiac Parasympathetic Nerve Activity (PNA) on HR

Increased blood pressure causes the brainstem baroreflex neural circuit to *decrease* SNA. Conversely, elevated blood pressure *increases* cardiac PNA. The inverse relationship within this latter nested cycle occurs because increased cardiac PNA *decreases* HR. The neurotransmitter released from the parasympathetic (i.e., vagal) nerve endings is acetylcholine (ACh), which acts through a *muscarinic receptor* on the cell membrane. Figure 13-5 shows the effects that electrically stimulating the right vagus nerve produces on arterial and left ventricular pressures and on HR. Stimulating the vagus nerve causes a large, sudden decrease in HR. Careful examination of the electrocardiogram (ECG) at a faster recording speed confirms that, in this example, an atrial depolarization (presumably originating in the sinoatrial [SA] node) preceded the QRS complex for each heart beat, so this is a *sinus bradycardia*. The vagal bradycardia resulted in an overall decrease in arterial blood pressure because it decreased CO (i.e., CO = HR × SV). This important physiologic relationship appears in the upper right quadrant of the complete cycle diagram for the arterial baroreflex (Figure 13-6).

Cycle Diagram of the Arterial Baroreflex

The individual components of the baroreflex that were developed above are assembled in Figure 13-6 to show the overall cycle diagram. Only the elements in the lower right quadrant have not been examined individually; a discussion of these must await the development of a few more concepts later in this chapter. Nonetheless, the overall impact of the diagram is clear: *any perturbation that acts to increase or decrease arterial*

FIGURE 13-5 ▶

Cardiovascular Response to Increased Parasympathetic Nerve Activity. The arterial blood pressure (BP), left ventricular pressure (LVP), electrocardiogram (ECG), and heart rate (HR) recordings are from an anesthetized dog. The right vagus nerve in the neck was electrically stimulated at moderate intensity; the beginning and end of the 30-second stimulation are indicated on the time scale (bottom). The increase in parasympathetic activity to the sinoatrial node slowed HR as indicated by the decreased number of heartbeats per minute (bpm). Blood pressure decreased because of the decrease in cardiac output caused by the vagal bradycardia. All variables recovered quickly to prestimulus control upon cessation of the stimulus.

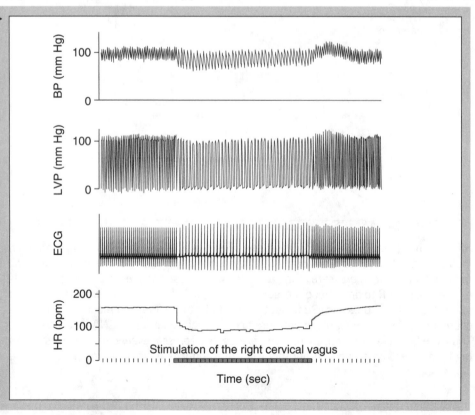

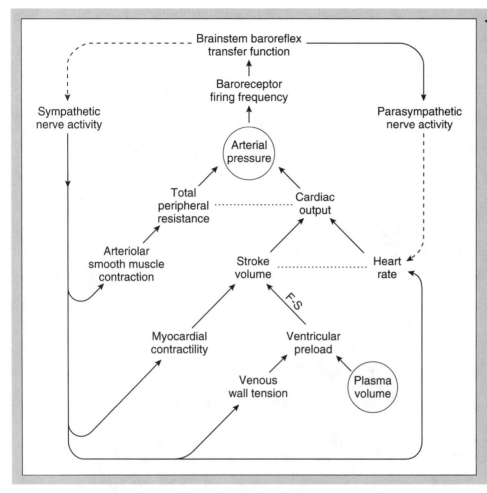

FIGURE 13-6
Comprehensive Cycle Diagram of the Arterial Baroreflex. Notice how the elements shown in Figure 13-1 form the basis of the complete cycle. Each loop includes one inverse relationship. The various loops of the cycle are "nested," thereby increasing the overall stability of blood pressure. This nesting may obscure disease processes within one of the components (see Chapter 7). For example, if the ability of the sympathetic nervous system to increase myocardial contractility is compromised by disease, the relationship between ventricular preload and stroke volume (SV) [i.e., the Frank-Starling relationship] may be able to maintain SV and will, therefore, continue to confer some stability on arterial pressure. The lower right quadrant of the figure represents the influence of blood volume on arterial pressure, which is explained further in Figures 13-9 and 13-10. F-S = Frank-Starling relationship. (Source: This cycle diagram was developed by Dr. Joseph Engelberg, Department of Physiology, University of Kentucky College of Medicine, Lexington, Kentucky.)

pressure transiently is counteracted by the reflex responses within the total cycle so that beat-to-beat blood pressure fluctuations are minimized.

Central Nervous System (CNS) Pathways Mediating the Arterial Baroreflex

Many different regions within the CNS are involved in the baroreflex regulation of arterial blood pressure, and it would be a mistake to think that all the relevant neurons are located wholly within one particular region of the brain. In Chapter 7, Figure 7-3 emphasizes this broadly integrative nature of the nervous regulation of blood pressure. Nonetheless, a group of interconnected neurons located within the medulla oblongata of the brainstem is clearly indispensable for operation of the baroreflex.

The easiest way to understand the organization of this network is to identify first the cells that receive afferent projections from the baroreceptors. In this regard, it is now well established that the afferent nerves originating from the carotid sinus, the aortic arch, the cardiopulmonary receptors, and the chemoreceptors (see Chapter 19) project to the *nucleus of the solitary tract* (or NTS, from "nucleus tractus solitarius"). The NTS is located in the dorsomedial portion of the medulla oblongata. Neurons within the NTS both send axons to, and receive fibers from, numerous areas of the brainstem. In particular, the NTS projects to a group of cells in the central portion of the medulla known as the *nucleus ambiguus*. Electrical stimulation of cells in and around the nucleus ambiguus slows the HR because the parasympathetic preganglionic neurons innervating the SA node are located there. The left portion of Figure 13-7A diagrams the parasympathetic pathways of the baroreflex within the brainstem. It is not known with certainty how many neurons are actually involved in this simplest of the central baroreflex "circuits."

With respect to the sympathetic outflow from the brain, neurons in the *rostral ventrolateral medulla* (RVLM), especially adrenergic cells in the subretrofacial nucleus, are the source of the *sympathoexcitatory pathway* to the sympathetic preganglionic

NTS is a favorite structure of first-year neuroanatomy students because the nucleus and its associated tracts have an unmistakable doughnut-like appearance when viewed under the microscope in appropriately stained sections of the medulla. Chapter 19 explains the involvement of NTS in the regulation of respiration and emphasizes the very close interaction between cardiovascular and pulmonary regulation at multiple sites within the CNS.

FIGURE 13-7 ▶

Central Nervous System Baroreceptor Pathways. *(A) This is a simplified diagrammatic representation of the major pathways involved in the arterial baroreflex. The somata of the sensory fibers innervating the arch of the aorta and carotid sinus are located in sensory ganglia (nodose and petrosal ganglia, respectively). Afferent signals from these, and other, receptors project to the nucleus tractus solitarius (NTS). Cells within the NTS project axons to neurons in and around the nucleus ambiguus, which, in turn, is the source of the cardiac vagal preganglionic efferent nerves. Neurons within the rostral ventrolateral medulla (RVLM) provide a tonic descending sympathoexcitatory outflow to the intermediolateral column of the spinal cord. Interruption of these pathways decreases arterial blood pressure. The activity of cells within RVLM is inhibited by a pathway from the caudal ventrolateral medulla (CVLM); the CVLM is excited by cells within the nucleus ambiguus. In addition, a descending pathway from cells within the raphe nuclei of the brainstem (not shown) inhibit sympathetic preganglionic neurons in the intermediolateral column. (B) This figure uses an outline of the rat brain to show some of the inputs to vasopressor neurons within RVLM. These include tracts from the periaqueductal gray, paraventricular nucleus, and the lateral hypothalamic area. Cells within the RVLM give rise to the descending sympathoexcitatory pathway (thick line) to the intermediolateral column of the spinal cord. Pathways in A and B from one region to another are not necessarily monosynaptic. (Sources: Panel A was adapted with permission from Svend AF, Gordon FJ: Amino acids as central neurotransmitters in the baroreceptor reflex pathway.* News Physiol Sci *9:244, 1994. Panel B was adapted with permission from Dampney R: The subretrofacial nucleus: its pivotal role in cardiovascular regulation.* News Physiol Sci *5:65, 1990.)*

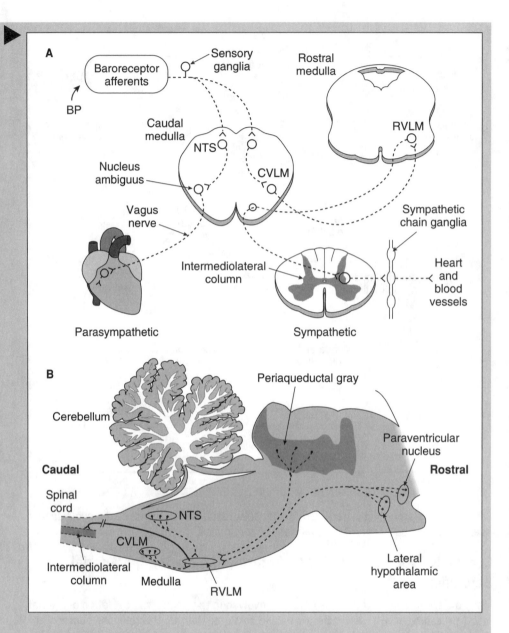

neurons in the *intermediolateral column of the spinal cord* [7]. For this reason, this area of the medulla has historically been known as the *vasomotor center*. Microinjection of excitatory amino acids (e.g., L-glutamate) into the RVLM increases SNA and causes blood pressure to increase. It is especially interesting to note that the NTS also sends fibers to the *caudal ventrolateral medulla* (CVLM). Activating CVLM neurons decreases blood pressure. Stated as simply as possible, an increase in baroreceptor input to the NTS increases cardiac PNA by activating cells in the nucleus ambiguus. In addition, the rise in afferent input to the NTS also excites the CVLM, which, in turn, *inhibits* sympathoexcitatory output from the RVLM to the spinal cord. The activation of the nucleus ambiguus slows HR directly, whereas the other actions decrease HR, CO, and peripheral vascular vasomotor tone by withdrawal of tonic SNA. Naturally, opposite changes occur when blood pressure within the carotid sinus drops.

The simple outline given above barely begins to grapple with the complex neuronal circuits responsible for the regulation of arterial pressure. In particular, a number of pathways shown in Figure 13-7B descend from "higher" regions of the brain to the

RVLM. A later section of this chapter (see Central Nervous System Regulation of Blood Volume) explains that neurons within the *paraventricular nucleus* and *lateral hypothalamus* subserve the regulation of body fluid volume. Cells located within the midbrain *periaqueductal gray* appear to mediate pressor responses associated with defensive behavior. Physiologists are learning the functional importance of these descending pathways, and they are identifying the neurotransmitters involved at different synapses within the many pathways [8]. As investigators learn more about these pathways, it seems inevitable that new and more effective therapies will be developed to treat disorders of blood pressure regulation. The interested student may consult a number of very informative reviews of the central neural regulation of cardiovascular function for additional details [7–11].

Blood Pressure Lability in the Absence of the Arterial Baroreflex

It is possible to eliminate the arterial baroreflexes in animal experiments by destroying the ability of the baroreceptors to signal the prevailing blood pressure to the brain. This is usually accomplished by cutting the nerve fibers from the carotid sinuses and aortic arch in anesthetized subjects. The reflex feedback loop is "opened" in animals that have this sinoaortic denervation. Figure 13-8A is a recording of mean arterial pressure in an awake rat with normal baroreflex control of blood pressure. Although there were brief moments when the pressure either increased or decreased, the blood pressure mostly was stable and remained within a restricted range. Figure 13-8B shows an analogous pressure recording from a rat whose baroreflex was eliminated by sinoaortic denervation. This animal's arterial pressure fluctuated over a wide range. In other words, arterial pressure was highly *labile* in rat B, whose baroreflex was not functioning. Figure 13-8C is a *frequency histogram* showing the distribution of mean arterial pressure in these two animals. The sharp peak for the normal rat shows that mean blood pressure for almost every beat was at, or very close to, the grand average of 100 mm Hg. Conversely, the frequency distribution for the rat with an interrupted baroreflex was much broader because of the increased lability, although rat B's grand average pressure of 106 mm Hg did not differ notably from that of rat A. Other experiments confirm that *the baroreflex minimizes beat-by-beat, moment-to-moment increases or decreases in arterial blood pressure* [13].

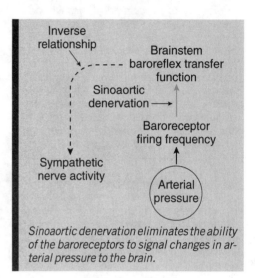

Sinoaortic denervation eliminates the ability of the baroreceptors to signal changes in arterial pressure to the brain.

FIGURE 13-8 ▶

Buffering of Moment-to-Moment Fluctuations in Arterial Blood Pressure by the Baroreflex. *(A) This figure shows a portion of an 8-hour continuous recording of arterial blood pressure in an awake rat with an intact, normally functioning baroreflex. The pressure was recorded through an arterial catheter while the animal was left undisturbed in its cage. The systolic and diastolic pulsations that occurred with each heartbeat were electronically filtered to produce this recording of mean blood pressure. The rat's overall mean arterial pressure was relatively stable, although there were occasional small increases and decreases. [Note that the calibration of the blood pressure scale is the same in panels A and B.] (B) This figure shows a similar recording, except the arterial baroreflex was eliminated in this rat by denervating the left and right carotid sinus and the arch of the aorta. Arterial blood pressure fluctuated widely in the baroreflex-denervated rat, although, over the course of the total recording, average pressure was not markedly different in the subjects in panels A and B. (C) This graph plots the number of beats, expressed as a percentage of the total heartbeats (y-axis) that had a given blood pressure. The tall, narrow trace is from the data in panel A, and it shows that blood pressures for most heartbeats were very close to a central value (i.e., grand average) of 100 mm Hg. The broad, lower tracing is from the data in panel B; sinoaortic denervation caused a marked dispersion of pressures, although the grand average of 106 mm Hg was not markedly different than for the baroreflex-intact rat. This technique was developed by Brown and colleagues to quantify blood pressure fluctuations [12]. (Source: These data were provided courtesy of Dr. David Brown, Center for Biomedical Engineering, University of Kentucky College of Medicine, Lexington, Kentucky.)*

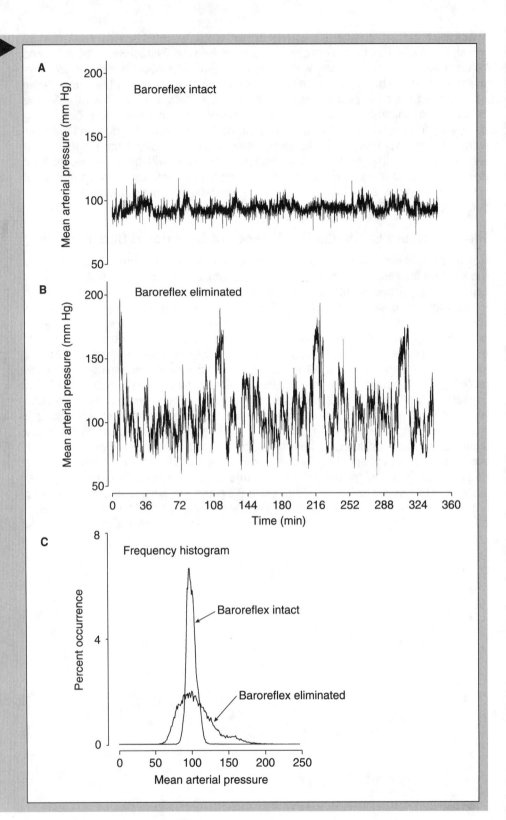

CARDIOPULMONARY REFLEXES

The physiologic role of cardiovascular reflexes that are triggered by afferent information coming from receptors within the atria, the ventricles, and the pulmonary vasculature is still uncertain in many ways. These afferent or sensory nerves originate from what are collectively known as *cardiopulmonary receptors*. Their primary or at least their best-understood function appears to be the *regulation of total blood volume*. Nonetheless, the possibility that cardiopulmonary receptors cooperate with the baroreflex to regulate arterial pressure cannot be dismissed [14].

Mechanoreceptors and Chemoreceptors in the Heart

Afferent nerves with sensory fibers in the heart project to the brainstem by way of the vagus nerves and to the spinal cord via the sympathetic nerves (see Figure 7-3). In general, the receptor nerve endings for *myelinated vagal afferents* are located primarily in the atria. These receptors discharge either during atrial systole (type A pattern), during atrial filling (type B pattern), or during both phases of the atrial cycle. Most *unmyelinated vagal afferents* originate from within the left ventricle. Vagal afferent fibers may be either *mechanosensitive* (i.e., responding to changes in the stretch on the ventricular muscle fibers or to changes in the force the fibers generate) or *chemosensitive*. Most receptor endings for cardiopulmonary *sympathetic afferent* fibers are unmyelinated and originate from sensory endings in the left ventricle. These "sympathetic afferents" often respond to both mechanical and chemical stimuli.

Several reflexes have been described in anesthetized animals that are associated with activation of cardiopulmonary sensory fibers, but, in many cases, their significance has not been definitively demonstrated in humans. It seems certain, however, that there are sensory fibers that respond to the chemical and mechanical changes that occur within the heart during myocardial ischemia (i.e., a "heart attack"). These sensory fibers or other receptors are presumably responsible for the painful sensation of *angina pectoris* that often accompanies episodes of myocardial ischemia. Finally, increases in cardiac SNA that may occur during myocardial ischemia are thought to originate, at least in part, from reflexes activated by the cardiopulmonary receptors. This increased SNA may trigger ventricular ectopic beats (see Chapter 8). See Thames and colleagues [15] as well as Smith and Thames [16] for recent reviews of the physiology to the cardiopulmonary receptors.

Cardiopulmonary Reflexes Contributing to Blood Volume Regulation

Arterial baroreceptors and cardiopulmonary afferent fibers converge on the same general pool of neurons within the brainstem, and it seems likely that they cooperate in some way in the overall regulation of blood pressure [14]. The specific role of atrial receptors in regulating extracellular volume has been studied for many years, although this issue has not yet been resolved [17]. The B-type receptors mentioned above send information to the CNS on atrial volume. The effects of activation of these atrial volume receptors (sometimes called low pressure receptors) have been studied by immersing humans in water. This causes blood that is normally pooled by gravity in the lower extremities to shift into the thorax, engorging the heart. Water immersion causes a fairly rapid increase in urine production (*diuresis*) and a *natriuresis* (increased renal excretion of salt). This increased loss of body salt and water eventually decreases extracellular fluid volume, including blood volume, unless compensatory responses are activated. Animal experiments indicate that the diuretic effect depends on those myelinated vagal afferent fibers from the heart, although the arterial baroreceptors can also participate. Plasma levels of *vasopressin*, also known as *antidiuretic hormone* (ADH), decrease, which contributes importantly to the diuresis.

The cycle diagrams in Figure 13-9 summarize the role of atrial receptors in the regulation of plasma volume. This figure shows multiple nested feedback cycles that enhance overall stability of blood volume as discussed in Chapter 7. The cycles in Figure 13-9 help complete the explanation of the lower right quadrant of Figure 13-6.

The term "angina pectoris" is derived from the Latin angere, *meaning choking, and* pectoris, *meaning breast or chest. The feeling of chest pain occurs when the myocardium's need for oxygen is not being met by delivery of adequate oxygenated blood. The resulting accumulation of metabolites and acidosis activates local chemoreceptors. Cardiologists now recognize, however, that not all myocardial ischemia produces anginal pain; an individual may not even be aware of this so-called **silent ischemia**.*

Blood also shifts from the lower body into the chest in astronauts exposed to "microgravity." On earth, gravity pools a portion of the blood in the lower body. Once in orbit, a significant shift in blood from the lower body into the thoracic cavity occurs quickly. This shift results in a fairly rapid contraction of total body fluid volume and of blood volume. Over several days of weightlessness, a state called "cardiovascular deconditioning" can result in severe orthostatic intolerance upon reentry. NASA currently encourages astronauts to consume a salt-water solution prior to reentry to increase blood volume temporarily.

***Vasopressin**, or **ADH**, acts on the kidneys to retain water (an antidiuresis). The hormone is synthesized by neuroendocrine cells in the supraoptic and paraventricular nuclei of the hypothalamus (see Figure 13-9). It is transported from the hypothalamus to the posterior pituitary gland, where it is released into the capillaries of the pituitary portal system when appropriate neural stimulation occurs. The release of ADH is also regulated by changes in plasma osmolality, atrial natriuretic peptide, angiotensin II, pain, and perhaps other factors [18].*

FIGURE 13-9 ▶

Atrial Reflexes Contributing to Regulation of Plasma Volume. Reflexes originating from receptors within the atria contribute to the regulation of renal salt and water metabolism (i.e., retention or loss). Other influences, including the arterial baroreflex, also help regulate renal function. The outer loop depends on principles summarized in Chapter 12 concerning filtration of water from capillaries, including the glomerular capillaries, into the interstitial space. The middle loop indicates how the kidney's production of renin, which controls the conversion of angiotensinogen to angiotensin I, ultimately influences the kidney's retention of Na+ by means of the hormone aldosterone. The inner loop depends on the ability of antidiuretic hormone (ADH) to increase the kidney's retention of water. In addition to the pathways shown here, the concentration of ADH in the plasma is detected by neurons within the brain that also help maintain salt and water balance (see Figure 13-10).

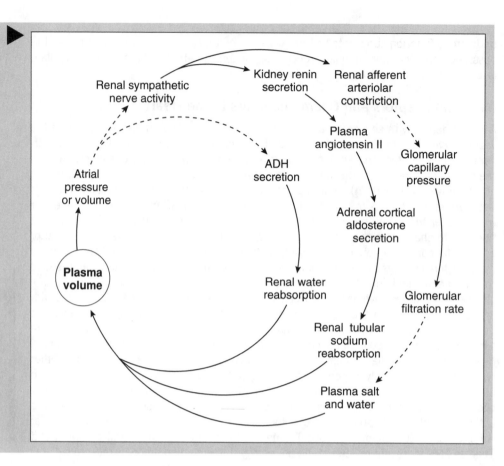

The capillaries of most regions of the brain have endothelial cells whose structure (e.g., intercellular tight junctions, absence of fenestrations) limits the exchange of substances between the blood and parenchyma of the brain. These endothelial cells allow lipid-soluble substances, including oxygen and carbon dioxide, to pass easily. Some other substances, such as glucose and amino acids, have specific transporters, but large molecules such as proteins and many exogenous drugs are excluded by the blood–brain barrier. The blood–brain barrier is absent in the circumventricular organs. Capillaries in these latter areas have "windows," known as fenestrations, that allow larger molecules to pass into the parenchyma of the brain.

CNS REGULATION OF BLOOD VOLUME

The reflexes described in Figure 13-9 do not include several additional mechanisms that also regulate extracellular fluid volume. These mechanisms rely on regions of the CNS that lack the *blood–brain barrier*. These areas of the brain are generally located along the midline around the third and fourth cerebral ventricles and are collectively referred to as *circumventricular organs*. The relative lack of a blood–brain barrier within these regions allows some larger proteins and hormones to gain access to neurons within the brain itself. Once inside the brain, they can trigger mechanisms to increase salt and water intake or diminish their loss.

Angiotensin II plays a particularly important role within the CNS in blood volume regulation beyond those effects on renal function shown in Figure 13-9. Figure 13-10 includes the effects of changes in plasma levels of angiotensin II upon the brain's control of drinking, upon its production of vasopressin, and upon its control of the autonomic nervous system. The illustration shows that certain neurons within the circumventricular region have receptors that detect the changes in plasma angiotensin II produced as a result of the homeostatic cycles in Figure 13-9. Physiologists have mimicked these changes by injecting minute amounts of angiotensin II into the subfornical organ of experimental animals and found that this injection induces drinking [19]. This *dipsogenic* action of angiotensin II helps restore extracellular fluid volume when total body water is depleted. In addition, at least some of the components of the renin-angiotensin system are actually synthesized within the brain [20]. Cells within the subfornical organ and the organum vasculosum of the lamina terminalis (OVLT), a region that is virtually surrounded by cerebrospinal fluid on two sides, appear to act as osmoreceptors or perhaps as sodium (Na+) receptors [21]. Neurons in these regions are excited when the plasma becomes more concentrated (i.e., its osmolality increases) because of decreased water or increased plasma electrolytes. This activates behavioral as well as physiologic mechanisms to restore normal blood volume and osmolality.

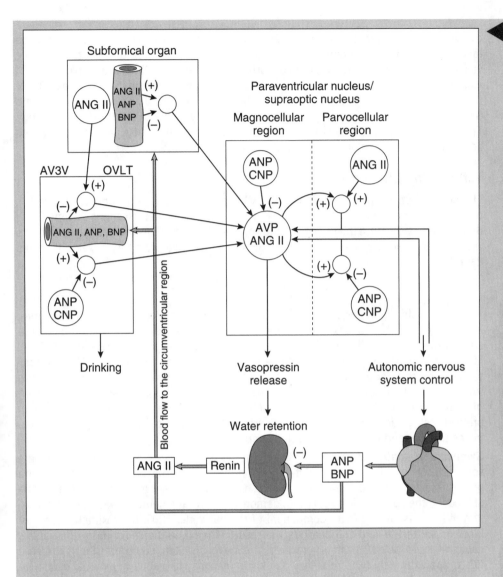

FIGURE 13-10
Schematic Summary of the Regulation of Salt and Water Metabolism and Autonomic Nervous System Activity. The kidney secretes renin (see Figure 13-9) in response to a decrease in renal afferent arteriolar pressure, a decrease in Na^+ load, or increased sympathetic nervous activity. Renin is an enzyme that controls the conversion of angiotensinogen to angiotensin I, which is then converted to angiotensin II (ANG II). ANG II plays a major role in controlling cardiovascular and renal function in addition to the actions shown here. The atrial myocytes release natriuretic peptide into the blood in response to increased wall stress caused by elevated plasma volume; atrial natriuretic peptide (ANP) inhibits (−) renal reabsorption of salt and water. The plasma concentrations of ANG II, ANP, and brain natriuretic peptide (BNP) are sensed by cells in the circumventricular region of the brain, including the subfornical organ, the anteroventral third ventricular (AV3V) region, and the organum vasculosum of the lamina terminalis. This information is transmitted to the large cells of the paraventricular region that secrete arginine vasopressin also known as antidiuretic hormone (ADH), which promotes renal water retention. Other neurons in the parvocellular region influence the autonomic outflow from the brain. Finally, the subfornical organ also projects to the AV3V region, which influences drinking behavior. CNP = central natriuretic peptide. (Source: Adapted with permission from Yamashita H, Kannan H: Inhibition of hypothalamic neurons by the atrial natriuretic peptide family. News Physiol Sci 7:78, 1992.)

Figure 13-10 also indicates the central importance of the *anteroventral third ventricular* (AV3V) region in the maintenance of fluid and electrolyte balance. The AV3V region appears to function in many ways like a "drinking center." Rats with lesions of this area virtually cease drinking and die of dehydration within a few days [22]. The AV3V region receives projections from the subfornical organ, which may partially explain the *adipsia* (failure to drink) after lesioning this region. Angiotensin II also binds to receptors within the subfornical organ, as do members of the natriuretic polypeptide family. Neurons within the AV3V region project to the paraventricular nucleus (where they influence the production of ADH by the magnocellular neurons) as well as to the parvocellular region (where they influence the autonomic regulation of cardiopulmonary function). Because the paraventricular region is the source of the ADH shown in Figure 13-9, the homeostatic mechanisms in these two figures are actually nested cycles functioning synergistically to control blood pressure, blood volume, and CO.

Atrial natriuretic polypeptide was first identified in the mammalian atria. It is secreted by specialized myocytes in the atria in response to high cardiac-filling pressures. It enhances the renal excretion of salt (a natriuresis) and relaxes vascular smooth muscle. The function of brain natriuretic polypeptide seems to relate to pathologic states such as heart failure [21]. The most recently identified member of the family is central natriuretic peptide, which is found in the CNS. It, too, has a natriuretic action, but its physiologic role is not clear.

ROLE OF THE VENOUS SYSTEM: MATCHING CARDIAC OUTPUT AND VENOUS RETURN

The lower right quadrant of Figure 13-6 recognizes the contribution of the venous system in the ultimate regulation of arterial blood pressure, but the relative importance of the venous system and the precise physiologic mechanisms whereby the veins contribute to overall circulatory regulation has been widely debated. The veins would seem to be ideally designed and anatomically situated to play an important role. First, the systemic veins are much more compliant than the arteries, so they can adapt readily to changes in volume. Second, the venous system may contain at any given moment as much as 70% of the total blood volume. Third, this "pool" of blood can be "mobilized" centrally (i.e., into the thoracic cavity) to increase the amount of blood available to the heart for pumping. The following sections explain the current understanding of how the venous system contributes to the regulation of CO and arterial blood pressure.

Venous Compliance

The concept of compliance developed in Chapter 3 is essential to understanding the physiology of the venous system. Recall that the compliance of the venous system (C_v) is determined by dividing the change in the volume of blood in the veins (ΔV_v) that occurs with a given change in venous pressure (ΔP_v). A simple algebraic rearrangement of this definition yields:

$$\Delta V_v = C_v \times \Delta P_v$$

The term **venous pressure** has been used rather loosely in physiology. **Central venous pressure** is measured in the great veins near their juncture with the heart. Central venous pressure changes noticeably during the respiratory cycle because these vessels are thin walled, distensible, and surrounded by the intrapleural pressure that changes with inspiration and expiration (see Chapter 15).

This relationship is important for the regulation of cardiac preload, CO, and, therefore, arterial pressure, because C_v is very large (more than 10 times greater than the compliance of the systemic arteries). This is especially true of the splanchnic circulation [23]. Moreover, the one-way valves in the veins prevent blood from flowing "backwards" towards the capillaries so that, once on its way from the veins, the blood must move toward the heart. *Therefore, a very small change in venous pressure results in a large shift of blood to the heart.* Once the blood is delivered to the heart, the resulting increase in preload assures an increase in SV. There are at least four important physiologic mechanisms that depend in some way on this simple equation.

Sympathetic Control of Venomotor Tone. The peripheral veins, especially those of the splanchnic and cutaneous circulation, are innervated by the sympathetic nerves and possess α-adrenergic receptors. Decreasing carotid sinus pressure decreases the volume of blood in the splanchnic circulation, demonstrating that a neurally mediated mobilization of blood is an important component of the baroreflex [24]. Approximately 350 ml blood is shifted toward the heart as the result of maximal constriction of the venous capacitance vessels [23]. In other words, the nervous system could transiently increase CO by approximately 50% relatively quickly in response to a sudden external challenge (e.g., being threatened) by shifting this volume of blood to the heart. This is put into a broader context when considering the effect of SNA on the vascular function curve (sometimes called the venous return curve; see below).

Passive Effects on Venous Capacity: The Effects of Gravity and the Muscle Pump. The venous *transmural pressure* (see Chapter 3) significantly affects the volume of blood contained within the veins. When humans assume the upright posture, the pressure in the vessels of the abdomen and in the *dependent limbs* increases significantly. In effect, the weight of the blood contributes to the intraluminal pressure (see the discussion of *hydrostatic pressure* in Chapter 3). The volume of blood that "falls" into the lower body is blunted by the pressure applied to the external walls of the vessels by the viscera and muscles, but transmural pressure increases nonetheless. The resulting increase in V_v decreases venous return, at least for a few moments, with a resultant decrease in ventricular preload (Figure 13-11). Some individuals experience *syncope* (i.e., they faint) as a result of this *postural hypotension*. The reflex increase in venomotor tone shown in the lower right quadrant of Figure 13-6 that results from the decline in arterial pressure is an important component of the overall maintenance of blood pressure in these situations. The opposite situation occurs during exercise. Those vessels surrounded by skeletal muscle experience a compressive force during exercise. In effect, the extraluminal pressure on the veins increases, so the transmural pressure decreases, and venous blood is shifted centrally. This *muscle pump* plays a significant role in quickly increasing the blood available to the heart during exercise [25].

Respiratory Pump. During *inspiration*, intrapleural pressure (P_{pl}) becomes more negative. This assists the filling of the heart by increasing the pressure difference across the walls of each chamber (i.e., the transmural pressure). Moreover, contraction of the

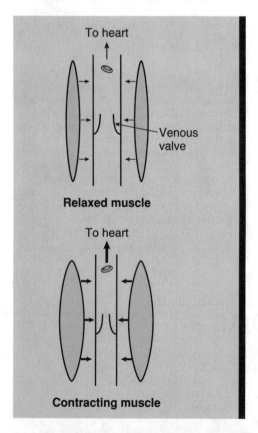

To heart

Venous valve

Relaxed muscle

To heart

Contracting muscle

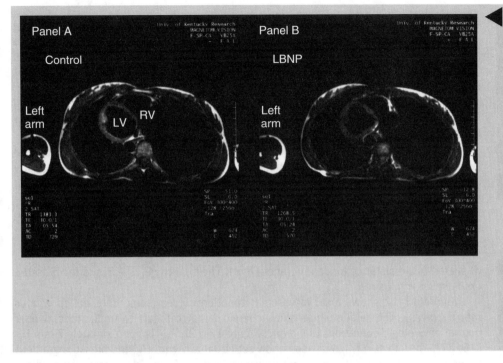

FIGURE 13-11
End-Diastolic Ventricular Size of the Human Heart before and during Pooling of Blood in Lower Body. A volunteer in the supine position was fitted with a lower body negative pressure (LBNP) device. The photographs were made using magnetic resonance imaging, and they show a cross section of the subject's body through the heart. In panel A, no negative pressure was applied to the lower body, so blood was distributed normally for a person in the horizontal position. Panel B was made during the application of the LBNP device, which caused blood to pool in the lower body, similar to what occurs in going from the supine to the standing position. Note the decrease in ventricular volume that occurred as a result of the inhibition of ventricular filling. RV = right ventricle; LV = left ventricle. (Source: The photographs were provided by L. Hilaire, J. Evans, C. Knapp, and J. Kirsch, Center for Biomedical Engineering, University of Kentucky College of Medicine, Lexington, Kentucky.)

diaphragm compresses the contents of the abdomen, increasing intra-abdominal pressure. This decreases the transmural pressure within the abdominal vessels and, because of the one-way valves of the veins, assists movement of the blood into the thoracic cavity. During *expiration*, P_{pl} becomes less negative, which one might think would move blood out of the chest. In fact, however, the retrograde flow of blood is impeded by the action of the venous valves. This total process is known as the *respiratory pump* and assists the return of blood to the right heart.

Vascular Function Curve and the Control of CO

The recognition that the pumping action of the heart and the flow of blood through the peripheral circulation (and the pulmonary circulation) are tightly coupled and highly coordinated has produced one of the major conceptual advances in the understanding of the control of CO and arterial blood pressure. Much of the credit for these developments belongs to Dr. Arthur Guyton and his colleagues [26, 27], who developed the concepts of *venous return* and of the *vascular function curve*. At the center of these concepts is the immutable fact that, *in the steady state, CO equals venous return*.

A very simple way to understand these relations is to compare the "voyage" of the blood around the circulation to the orbit of a comet around the sun. At some point far out in space, the comet reaches its furthest distance from the sun (apogee) and starts its return trip. Likewise, one can imagine that at some point near the capillaries the blood also starts its return trip to the heart. As is explained below, the return trip can be considered to start where blood pressure falls below mean circulatory pressure.

Mean Circulatory Pressure. The simple model of the circulation in Chapter 3, Figure 3-4 demonstrated that the pressure inside the arteries and veins was *equal* when the pump was off and that this pressure was *not zero*. Although this latter fact may not have been obvious at first, it is clear upon reflection that the pressure in the fluid filling any elastic (i.e., compliant) container, such as the circulation, must be greater than zero, as long as the volume of fluid exceeds the amount needed to fill the container (i.e., the unstressed vascular volume). The concept of *mean circulatory pressure* (P_{mc}) can be visualized by imagining what would happen if the heart were suddenly to stop pumping, and there were no reflexes. It is easy to see that arterial pressure would fall rapidly, but it takes some thought to realize that *central venous pressure* would gradually *rise*. At least in theory the two pressures would converge at a value equal to P_{mc}. P_{mc} is, therefore, the pressure that would be measured in the circulation if one could instantaneously stop the heart and immediately redistribute blood around the circulation at the new equilibrium. P_{mc} is determined by the total volume of blood in the system and the overall compliance of the

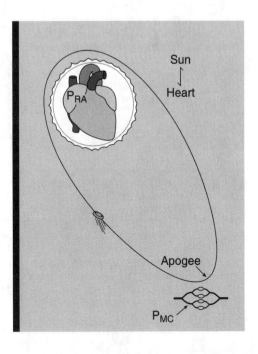

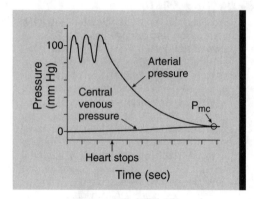

This equation is another example of a hydraulic equivalent to Ohm's law, where VR
is a flow rate in liters/minute. The resistance to venous return, which equals
1/k, is small, although changes in its value
are physiologically significant.

arterial and venous systems. In a sense, therefore, one can regard the blood as crossing from the arterial "side" of the circulation to the venous "side" of the circulation at the point where blood pressure falls just below P_{mc}. The value of P_{mc} in the control state is generally given as approximately 7 mm Hg. This is the basis for an important concept called the *pressure gradient for venous return*.

Pressure Gradient for Venous Return. As with any fluid flow, there must be a pressure difference that drives the flow of blood back to the heart, or venous return (VR). Given that the return voyage starts at a pressure equal to P_{mc}, the only remaining issue is the pressure at the end of the journey. Sometimes this end pressure is simply called central venous pressure, but it seems pedagogically advantageous to be more precise and specify it as right atrial pressure (P_{RA}) since this is the pressure at the end of the journey, that is, the entrance to the heart. It is an easy task to construct the equation for the vascular function curve as developed by Guyton and colleagues [26, 27] once one accepts these designations:

$$VR = k(P_{mc} - P_{RA})$$

where "k" is a resistance (or conductance) term. The quantity $P_{mc} - P_{RA}$ is *the pressure gradient for venous return.*

Figure 13-12 shows a set of vascular function curves (sometimes called *venous return curves*). The relationships shown here are not difficult to understand. Under normal physiologic conditions (*solid line*, Figure 13-12), P_{mc} is approximately 7 mm Hg [26, 27]. Therefore, if P_{RA} were somehow set equal to 7 mm Hg, the pressure gradient would be zero. As a result, venous return would be zero. As P_{RA} decreases, the gradient increases, and venous return must increase. In fact, recall from the discussion of Chapter 3, Figure 3-4 that right atrial pressure *decreased* when the pump was turned on. If P_{RA} were to fall below P_{pl}, the transmural pressure across the venous wall would no longer exceed 0 mm Hg. This limits further increases in venous return and explains the flattening of the curve at low P_{RA} values. Increasing venomotor tone (or increasing blood volume) shifts the curve to the right (i.e., increases P_{mc}). Decreased blood volume or decreased venomotor tone has the opposite effect.

FIGURE 13-12
Relationship Between Venous Return (VR) and Right Atrial Pressure (P_{RA}). The vascular function curve is a graphic representation of the equation $VR = k(P_{mc} - P_{RA})$, where k represents hydraulic conductance (assumed for the moment to be constant) and P_{mc} is the mean circulatory pressure. If P_{RA} decreases from a positive value, the pressure gradient for VR increases. This explains the increase in VR as P_{RA} decreases from 7 mm Hg toward 0 mm Hg. Adding blood to the circulation or decreasing the compliance of the venous system by venoconstriction shifts the curve to the right.

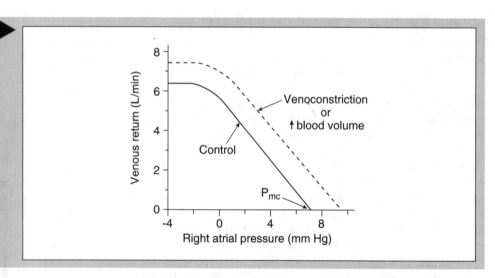

Although Starling's law of the heart has
been presented in terms of left ventricular
function, the concepts are equally valid for
the right ventricle. In this case, right ventricular CO would appear on the y-axis and
right ventricular preload on the x-axis. In
fact, it really does not matter whether Starling's law of the heart is discussed in terms
of the right or left ventricle because, in the
steady state, right ventricular SV and left
ventricular SV are equal.

Coupling of the Frank-Starling Relationship and of the Vascular Function Curve. Starling's law of the heart relates CO and ventricular preload. Figure 13-13 shows the coupling of CO, as represented by Starling's law of the heart, and of venous return, as represented by the vascular function curve. Because CO equals VR (in the steady state), the ordinate (y-axis) in this graph can legitimately be used to plot either variable. Likewise, the usual designation for the abscissa (x-axis) is end-diastolic pressure; however, because the atrioventricular valves are open during diastole, right atrial pressure and right ventricular pressure are essentially the same during the filling phase of the cardiac cycle. Therefore, the abscissa can legitimately be used to plot either variable. *This is why Starling's law of the heart and the vascular function curve can be plotted on the same coordinates.* It is quickly obvious from Figure 13-13 that *CO and venous return* are equal at only one point: the intersection of the two curves. In the steady state, therefore, the values of CO and venous return must conform to this operating point.

Control of CO and Venous Return. One of the major questions dealt with in this and preceding chapters has been "What controls CO?" A more complete answer to that question can now be given. Figure 13-14 shows a set of Starling vascular function curves for an individual at rest (*solid lines*) and for a state of elevated SNA (*broken lines*). Notice the following specific points:

- The increase in SNA shifted the Starling curve upward and to the left, in accordance with the definition of an increase in contractility (see Chapter 10).
- The increase in SNA also shifted the vascular function curve to the right, as reflected in an increase in P_{mc}; this conforms with the known effects of increased venomotor tone on venous compliance.
- CO, as indicated by the intersection of the Starling curve and the vascular function curve, increased as a result of the elevated SNA, in this case with only a small increase in preload.

Because the cardiovascular system is a closed loop—a *circulation*—it makes no sense to ask whether the action of the nervous system on the heart or on the vasculature was responsible for the increased CO and venous return. The salient point is that *the nervous system is able to use both the intrinsic and extrinsic properties of circulatory function to assure that the needs of the tissues for increased delivery of oxygenated blood are met.*

Students are often confused because Figure 13-13 shows that an increase in P_{RA} increases CO/VR in one situation (Starling's law of the heart) and decreases them in another (the vascular function curve). How can both be true at the same time? Actually, this results from a balance of forces, which is not at all unusual in everyday experience. For example, increasing the gas delivered to an airplane engine tends to increase the speed of the plane. Conversely, the plane encounters increased resistance from the air as its speed increases because of the increased fuel delivery; this tends to impede the plane's speed. The actual new forward velocity of the plane (and the actual value of CO and VR at any given P_{RA}) results from a balance between these opposing forces. Only in space, where there is no opposing resistive force, will the steady burn of a rocket engine produce a continuously increasing speed.

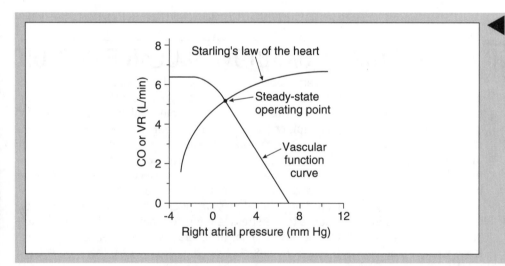

FIGURE 13-13
Steady-State Relationship Between Starling's Law and the Vascular Function Curve. *Because the circulation is a closed system, venous return (VR) and cardiac output (CO) must be equal over the long run. Therefore, the steady-state values of CO and VR are given by the point of intersection of these two curves. These concepts were developed by Dr. Arthur Guyton and colleagues [26, 27].*

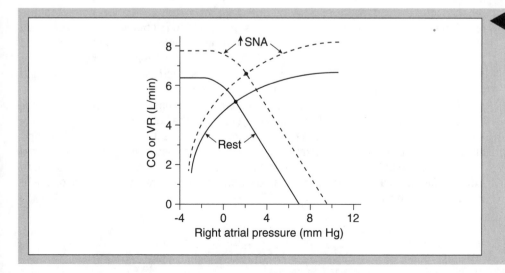

FIGURE 13-14
Effect of an Increase in Sympathetic Nervous Activity (SNA) on the Relationship Between Starling's Law of the Heart and the Vascular Function Curve. *At rest, when SNA is relatively low, the Frank-Starling relationship and the vascular function curve intersect at the point shown by the two solid lines. Increased levels of SNA shift both curves upward so that the steady-state operating point for VR and CO is elevated. If the increase in SNA was associated with exercise, this example would show how the nervous system coordinates cardiac and vascular performance to meet the needs of the circulation for increased delivery of oxygenated blood.*

LONG-TERM REGULATION OF ARTERIAL BLOOD PRESSURE

"Plasma volume" is shown at the bottom right of Figure 13-6 with no inputs, as though it played no active role in the regulation of arterial blood pressure. However, nothing could be further from the truth. Indeed, Figure 13-9 shows three nested cycles that help regulate plasma volume. Consequently, this latter diagram begins to show how plasma volume is actually an active partner in the regulation of arterial pressure. There is, moreover, an additional mechanism, called *pressure diuresis*, whereby the kidney contributes to the regulation of arterial pressure by means of changes in plasma volume [27]. Pressure diuresis means that an increase in the blood pressure perfusing the kidney causes an increase in urine formation. The *increase* in urinary water (and salt) loss from the body *decreases* plasma volume; this critical inverse relationship allows the cycle to help stabilize pressure. The direct relationship between renal perfusion pressure and urinary volume output is intrinsic to the way the kidney operates. The mechanism involves changes in the tubular reabsorption of Na^+ and water (see Chapter 7, Figure 7-2A). Pressure diuresis endows the circulation with a long-term stability independent of the nervous or endocrine systems.

Figure 13-6 diagrams the neurally mediated baroreflex, and so it intentionally does not include pressure diuresis. However, all that would have been required to include this mechanism is a *dashed arrow* from "arterial pressure" to "plasma volume." Therefore, it should now be clear that plasma volume, by virtue of multiple neural, hormonal, and intrinsic regulatory pathways, plays a critically important role in the regulation of arterial pressure and CO.

OPEN-LOOP REGULATION OF CARDIOVASCULAR FUNCTION

There are circumstances, which are probably more common than realized, when the CNS does not depend exclusively on biofeedback reflexes to regulate cardiopulmonary function. This is sometimes referred to as a *feed-forward* mechanism (see Chapter 1), sometimes as an *open-loop* control, or sometimes as *central command*. Figure 13-15 shows SNA and changes in mean arterial blood pressure (ΔmBP) recorded from a rat trained in an emotional conditioning test. The rat was resting quietly prior to the beginning of the behavioral challenge. The onset of the stress stimulus evoked a sudden, large burst of nerve activity that *preceded* an increase in arterial blood pressure. This temporal relationship, and the lack of any drop in blood pressure prior to the burst in nerve activity, indicates that this initial response to the stress stimulus did not behave like a biofeedback mechanism. Instead, the sudden burst has the characteristics expected of an open-loop response produced by the CNS independently of the baroreflex or other biofeedback mechanisms [28]. SNA decreased briefly after its initial increase; however, within 2–3 seconds after the sudden burst, SNA increased approximately 27% above control for the remainder of the stress. Likewise, blood pressure started to fall but was then moderately elevated along with the increase in SNA. One reasonable interpretation of these data is that the initial open-loop response was followed almost immediately by an upward *resetting* of the baroreflex (i.e., producing the sustained increase in SNA) so that blood pressure remained elevated during the later seconds of the stress.

This experiment illustrates the complicated interactions that undoubtedly occur between the "higher" centers of the nervous system and the homeostatic reflexes in daily life [25, 29]. Figure 13-16 summarizes the probable interaction of the open-loop and biofeedback pathways in the regulation of arterial blood pressure. As Chapter 1 explains, the combination of these two mechanisms permits the body to adjust blood pressure to external and internal challenges more rapidly and more effectively than the use of one or the other system alone.

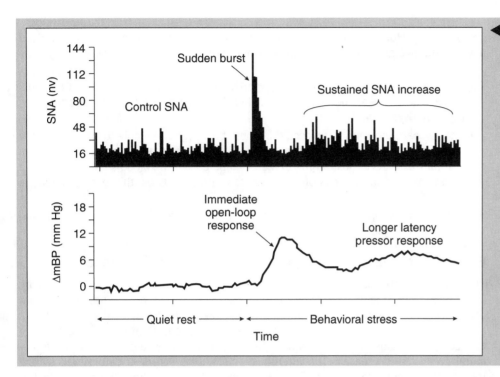

FIGURE 13-15
Sympathetic Nerve Activity (SNA) and Changes in Mean Arterial Blood Pressure (ΔmBP) during Sudden Behavioral Stress in the Rat. Pavlovian conditioning was used to train the rat in an acute stress paradigm [28]. Multifiber SNA was recorded as in Figure 13-3. The calibration marks on the x-axis designate 3-second intervals. There was a sudden, intense burst of SNA within approximately 0.5 seconds after the beginning of the stressful stimulus. This barrage of nerve impulses was followed almost immediately by an initial increase in arterial blood pressure. This first sequence of events represents an open-loop response because it did not depend on earlier changes in blood pressure that were fed back into the neuronal circuits of the baroreflex. SNA and blood pressure dropped momentarily, but then they increased again, perhaps because the baroreflex was reset to regulate arterial pressure at a higher level during the stress.

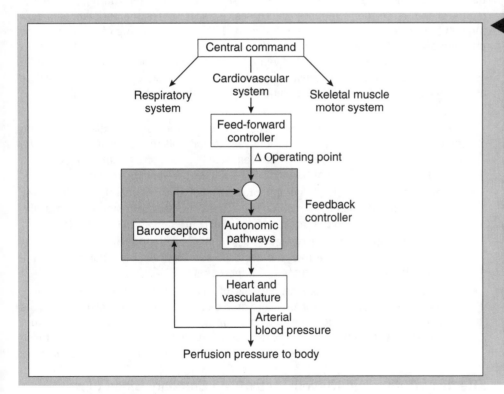

FIGURE 13-16
Scheme for the Coordination of Open-Loop and Baroreflex Feedback Mechanisms for the Regulation of Blood Pressure during Exercise. The model shows how the brain provides efferent nervous activity to the skeletal muscles to produce the exercise and to the respiratory system to increase ventilation. It also formulates an open-loop, or feed-forward output to regions within the brain controlling blood pressure. This model assumes that these influences are exerted by changing the set point of the baroreflex, although other mechanisms are possible. That portion of the picture enclosed within the shaded box is a simplified version of Figure 13-6. Blood pressure is the output from the heart and vasculature (i.e., the effectors) and is "fed back" via the baroreflex. Blood pressure also constitutes the pressure that perfuses blood through the entire circulation. (Source: Adapted with permission from Rowell LB: Human Cardiovascular Control. New York, NY: Oxford University Press, 1993, p 463.)

AUTONOMIC NEURAL INFLUENCES ON CORONARY VASCULAR FUNCTION

Blood flow through the coronary vessels is regulated by the same influences explained in Chapter 12 for other regional circulations. In fact, *coronary blood flow in people who do not have severe coronary artery disease is increased by vasodilation or decreased by vasoconstriction in proportion to metabolic requirements of the myocardium for oxy-*

The venous blood draining most circulations contains significant residual amounts of oxygen (i.e., only approximately 20%–25% of the oxygen originally present in the arterial blood is used). Therefore, organs other than the heart can meet increased metabolic demands, at least partially, by extracting a relatively greater percentage of the oxygen contained in the blood perfusing their capillary beds.

genated blood. However, there are some special considerations relevant to coronary blood flow and its regulation that have critically important clinical implications:

- The myocardium cannot sustain an oxygen debt for any extended period of time. This is because the heart never rests and, therefore, has only a limited opportunity to repay an oxygen debt.
- The myocardium cannot increase the amount of oxygen available to it by increasing its extraction of oxygen from the arterial blood. This is because the myocardium normally extracts almost all the oxygen available from the blood so that the oxygen content of coronary venous blood is very low; in other words, the *extraction ratio* is very high.
- Blood flow through the coronary vessels supplying the left ventricle is *low* during *systole* and higher during diastole because of the throttle effect.

Effect of Extravascular Compression on Left Coronary Blood Flow

The *throttle effect* occurs because the coronary vessels within the left ventricular wall are surrounded by muscle. When the myocardium contracts, it compresses these vessels and decreases their internal diameter. In other words, the pressure outside the blood vessels rises during systole because of the muscle's contraction. Therefore, the difference between the intraluminal pressure and the extraluminal pressure—that is, the transmural pressure—decreases. The internal diameter of a vessel is determined by the transmural pressure (see Chapter 3), so as transmural pressure drops during systole, the radius of the vessel concomitantly decreases. This increases the resistance to flow through the vessels, and flow decreases. Figure 13-17 is a recording of left ventricular pressure and the flow of blood through the left circumflex coronary artery. Circumflex coronary flow decreases at the onset of ventricular contraction and remains low throughout systole. Peak flow to the left ventricular myocardium occurs early in diastole. There are several clinically relevant consequences of the throttle effect:

*The **throttle effect** is not unique to the left ventricle. Flow also decreases momentarily through arterial vessels within skeletal muscle as it contracts. This is the reason why sustained isometric exercise can cause arterial blood pressure to increase, sometimes remarkably so. In phasic exercise, however, the contractions are usually of short duration, so the resulting oxygen debt can be repaid during periods of rest. The effects of extravascular compression are much lower in the right ventricle than in the left ventricle. In fact, because right ventricular pressure is generally 40 mm Hg or less, the corresponding intramyocardial pressure is always less than the pressure inside the larger coronary arteries. Therefore, the flow through the vessels supplying the right ventricle is more like that of the general circulation because it is high during systole and drops during diastole.*

- The extravascular compression is less severe within the subepicardial muscle and increases across the width of the left ventricular wall to high values nearer the subendocardium. Therefore, the left ventricular subendocardium experiences a much greater drop in flow during systole than does the subepicardium.
- Systole occupies a relatively greater proportion of the total cardiac cycle during tachycardia as compared to resting HR. Therefore, the decrease in myocardial perfusion attributable to the throttle effect is accentuated at high HRs.
- The positive inotropic effects of elevated SNA increase the magnitude of the extravascular compression. Therefore, the decrease in myocardial perfusion attributable to the throttle effect is accentuated with increases in SNA.
- The pressure inside the coronary vessels of people with severe coronary artery disease is decreased due to the pressure drop caused by the atherosclerotic plaques (i.e., similar to the obstruction in the community water supply in Chapter 3, Figure 3-1). Therefore, the effects of the extravascular compression can be serious in these individuals, especially in the innermost layers of the left ventricular myocardium.

*Because of the greater extravascular compression near the subendocardium, a myocardial infarction in persons with coronary artery disease can be restricted to this region, sparing more superficial muscle. In other cases, the infarction involves the entire thickness of the wall within the affected region. These are called **transmural infarctions**.*

Effects of Autonomic Nervous Activity on Coronary Blood Flow

The coronary arterioles are innervated by α-adrenergic vasoconstrictor fibers. These nerves can momentarily decrease coronary flow, but generally within seconds the increase in myocardial metabolic demand that accompanies elevated cardiac sympathetic drive augments coronary flow. Animal studies have shown transient increases in coronary vascular resistance during behavioral stress attributable to increased sympathetic vasoconstriction [30]. Scientists are now testing the hypothesis that neurally mediated coronary vasoconstrictor effects, such as might occur during behavioral stress, may be dangerous in people with advanced coronary artery disease and might help trigger myocardial infarctions in some of these individuals [31, 32]. Interested students should refer to Feigl [33] for further analysis of adrenergic coronary vasoconstriction.

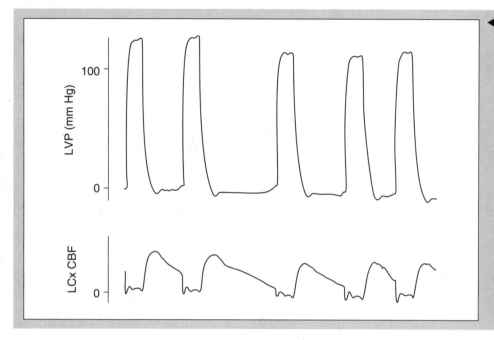

FIGURE 13-17
Simultaneous Recordings of Left Ventricular Pressure (LVP) and Blood Flow Through the Left Circumflex Coronary Artery. The recordings were made in a dog with a normal coronary circulation using a flow probe placed around the left circumflex coronary artery and a pressure transducer inserted inside the left ventricular cavity. The systolic throttle effect decreased left circumflex coronary blood flow (LCx CBF) during systole.

SUMMARY

Blood pressure, CO, and many other cardiovascular variables are carefully controlled by neurohumoral regulatory mechanisms and by the intrinsic properties of the heart and circulation. Together, these stabilize the cardiovascular system even in the face of serious challenges. More specifically, the arterial baroreceptors buffer moment-to-moment changes in blood pressure, resulting from changes in posture or other sudden perturbations. The baroreceptors accomplish this by making appropriate adjustments in the heart's pumping ability and by controlling the operating characteristics of the peripheral vasculature. One of the body's marvels is how the autonomic nervous system and intrinsic properties of the circulation match venous return and CO. The regulation of total blood volume is also an essential aspect of the overall control of cardiopulmonary function, particularly regarding the long-term maintenance of normal arterial blood pressure. Physicians must consider all aspects of the regulation of the heart and circulation when evaluating the cardiovascular status of their patients, especially those patients with coronary artery disease [34]. Therapy targeted at a single cardiovascular entity may not ultimately be in the best interest of the patient because it may ignore other pathologic processes that are hidden by the adaptive properties of the cardiopulmonary system.

RESOLUTION OF CLINICAL CASE

Peripheral blood pooling caused by gravity upon standing explains why even completely normal people may occasionally experience *orthostatic hypotension* that results in a feeling of faintness. The circulation has several physiologic defenses against this *postural hypotension*. First, the myocardium's compliance is normally sufficiently high so that a moderate decrease in filling pressure does not dramatically compromise preload. In addition, the baroreflexes normally minimize the *depressor* effect of standing. Figure 13-18 shows the cardiovascular response of a healthy individual to lower body negative pressure, a procedure that mimics the effects of suddenly standing upright.

The patient has a disease process called *amyloidosis* in which a protein (amyloid) is deposited in the extracellular matrix beneath the endothelium of capillaries; in the walls of arterioles; and in the intercellular matrix of skeletal muscle, the heart, peripheral nerves, and other organs. The ventricular hypertrophy seen during the echocardiographic

FIGURE 13-18 ▶

Cardiovascular Response of a Healthy Person to Lower Body Negative Pressure (LBNP). Blood pressure (BP) was measured noninvasively using a probe placed on the subject's finger. Likewise, flow through the root of the aorta (Ao flow), equivalent to left ventricular stroke volume, was measured by a beam of ultrasound from a probe placed at the suprasternal notch. The individual was initially supine and resting quietly; no LBNP was applied (0–6 sec). LBNP was then initiated to simulate the pooling of blood that occurs upon standing from the prone position. Note the drop in Ao flow and BP that started to occur at approximately 14–15 seconds. The increase in heart rate (HR) is a reflex response that started to restore BP toward normal levels by approximately 24 seconds. (Source: These data were provided courtesy of Ms. Joyce Evans and Dr. David Brown, Center for Biomedical Engineering, University of Kentucky College of Medicine, Lexington, Kentucky.)

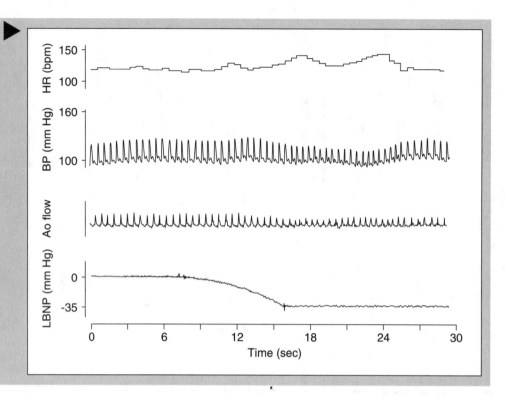

*This is a clinical example where pressure is measured in centimeters of blood rather than millimeters of mercury. Blood does not normally engorge the jugular vein in the upright or sitting position. The jugular veins of this patient, however, were filled with blood to a height of 8 cm above the heart because of the backup of blood into the veins known as **venous congestion**.*

examination is due to the accumulation of this insoluble, fibrillar, noncontractile protein. Although infiltration of the heart by amyloid protein may cause systolic dysfunction (leading to congestive heart failure), in this patient, the cardiac manifestation of the disease process is primarily in diastolic function: *increased passive stiffness of the myocardium decreases the compliance of the ventricle during filling.* As a result, the stiff muscle does not adequately accommodate venous return, thereby limiting filling (i.e., preload) and, in turn, CO. *The normal hemodynamic response to a low ventricular compliance would be for blood to "back up" or congest in the veins.* This, in turn, increases venous pressure and explains the jugular venous pressure of 8 cm.

Amyloid infiltration can also affect the autonomic nervous system. The failure of this patient's HR to increase upon standing demonstrates an *autonomic neuropathy* secondary to the amyloidosis. As a result, the baroreflex was unable to compensate effectively for the posturally induced decrease in venous return.

Finally, amyloid deposition in the kidney disrupts the glomerular capillary and allows plasma proteins to leak into the urine. This nephrotic syndrome may upset the balances of forces favoring filtration and absorption of fluid and dramatically compromise the maintenance of normal blood volume. In addition, the kidney's production of erythropoietin becomes inadequate to maintain normal red blood cell production, which explains the patient's low hematocrit.

Effective treatment of an individual with this degree of compromise in so many important adaptive mechanisms is difficult, if not impossible. The physician soon finds himself or herself facing the dilemma explained in Chapter 7, where feedback systems are no longer effective in countering external or internal challenges. This causes rapid disintegration of the organism, terminating in death [35].

REVIEW QUESTIONS

Directions: For each of the following questions, choose the **one best** answer.

1. Which one of the following statements regarding the neural control of the circulation is correct?

   (A) Increasing sympathetic adrenergic tone causes vascular smooth muscle to contract via activation of β_2-muscarinic receptors

   (B) The primary control of blood flow through the healthy coronary circulation is by sympathetic, β-adrenergic vasodilation

   (C) Physiologic levels of circulating catecholamines tend to produce vasoconstriction, especially in skeletal muscle, via activation of muscarinic receptors

   (D) Increasing the blood pressure inside the carotid sinus tends to decrease activity in the carotid sinus nerve

   (E) Increases in cardiac parasympathetic nerve activity caused by elevated pressure inside the carotid sinus tend to depress the slope of the pacemaker potential in SA-nodal cells

2. Which one of the following statements regarding the figure below is correct?

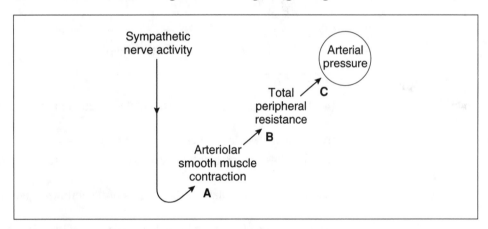

   (A) The classic neurotransmitter employed at *A* is norepinephrine, which acts on α_1-adrenergic receptors located on the cell membrane of vascular smooth muscle cells

   (B) The arrow indicated by *B* indicates that an increase in the radius of an arteriole increases the resistance to the flow of blood through the vessel

   (C) The arrow at *B* represents Starling's law of the heart

   (D) The arrow at *C* is based on the mathematical equation that blood pressure equals stroke volume multiplied by total peripheral resistance, the product of which is divided by heart rate [i.e., BP = (SV × TPR)/HR]

   (E) The arrow at *C* must be dashed if these relationships are to be part of a homeostatic cycle

3. Which one of the following anatomic locations would be the most critical area in the brain for the determination of the set point or operating point of the baroreflex?

    (A) Brainstem

    (B) Central nucleus of the amygdala

    (C) Basal ganglia

    (D) Adenohypophysis

    (E) Accessory motor cortex

4. Which one of the following statements regarding the figure below is most accurate?

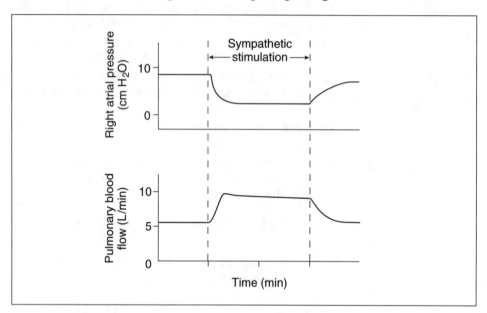

    (A) The increase in pulmonary blood flow is due to the Frank-Starling mechanism

    (B) Right ventricular preload increased during the stimulation

    (C) The pressure gradient for venous return probably increased during the stimulation

    (D) During the stimulation, the volume of blood in the great veins must have increased

    (E) Aortic blood flow must have decreased during the stimulation

5. A decrease in mean arterial blood pressure tends to result in a reflex

    (A) decrease in heart rate (HR) and increase in vascular smooth muscle contraction

    (B) tachycardia and increased left ventricular stroke volume (SV)

    (C) increase in the activity in the cardiac branches of cranial nerve X

    (D) decline in ventricular inotropism

    (E) bradycardia and an increase in left ventricular afterload

6. Which one of the following statements regarding the simple model of the circulation shown below is most accurate?

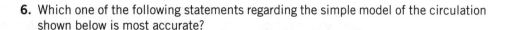
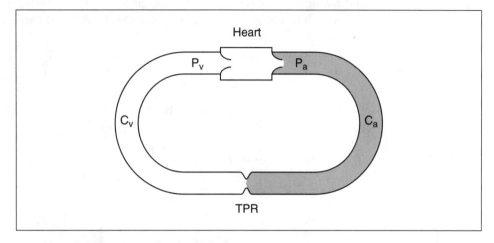

(A) When the pump is off, the compliance of the arteries (C_a) equals the compliance of the veins (C_v)

(B) When the pump is off, the pressure in the arteries (P_a) and in the veins (P_v) would have an equal value determined by the volume of fluid in the heart and the total peripheral resistance (TPR)

(C) When the pump is first turned on, P_a decreases modestly, whereas P_v increases slightly

(D) When the pump is turned on, the volume of blood in the arteries (*stippled*) increases, whereas the volume of blood in the veins (*clear*) decreases

(E) $C_v = C_a = 7$ mm Hg

7. Which one of the following statements about chronic hypertension is correct?

(A) It forces the heart to eject a given volume of blood at an increased rate of oxygen consumption

(B) The baroreflex is responsible for producing a chronic hypertension

(C) It is relatively less dangerous in persons with coronary artery disease

(D) The most effective method of treatment is administration of an α-adrenergic agonist

(E) Restricting the salt intake of a person with chronic hypertension tends to increase his or her mean circulatory pressure (P_{mc})

8. Which one of the following statements about the coronary circulation is correct?

(A) Coronary blood flow is normally controlled primarily by β-adrenergic receptors on coronary arteriolar vascular smooth muscle

(B) The coronary circulation normally receives more than 35% of the total cardiac output

(C) The oxygen content in blood drawn from the coronary sinus is lower than in mixed venous blood

(D) During exercise the highest rate of blood flow through the right coronary vessels occurs during late diastole

(E) Coronary vascular resistance is abnormally low in persons with advanced coronary artery disease

9. Assume that the heart and circulation were originally functioning at point A in the figure below and that increased sympathetic nervous activity (SNA) suddenly shifted the Starling curve upward so that cardiac output (CO) abruptly increased to the value at B. Which one of the following best describes what would happen in the next few beats if the increased inotropism were maintained?

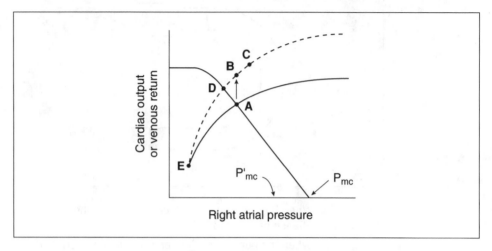

(A) CO would remain at B until the pressure gradient for venous return increased enough to return CO to A

(B) Mean circulatory pressure would decrease from P_{mc} to P'_{mc} so that CO would return to A

(C) CO would increase to C for a few beats until a decrease in venous return forced CO back to A

(D) Over a few beats, the increase in stroke volume would decrease right atrial pressure (P_{RA}) so that the heart would function at a new steady value equal to point D

(E) The heart would gradually move to point E and stop in asystole

ANSWERS AND EXPLANATIONS

1. The answer is E. The reflex response to an increase in intrasinus pressure is an increase in parasympathetic nerve activity that slows HR by depressing the spontaneous depolarization in SA-nodal pacemaker cells (see Figure 13-6). Coronary blood flow in the healthy person is primarily regulated by metabolic factors to meet myocardial oxygen demand, not by the autonomic nervous system (B). Physiologic levels of circulating epinephrine primarily produce vasodilation by activating β-receptors, especially in skeletal muscle (C).

2. The answer is A. The arrow at B indicates that smooth muscle contraction increases total peripheral resistance; this represents Poiseuille's law (B and C). These relationships are only a component of a feedback cycle; a complete cycle must be "closed" and have an odd number of inverse relationships to be homeostatic.

3. The answer is A. Although many areas of the brain participate to some degree in the regulation of blood pressure, the brainstem is the crucial region for mediating the baroreflex. The hypothalamus also interacts strongly with the medulla in modulating the baroreflex.

4. The answer is C. The heart transferred more blood from the right atrium into the pulmonary circulation during the sympathetic stimulation, so right atrial pressure decreased. This increases the pressure gradient for venous return and must have helped increase venous return to match the augmented right ventricular stroke volume. The decrease in right atrial pressure indicates a decrease in right ventricular preload (B) and a decrease in the volume of blood in the great veins (D). It is very likely that aortic flow also increased (E), or blood would have congested within the lungs.

5. The answer is B. When arterial blood pressure decreases, the pressure inside the carotid sinus decreases. The fall in carotid sinus pressure is signaled to the brain, which, in turn, produces an increase in sympathetic nerve activity (SNA). The rise in SNA increases HR and SV. This sequence of events is portrayed in Figure 3-6.

6. The answer is D. With each stroke volume, the heart translocates blood from the low-pressure side of the circulation to the high-pressure side (D). When the heart stops, therefore, it swells in size as blood accumulates within it. When the pump is off, P_a and P_v are equal (that value being the mean circulatory pressure—P_{mc}), which is determined by total blood volume and the overall compliance of the heart and circulation (B). The P_{mc} (not C_a or C_v) is normally approximately 7 mm Hg (E).

7. The answer is A. This decrease in efficiency and increase in metabolic load is one of the reasons that chronic hypertension is so deleterious, especially in persons with coronary artery disease which makes option C incorrect. It is unlikely that the baroreflex is directly responsible for hypertension (B). Physicians should be careful about exposing patients with high blood pressure to α-adrenergic agonists, which would further exacerbate their problems.

8. The answer is C. The coronary circulation normally has a very high oxygen extraction ratio. People with coronary artery disease may be able to maintain adequate blood flow to the myocardium at rest by vasodilating the peripheral coronary vessels. However, this leaves them with little or no vasodilatory reserve during exercise or other such challenge.

9. The answer is D. If it were possible for CO to increase instantaneously to the value at B in response to an increased sympathetic drive, end-systolic volume must decrease (see, point 9 in Chapter 10, Figure 10-7). The heart would, in effect, decrease its volume and P_{RA}, until it was able within a few heartbeats to operate at a new steady-state value at D. This shift is often shown as a series of progressive, stair-step changes extending from B to D.

REFERENCES

1. Hering HE: *Die Karotidsinus Reflexe auf Herz und Gefasse.* Leipzig, Ger: D. Steinkopff, 1927.
2. Heymans C: *Le Sinus Carotidien.* London, UK: H. K. Lewis, 1929.
3. Koch E: *Die Reflektorische selbsteuerung des Kreislaufes.* Leipzig, Ger: D. Steinkopff, 1931.
4. Randall WC, Wurster RD, Randall DC, et al: From cardioaccelerator and inhibitory nerves to a "heart brain." In *Nervous Control of the Heart.* Edited by Shepherd JT, Vatner SF. Amsterdam, Neth: Harwood Academic, 1996, pp 173–199.
5. Bronk DW, Stella G: The response to steady pressures of single end organs in the isolated carotid sinus. *Am J Physiol* 110:708–714, 1935.
6. Franz GN, Scher AM, Ito CS: Small signal characteristics of carotid sinus baroreceptors of rabbits. *J Applied Physiol* 30:527–535, 1971.
7. Dampney R: The subretrofacial nucleus: its pivotal role in cardiovascular regulation. *News Physiol Sci* 5:63–67, 1990.
8. Sved AF, Gordon FJ: Amino acids as central neurotransmitters in the baroreceptor reflex pathway. *News Physiol Sci* 9:243–246, 1994.
9. Loewy AD, Spyer KM: *Central Regulation of Autonomic Function.* New York, NY: Oxford University Press, 1990.
10. Spyer KM: Central nervous mechanisms contributing to cardiovascular control. *J Physiol* 474:1–19, 1994.

11. Dampney RAL: Functional organization of central pathways regulating the cardio-vascular system. *Physiol Rev* 74:323–364, 1994.

12. Brown DR, Cowley AW: Computer analysis of continuous data collection. *J Miss Acad Sci* 17:65, 1971.

13. Cowley AW, Liard JF, Guyton AC: Role of the baroreceptor reflex in daily control of arterial blood pressure and other variables in dogs. *Circ Res* 32:564–576, 1973.

14. Persson PB, Ehmke H, Kirchheim HR: Cardiopulmonary-arterial baroreceptor interaction in control of blood pressure. *News Physiol Sci* 4:56–59, 1989.

15. Thames MD, Smith ML, Dibner-Dunlap ME, Minisi AJ: Reflexes governing autonomic outflow to the heart. In *Nervous Control of the Heart*. Edited by Shepherd JT, Vatner SF. Amsterdam, Neth: Harwood Academic, 1996, pp 295–327.

16. Smith ML, Thames MD: Cardiac receptors: discharge characteristics and reflex effects. In *Neurocardiology*. Edited by Armour JA, Ardell JL. New York, NY: Oxford University Press, 1994, pp 19–52.

17. Share L: Control of vasopressin release: an old but continuing story. *News Physiol Sci* 11:7–13, 1996.

18. Hirsch AT, Levenson DJ, Cutler SS, et al: Regional vascular responses to prolonged lower body negative pressure in normal subjects. *Am J Physiol* 257:H219–H225, 1989.

19. Simpson JB, Routtenberg A: Subfornical organ: site of drinking elicited by angiotensin II. *Science* 181:1172–1175, 1973.

20. Moffett BR, Bumpus FM, Husain A: Cellular organization of the brain renin-angiotensin system. *Life Sci* 41:1867–1879, 1987.

21. Yamashita H, Kannan H: Inhibition of hypothalamic neurons by the atrial natriuretic peptide family. *News Physiol Sci* 7:75–79, 1992.

22. Johnson AK, Loewy AD: Circumventricular organs and their role in visceral functions. In *Central Regulation of Autonomic Functions*. Edited by Lowey AD, Spyer KM. New York, NY: Oxford University Press, 1990, pp 247–267.

23. Hainsworth R: The importance of vascular capacitance in cardiovascular control. *News Physiol Sci* 5:250–254, 1990.

24. Brunner MJ, Greene AS, Frankle AE, et al: Carotid sinus baroreceptor control of splanchnic resistance and capacity. *Am J Physiol* 255:H1305–H1310, 1988.

25. Rowell LD: *Human Cardiovascular Control*. New York, NY: Oxford University Press, 1993.

26. Guyton AC, Jones CE, Coleman TG: *Circulatory Physiology: Cardiac Output and Its Regulation*, 2nd ed. Philadelphia, PA: W. B. Saunders, 1973.

27. Guyton AC, Coleman TG, Cowley AW: A system analysis approach to understanding long-range arterial blood pressure control and hypertension. *Circ Res* 35:159–176, 1974.

28. Randall DC, Brown DR, Brown LV, et al: Sympathetic nervous activity and arterial blood pressure control in the conscious rat during rest and behavioral stress. *Am J Physiol* 267:R1241–R1249, 1994.

29. Stella A, Golin R, Zanchetti A: Sympathorenal interactions in the control of cardiovascular functions. *News Physiol Sci* 5:237–241, 1990.

30. Billman GE, Randall DC: Mechanisms mediating the coronary vascular response to behavioral stress in the dog. *Circ Res* 48:214–223, 1981.

31. Kamarck T, Jennings JR: Biobehavioral factors in sudden cardiac death. *Psychol Bull* 109:42–75, 1991.

32. Verrier RL, Dickerson LW, Nearing BD: Behavioral states and sudden cardiac death. *PACE* 15:1387–1393, 1992.

33. Feigl EO: The paradox of adrenergic coronary vasoconstriction. *Circulation* 76:737–745, 1987.

34. Engelberg J: *The Nature of Integrative Study*. Stillwater, OK: New Forums Press, 1994.

35. Engelberg J: On the dynamics of dying. *Integrative Physiol Behav Sci* 32:143–148, 1997.

14 THE RESPIRATORY PUMP

INTRODUCTION OF CLINICAL CASE

A soldier was brought directly from the battlefield to a medical unit. He was unconscious and in obvious respiratory distress and exhibited very little muscle movement. The medics related that the patient was the only survivor found in the immediate area. His arterial blood gases revealed a Pa_{O_2} of 50 mm Hg and a Pa_{CO_2} of 75 mm Hg. Normal reflexes were greatly diminished. Physical examination revealed no apparent injuries that suggested damage to the brainstem. Administration of 100% oxygen was considered, but artificial ventilation was chosen instead.

INTRODUCTION

The respiratory pump is composed entirely of striated muscle innervated by the somatic nervous system. Each muscle fiber is part of a motor unit and possesses a neuromuscular junction with cholinergic receptors to bind the neurotransmitter acetylcholine (ACh). Al-

> **Case Relevance**
> One cause of respiratory muscle weakness is failure of the myoneural junction.

though smooth muscle is important in controlling airway diameter, it does not play a role in generating the pressures required for movement of air. As discussed in Chapter 5, the respiratory pump is often regarded as two separate pumps: one for inspiration and one for expiration. These pumps are responsible for maintaining appropriate ventilation and lung volumes.

LUNG VOLUMES

The size and shape of the lungs are determined by their elastic properties, the distending forces exerted by the respiratory musculature, and the structures of the rib cage and abdomen. During the respiratory cycle, muscular contractions are responsible for changing the shape of the thoracic cavity and subsequently the lungs. Lung volume changes cause changes in pressure, which in turn cause *ventilation* or the movement of air. These volumes are measured with a *spirometer*. The names of the various components of ventilation seen in typical spirometer recordings are shown in Figure 14-1. The fundamental units that are not further subdivided are defined as *volumes; capacity* refers to the addition of two or more volumes.

FIGURE 14-1 ▶
Spirometer Tracing of Important Lung Volumes and Capacities from a Typical Young Adult Man. *Inspiratory volumes are illustrated as upward deflections. Three normal tidal breaths are followed by a maximal inspiration and a 5-second breathhold, before proceeding with a maximal forced expiratory effort. FEV_1 = forced expiratory volume in 1 second; IRV = inspiratory reserve volume; V_T = tidal volume; ERV = expiratory reserve volume; RV = residual volume; IC = inspiratory capacity; FRC = functional residual capacity; VC = vital capacity; FVC = forced vital capacity.*

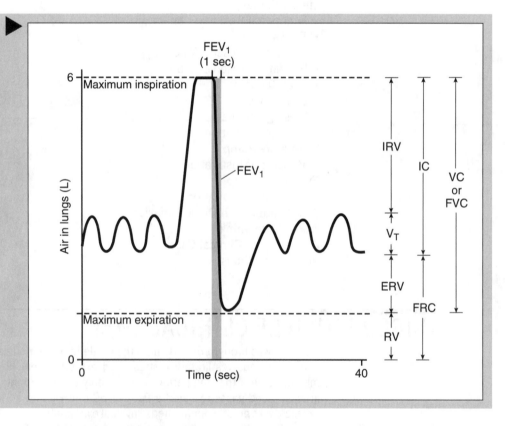

Functional Residual Capacity

The functional residual capacity (FRC) reflects the amount of air normally remaining in the lung at the end of passive expiration. It is the sum of two volumes: the *residual volume* (RV) and the *expiratory reserve volume* (ERV). The RV is 1–1.5 L of air in the lungs that cannot be expired regardless of the strength of the exhalation. This volume prevents collapse of the alveoli and contributes to the reservoir function of the FRC. The ERV represents the lung volume that can be emptied beyond the limits of normal tidal volume by active contraction of the expiratory muscles to increase expiratory effort. With exercise, some of this volume is exhaled with each breath to increase the amount of air moved.

At rest with no respiratory muscle activity and with an open glottis, the lung elastic forces that tend to collapse the lung are balanced by the opposing forces exerted by the

At sea level, the inspired oxygen concentration (P_IO_2) is about 150 mm Hg. If lung volumes during expiration fell to 0, the Pao_2 could vary between 0 and 150! Instead, they tend to vary from about 95–105 during the breathing cycle.

chest wall and abdomen that act to expand the lung. At the end of a normal expiration, the balance between these forces develops a negative *intrapleural pressure* of 3–5 cm H_2O within the *intrapleural space*. "Intrapleural space" is a misnomer since the visceral pleura on the surface of the lung is separated from the parietal pleura lining the chest wall by only a very thin film of fluid that leaves no obvious "space." The pleura slide over each other with each breath. Inflammation of these tissues leads to the painful condition of *pleurisy*. The intrapleural pressure keeps the lung expanded at a total volume, the FRC. This capacity averages between 2 and 3 L in a healthy adult and is positively correlated with body size. This air serves as a reservoir for continued gas exchange during expiration and prevents large changes in the concentration of alveolar gases during the breathing cycle.

Tidal Volume

Tidal volume (V_T) is the amount of air moved by the lungs with each breath. In a resting adult, the mean V_T during quiet breathing, or *eupnea*, is approximately 0.5 L. V_T increases greatly when breathing is enhanced, such as during exercise.

Inspiratory Reserve Volume

The amount of air that can be inhaled in addition to the volume contained in the lungs at the end of a normal inspiration (when lung volume would be equal to FRC + V_T) is called the inspiratory reserve volume (IRV), a volume of 2–3 L in a normal adult. Although the respiratory muscles are capable of much greater contractions, and therefore considerable enlargement of the lungs, the human body does not often use the full extent of its respiratory reserves because this is not energetically efficient. However, with increased demand for ventilation, the human body can and does use portions of this reserve to meet metabolic demands.

> *Case Relevance*
> *When resting ventilation is inadequate, one normally begins to use the IRV to increase oxygen intake. The patient in this clinical case may have maximal neural drive; however, the respiratory muscles are not contracting appropriately.*

Expiratory Reserve Volume

When expiratory muscles are recruited, lung volumes can be decreased below FRC to the RV. This volume of air is called the expiratory reserve volume (ERV), and it averages 1.0–1.5 L. Portions of this reserve volume contribute to the increased V_T during exercise.

Vital Capacity

The total amount of air that can be moved in a single respiratory cycle by the respiratory pump is called the vital capacity (VC). The VC averages 4–6 L and is equal to the sum of the ERV, V_T, and IRV. The VC is also positively correlated with body size and negatively correlated with age. The VC plus the RV equals the *total lung capacity* (TLC). Because this capacity can change with expiratory flow rates and pressures, the clinician tends to be interested in the *forced vital capacity (FVC)*, which represents the maximal amount of air moved by a forceful expiration. Some other clinically useful measures are: the forced expiratory volume in 1 second (FEV_1), which is the volume exhaled in the first second of a maximally forced expiration; and the ratio of FEV_1 to FVC, which indicates the fraction of the FVC exhaled in the first second of a forced expiration. A healthy patient typically has an FEV_1: FVC of 0.8 or higher; however, this number can fall to very low values with severe airway obstruction.

Dead Space

The air inspired with each V_T includes the previously expired "old" air that remained in the conducting airways plus the fresh air that enters the respiratory airways. The air that participates in this gas exchange is called *alveolar ventilation* ($\dot{V}_A$), and it is usually expressed as the volume of air moved into the alveoli per minute. At the end of inspiration, the air within the conducting airways and some of the air within the transitional airways (see Chapter 5) cannot participate in gas exchange. This "wasted" air is said to occupy the *dead space* or, more precisely, the *anatomic dead space*. The volume of this dead space (V_D) in an adult is approximately 150 mL. Sometimes unperfused alveoli cause further wasting of ventilation, known as *alveolar dead space*. The alveolar dead space plus the anatomic dead space constitutes the *physiologic dead space*.

> *In a normal adult at rest, anatomic dead space is approximately 150 mL, and physiologic dead space is increased by an alveolar dead space of only a few more milliliters. Physiologic dead space is the most meaningful parameter because it represents all of the wasted ventilation.*

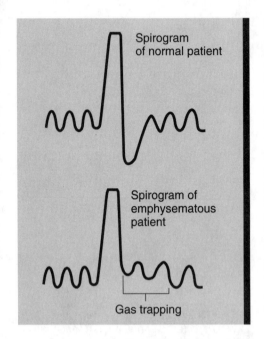

Spirogram
of normal patient

Spirogram of
emphysematous
patient

Gas trapping

Closing Volumes

Because of uneven transmural pressures within the lungs, some airways are likely to collapse as the lung volume decreases during a forced expiration. The pressure outside the small airways may exceed the pressure inside, creating a *Starling resistor* and compression of the airways. The air trapped within these collapsed airways increases the functional RV. The total amount of air in the lung at the end of a forced expiration is known as the *closing capacity*, which is the sum of the residual volume and the *closing volume*. For young, healthy individuals, the closing volumes are relatively small, and the closing capacity approximates the RV. With age, however, the closing volume may approach the ERV. Similarly, high closing volumes can be observed in disease states. To prevent this "gas trapping," many patients with emphysema exhale through pursed lips to maintain high pressures inside the airways during expiration. This decreases transmural pressures, thereby preventing airway collapse. Because of the extensive gas trapping (i.e., high closing volumes) that occurs with forced expiration in these patients, their measured FVC will be considerably smaller than their VC. If they are permitted to exhale their total VC slowly, the airways are more likely to remain patent, and the closing volume will be smaller. Unfortunately, the times when a larger VC is needed usually coincide with the need for faster, more vigorous breathing. Therefore, elevated closing volumes can pose a serious hindrance to adequate ventilation.

Minute Ventilation

Cardiac output = heart rate × stroke volume
Minute ventilation = respiratory frequency × tidal volume
Alveolar ventilation = respiratory frequency × tidal volume − volume of dead space

The volumes and capacities described above are determined from a single breath; however, the purpose of the respiratory pump is to move air continuously. Moving an adequate volume of air per minute is essential to meet metabolic demands. Similar to the cardiac output (CO) of the heart, the respiratory output is determined in liters per minute (L/min) and is the product of the amount moved with each pump stroke times the number of cycles per minute. The respiratory output is generally given as the *minute ventilation* ($\dot{V}_E$). Resting values of $\dot{V}_E$ are about 6 L/min and correlate with an average respiratory frequency (R_f) of 12 breaths/min and a V_T of 0.5 L ($\dot{V}_E = R_f \times V_T$). Because a portion of the V_T never leaves the dead space and therefore cannot contribute to gas exchange, $\dot{V}_E$ can misrepresent the useful ventilation. *Alveolar ventilation* ($\dot{V}_A$) describes only the useful ventilation and can be calculated as follows: $\dot{V}_A = R_f (V_T - V_D)$.

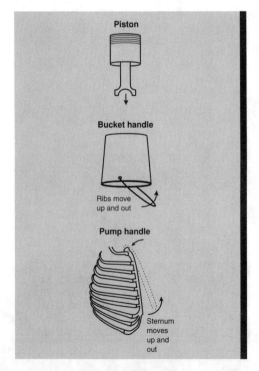

Piston

Bucket handle

Ribs move
up and out

Pump handle

Sternum
moves
up and
out

INSPIRATORY PUMP

The inspiratory pumping action uses three different motions. The primary pumping action during resting ventilation is due to the contraction of the diaphragm. As the diaphragm shortens, it tends to move downward like a piston, thereby decreasing intrapleural pressure. As a result, thoracic and lung volumes increase. The second type of motion is contributed by the intercostal musculature, which lifts the ribs. As the ribs are pulled closer together by the shortening of the intercostal muscles, they tend to rotate slightly in an anterior direction. This movement increases the anterior–posterior dimension of the chest and can be described as a "bucket-handle" motion. The third range of motion for the inspiratory pump is generated by the accessory muscles and the sternum. This "pump-handle" motion causes the sternum to be lifted and moved anteriorly, again increasing the volume of the chest. These three pumping actions typically work together to achieve chest and lung expansion. If movement in any group of muscles is prevented (i.e., by nerve damage, muscle weakness, restriction), a *paradoxical* movement of the chest and abdominal walls often occurs in which the action of one muscle group may "suck" in the inactive area. This is similar in concept to the lengthening of ischemic myocardium during systole described in Chapter 10. Such movements are easily observed in infants whose diaphragmatic contraction quite often causes the chest to move inward. These paradoxical breathing movements limit the total amount of ventilation despite increased work of breathing. In effect, some of the energy expended by the aggressively contracting muscle is wasted in stretching the noncontracting muscle.

Muscles of Inspiration

Diaphragm. The diaphragm typically contributes almost all of the resting ventilatory movements. It is composed of a large central tendon and two distinct muscles, the costal and crural diaphragm. The diaphragm is dome-shaped and depends on the liver and other abdominal contents for maintaining its initial length (see Chapter 4). Because of the mechanical coupling with abdominal contents and abdominal pressure, the activity of the diaphragm is greatly influenced by postural changes. When the body is in a supine posture, the abdominal contents push cephalically and increase the length of the diaphragm. However, when the body shifts to an upright posture, the abdomen expands as a result of the weight of the gut and effectively pulls down on the diaphragm, causing it to shorten. Fortunately, abdominal muscle tone limits the movement of the abdomen.

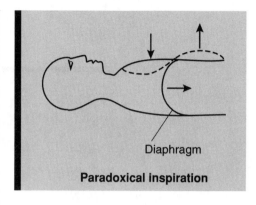

Diaphragm

Paradoxical inspiration

Intercostal Muscles. The external intercostals are generally considered to have an inspiratory function, although they also play an important role in maintaining normal posture. At rest in the supine position, they exhibit very little rhythmic respiratory-related activity; however, their activity can increase dramatically with increased respiratory drive (e.g., during exercise, hypoxia). They are innervated by the intercostal nerves, with the neuronal cell bodies in the ventral horns of the thoracic spinal cord. These motoneurons are driven by descending respiratory projections from the brainstem premotor neurons.

Accessory Muscles. The muscles of the neck and shoulder girdle can participate in inspiration by lifting the upper margin of the thorax. These muscles include the *scalenes* and the *sternocleidomastoids*. They are innervated by cranial motoneurons with axons in the spinal accessory nerve and by motoneurons in the upper cervical segments. Although these muscles have little rhythmic respiratory activity during resting ventilation, they are recruited with increased respiratory effort. In addition, these muscles can contribute significantly to ventilation in patients with cervical cord lesions.

EXPIRATORY PUMP

Expiration is generally passive since most of the driving force for expiration comes from stored energy in the elastic tissues of the expanded lung. Although expiratory-related muscles tend to exhibit some postural tone even at rest, there is little respiratory-related phasic activity until respiratory drive increases. As respiratory frequency increases, substantial recruitment of the expiratory muscles occurs to increase expiratory pressures and subsequently expiratory airflow. In addition, the expiratory musculature is very important in generating the rapid, high-pressure forces associated with vomiting and coughing. The *cough reflex* relies upon maximal airflow velocities to expel irritants from the airways.

Muscles of Expiration

Both the internal intercostal muscles and the abdominal muscles are part of the expiratory pump. They are innervated by motoneurons whose cell bodies are located in the ventral horns of the thoracic and lumbar spinal cord.

Internal Intercostals. These muscles have a low level of tonic activity with eupneic breathing. With increased respiratory drive, they increase their activity during expiration. Their expiratory-modulated activity is typically greatest in the most caudal intercostal spaces. As the intercostal muscles contract, they bring the ribs closer together and compress the rib cage, thereby decreasing thoracic volume and increasing alveolar pressure. This motor activity normally results in an increased expiratory flow rate and a decrease in end-expiratory volume.

Abdominal Muscles. Several sets of abdominal muscles can contribute to expiratory efforts by influencing pressure in the abdomen. Abdominal pressure is mechanically coupled to thoracic pressures through movement of the diaphragm. When abdominal muscles increase their contraction, the increased abdominal pressure tends to distend the diaphragm upward, again causing a decrease in thoracic lung volume. A low level of tonic activity is maintained in these muscles at all times for postural reasons. During eupnea, very little rhythmic respiratory activity occurs; however, these muscles are extensively recruited during the expiratory phase with increased ventilation.

COORDINATION WITH OTHER BEHAVIORS

In addition to their role in ventilation, all of these skeletal muscles participate in other motor acts. The muscles of the chest wall, abdomen, and shoulder girdle are very important in posture and movement. The coordination of these skeletal muscle functions with the ventilatory function is a complicated process regulated by the central nervous system. Even slight changes in posture require compensatory adjustments in respiratory muscle recruitment to maintain adequate ventilation.

Similarly, contraction of the diaphragm is very important in increasing abdominal pressure to provide a driving force for vomiting, coughing, and venous return. In addition, the Valsalva maneuver, which aids in defecation, also uses contraction of the diaphragm to increase abdominal pressure.

WORK OF BREATHING

During eupneic breathing, the respiratory muscles are controlled to produce the maximum alveolar ventilation with the minimum work. The diaphragm contracts during inspiration; however, most of the other respiratory muscles exhibit little or no rhythmic respiratory activity. They do, however, have some tonic activity, which is important for stabilizing the thorax and minimizing paradoxical movements. Total energy expenditure of the respiratory pump during eupneic ventilation is estimated to be only 1%–3% of the total oxygen consumption. However, with exercise, blood flow and metabolism of the respiratory musculature increase dramatically. Because of lowered ventilatory efficiency during hyperpneic ventilation (as a result of increased resistive and elastic work; see Chapter 15), the respiratory muscles require a disproportionate increase in blood flow. Oxygen consumption of these muscles may increase to 10%–15% of the total body oxygen consumption during strenuous exercise.

RESOLUTION OF CLINICAL CASE

Because the patient described at the beginning of the chapter sustained no apparent brainstem injury and given his inability to increase respiratory activity despite strong hypoxic and hypercapnic stimuli to breathe, the physician immediately suspected nerve gas poisoning. Most nerve gases act to block acetylcholinesterase activity, which then increases the ACh concentration. This in turn causes a depolarization block of cholinergic receptors. Because the respiratory pumps are composed of skeletal muscle using ACh as the exclusive neurotransmitter at the neuromuscular junction, nerve gases can effectively cause a respiratory muscle paralysis. With such poisoning, the central respiratory control system is likely to send a very strong signal through the respiratory nerves. However, very little of that signal is transmitted to the musculature because of the neuromuscular junction block. This produces a pronounced muscle weakness similar to that seen in myasthenia gravis. Because of muscle weakness, the patient was unable to make the necessary respiratory movements, and he was in danger of dying of asphyxia. Giving the patient 100% oxygen would have elevated the arterial oxygen levels and removed the hypoxic drive to breathe, probably resulting in an additional elevation of his $Paco_2$ level. Therefore, the correct decision was to ventilate the patient artificially to restore normal blood gas levels and then proceed to treat the effects of the neuromuscular blockade.

REVIEW QUESTIONS

Directions: For each of the following questions, choose the **one best** answer.

1. Functional residual capacity (FRC) is
    - **(A)** the volume in the lungs at the end of a normal inspiration
    - **(B)** the volume in the lungs when the inspiratory muscles are relaxed and the expiratory muscles are slightly contracted
    - **(C)** equal to the residual volume (RV) plus the expiratory reserve volume (ERV)
    - **(D)** usually less than 2.0 L
    - **(E)** the smallest lung volume

2. The respiratory muscles responsible for generating airway pressures have which of the following properties?
    - **(A)** They include both striated and smooth muscle
    - **(B)** They are innervated by cranial and spinal motoneurons
    - **(C)** They use multiple neurotransmitters at the neuromuscular junction
    - **(D)** They are used exclusively for respiratory-related efforts
    - **(E)** They are all recruited with every breath

3. Which of the following statements about expiration is true?
    - **(A)** Expiratory flow during resting ventilation is driven primarily by abdominal muscle contraction
    - **(B)** Expiratory muscles include the internal intercostals and abdominal muscles
    - **(C)** Expiratory muscles are innervated by cervical motoneurons
    - **(D)** Expiration is totally passive under all conditions
    - **(E)** Expiratory flow is usually more forceful than inspiratory flow

4. A patient suffering from an acute allergic reaction is likely to have
    - **(A)** a markedly reduced total lung capacity
    - **(B)** a decreased residual volume
    - **(C)** an increased forced expiratory volume in 1 second (FEV_1)
    - **(D)** a ratio of FEV_1 to forced vital capacity (FVC) that is less than 0.7
    - **(E)** a decreased closing volume

5. Which of the following volumes is largest in a healthy human?
    - **(A)** Expiratory reserve volume (ERV)
    - **(B)** Physiologic dead space
    - **(C)** Tidal volume (V_T)
    - **(D)** Closing volume
    - **(E)** Residual volume (RV)

6. Calculate the $\dot{V}_E$ and $\dot{V}_A$ for a patient with a respiratory frequency of 15 breaths per minute, a V_T of 0.8 L, and a V_{DS} of 150 mL.

	$\dot{V}_E$ (L/min)	$\dot{V}_A$ (L/min)
(A)	2.25	2.0
(B)	6.0	4.2
(C)	12	9.75
(D)	15	13
(E)	140	140

ANSWERS AND EXPLANATIONS

1. The answer is C. FRC is defined as the lung volume when all respiratory muscles are relaxed. This volume normally occurs at the end of expiration; by definition, it is equal to the RV + ERV.

2. The answer is B. The respiratory muscles that generate airflow are exclusively striated muscle. The accessory muscles are innervated by cranial motoneurons, while the diaphragm, intercostals, and abdominal muscles are innervated by motoneurons with cell bodies in the spinal cord. All motoneurons use acetylcholine at the neuromuscular junction. Because most of the respiratory muscles also play an important role in posture and movement, their activity must be coordinated between the respiratory drive and these other drives.

3. The answer is B. The internal intercostals and the abdominal muscles are the major expiratory-modulated muscles. They are innervated by motoneurons from the thoracic and lumbar segments. During eupnea, most expiratory flow results from energy stored in the lung elastic tissues; therefore, expiration is described as "passive." However, during deep breathing and forced expiration, expiratory muscles are recruited.

4. The answer is D. An allergic reaction causes a bronchoconstriction that dramatically increases airway resistance. Closing volumes are usually elevated, although most other lung volumes and capacities are relatively unaffected. The high airway resistance causes a dramatic fall in the FEV_1 and the FEV_1:FVC usually falls below 0.6.

5. The answer is A. In a healthy human, the closing volume is minimal. The physiologic dead space is approximately equal to the anatomic dead space (150 mL). The typical V_T is approximately 500 mL, RV is approximately 1000 mL, and ERV is approximately 1500 mL.

6. The answer is C. $\dot{V}_E = R_f \times V_T = 15/\text{min} \times 0.8\ \text{L} = 12\ \text{L/min}$. $\dot{V}_A = R_f (V_T - V_{DS}) = 15/\text{min}\ (0.8\ \text{L} - 0.15\ \text{L}) = 9.75\ \text{L/min}$.

15

MECHANICS OF THE RESPIRATORY CYCLE

INTRODUCTION OF CLINICAL CASE

A 50-year-old man presented with a complaint of dyspnea and excessive fatigue upon exertion. He had a history of chronic smoking and obesity. Respiratory frequency was approximately 32 breaths/min. He was observed to breathe at an elevated functional residual capacity (FRC) and to exhale through pursed lips. His pulse was 110, and his blood pressure was 135/90 mm Hg. No apparent cyanosis or clubbing was seen in the extremities. Blood gases were pH 7.40, Po_2 of 60 mm Hg, and Pco_2 of 52 mm Hg. Spirometry indicated a severe depression of his forced vital capacity (FVC) to 1.66 L, forced expiratory volume in 1 second (FEV_1) of 0.59 L, and relatively slow airflow velocities during tidal breaths. Total lung capacity (TLC) was 7.2 L. His lung compliance was elevated, and his chest wall compliance was decreased.

INTRODUCTION

The respiratory pumps described in Chapter 14 develop the various pressures that are essential for the flow of gases in and out of the lung. These *respiratory mechanics* are similar in many ways to the heart and cardiovascular mechanics described in the previous chapters. In addition to the active skeletal muscle contraction of the respiratory pump, the elastic properties of the chest and lung and the resistive properties of the airway and its smooth muscle are significant in regulating the flow of air.

The lung is a complex tissue with significant interactions occurring between pressures, volumes, airway resistance, and flow rates. All of these parameters are interdependent. To simplify some of the relationships, it is useful to examine the *static* properties of the lung, which can be measured when airflow is zero. This is accomplished experimentally by measuring parameters at a constant lung volume. However, normal lung function requires an almost continual change in lung volumes and pressures. Therefore, the *dynamic* properties observed during the breathing cycle may often vary considerably from those derived under steady-state conditions. Both static and dynamic properties are discussed below.

PRESSURES

Similar to the cardiovascular system, the various pressures related to respiratory pump function are usually referenced to ambient or *atmospheric pressure* (P_{atm}) and are therefore expressed as the *difference from ambient pressure* (see Chapter 3). Since most of the pressures are relatively small during resting ventilation, they are normally given in units of *cm H_2O*. At rest, the ambient pressure, or *mouth pressure* (P_m), is defined as 0 cm H_2O.

The pressure within the small airways and the alveoli is known as the *alveolar pressure* (P_A). At rest with an open glottis, P_A approximates atmospheric pressure. The difference between P_m and P_A during a breath is called the *transairway pressure*. This gradient provides the driving force for airflow. Therefore, if P_m is greater than P_A, air moves into the lung (i.e., inspiration), and if P_A is greater than P_m, expiratory airflow occurs. During deep breathing in a healthy human, the larger gradients result in faster flow rates. In normal breathing, P_m varies only slightly from 0 as a result of the movement of air; therefore, the major changes must occur in P_A.

The pressure inside the chest cavity between the parietal and visceral pleura is known as either the *intrapleural* or *pleural pressure* (P_{pl}). At rest, this pressure is negative, indicating that it is less than atmospheric pressure. The negative P_{pl} results from the elasticity of the lung and the chest wall, which are oriented in opposite directions at FRC. The natural tendency of the lung to collapse and the chest wall to expand is clearly seen in a *pneumothorax*. When the P_{pl} approximates atmospheric pressure because of perforation of either the visceral or parietal pleura, the chest wall expands and the lung collapses. Although the average resting P_{pl} is approximately −5 cm H_2O, it is significant that this pressure varies with position and gravity. In the upright position, the P_{pl} measured at the base of the lung is less negative than at the apex. The weight of the lung tends to distort the lung tissue so that more water and tissue fill the lower regions. This distortion leads to a more negative P_{pl} in the upper region (apex) and a less negative P_{pl} in the lower region (base). When an individual stands on his head, the P_{pl} around the base of the lung is more negative than the P_{pl} at the apex. Because the lung is primarily air filled, its specific density is considerably less than 1.0, and the difference between apical and basal P_{pl} is only a few cm H_2O (a small fraction of the 30-cm height of the lung).

The difference between P_A and P_{pl} is known as the *transpulmonary* or *transmural pressure* ($P_T = P_A − P_{pl}$). The P_T depends upon the elastic properties of the lung and is often used instead of P_{pl}. P_T is used for the sake of convenience: in most static measurements when P_A is equal to 0 (atmospheric pressure), the P_T is a positive number equal to $−P_{pl}$. Maximal inspiratory and expiratory transmural pressures depend on the strength of the respiratory muscles and are usually about 100 cm H_2O. This limits the individual's ability to overcome severe resistances or to breathe when chest movement is restricted (e.g., a person could probably breathe adequately if a small adult sat on his or her chest; however, the weight of a large adult could cause chest compression that could not be overcome, and hypoventilation would ensue).

$1 mm Hg = 1.34 cm H_2O = 13.4 mm H_2O$

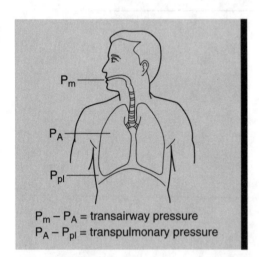

$P_m − P_A$ = transairway pressure

$P_A − P_{pl}$ = transpulmonary pressure

In a patient with emphysema, the loss of tissue around the small airways can result in collapse of the airways if the P_{pl} during expiration is greater than the P_A. By pursing the lips and limiting flow through the mouth, both P_m and P_A airway pressures are elevated to prevent collapse. The decreased elasticity of the lung results in an expansion of the chest and a symptom described as "barrel-chest."

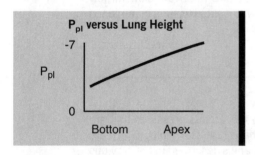

P_{pl} versus Lung Height

AIRWAY RESISTANCE

Resistive elements are found throughout the respiratory tree. In addition to the principles of resistance described in Chapter 3, the airways are subject to considerable distorting forces, causing the total lung resistance to change dynamically during the respiratory cycle. Mechanical factors and contraction of the bronchiolar smooth muscle both contribute to the regulation of airway resistance. Parasympathetic innervation via the vagus nerve stimulates the contraction, leading to bronchoconstriction and increased resistance. Asthma, allergens, cold, smoke, and inflammatory mediators are all potentially potent stimuli for bronchoconstriction. Exercise and psychologic factors can also initiate a bronchoconstrictive response. Drugs that prevent or reverse bronchoconstriction are important clinical tools in managing airway pathologies. These drugs include β_2-agonists, anticholinergics, corticosteroids, and antihistamines.

One of the major mechanical factors influencing airway resistance (R_{aw}) is the fact that the airways are located within the lung parenchyma and there are numerous attachments to the surrounding tissue that exert a significant traction on the airway wall. Because of this *tethering* effect, the radius of an airway is very responsive to changes in the lung volume. Figure 15-1 illustrates the dramatic effect of lung volume on airway resistance. This effect is especially prominent when the expiratory reserve volume (ERV) is utilized. As shown in the figure, airway resistance doubles as the lung volume decreases from FRC to residual volume (RV).

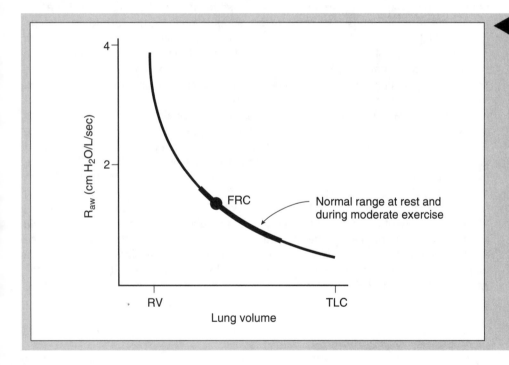

◀ **FIGURE 15-1**
Relationship Between Airway Resistance (R$_{aw}$) and Lung Volume. As the lung expands from residual volume (RV) to the functional residual capacity (FRC), there is a substantial decrease in R$_{aw}$. The traction of the lung parenchyma on the small airways as the lung expands results in increased diameter of the airways. The heavy portion of the line indicates the normal operating range of lung volumes for breathing during moderate exercise. The high-resistance areas of the curve are not normally used. TLC = total lung capacity.

Another major determinant of airway resistance is the pressure surrounding the airway. The structure of a normal bronchiole includes smooth muscle and connective tissue and, in the larger bronchioles, some cartilage. These components help to keep the airway patent. However, when $+P_{pl}$ is developed during forced expiration, pressures outside the airway may exceed the internal pressure, resulting in collapse of the airway. This type of resistive element, where an external force exceeds the internal pressure and causes narrowing of the vessel, is known as a *Starling resistor*. This phenomenon results in an elevated closing volume (see Chapter 14). In patients with diseases that destroy lung tissue, such as emphysema, the airways are much more susceptible to collapse.

A third important factor in determining airway resistance relates to the secretions of the respiratory tract. Fluid and mucous secretions are important protective mechanisms

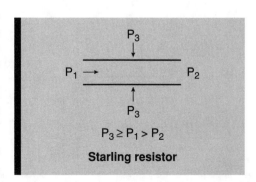

Starling resistor

that trap and remove particulates and bacteria from the lung. However, excessive secretions (or an impaired ability to move the secretions toward the pharynx) may cause mucus to accumulate in the airways and decrease the effective opening for gas flow.

FLOW

Within the small respiratory bronchioles and alveoli, very little bulk movement of air occurs, and most of the gases move by diffusive forces. However, throughout most of the *extra-alveolar* airways, there is significant airflow. In most of the larger airways, airflow is primarily laminar (see Figure 5-6). However, at airway bifurcations and with elevated flow velocities, the airflow can become turbulent. Turbulence can be detected clinically by the presence of lung sounds, and in some pathologies, there may be an obvious "wheeze" associated with turbulent airflow. Narrowing or partial obstructions of airways are important factors in creating high flow velocities.

During the course of a normal breath, the inspiratory muscles contract and cause the thoracic cavity to expand. As the chest wall moves away from the lung, the P_{pl} becomes more negative, and the transmural pressure increases. The absence of a pleural space keeps the lung closely apposed to the chest wall, and the lung inflates. P_A becomes negative as the air in the alveoli now occupies the greater lung volume. The pressure gradient from the mouth "pushes" air into the region of lower pressure until P_A equals P_m. At this point, airflow ceases. At the end of inspiration as the inspiratory muscles relax, the chest wall returns toward its "resting" state, and the thoracic cavity decreases in size, resulting in opposite changes in pressures throughout the respiratory system.

The relationships between the various pressures, flows, and volumes associated with a normal breath are shown in Figure 15-2. This figure is the respiratory equivalent of the Wiggers diagram (Chapter 9, Figure 9-2), illustrating the important relationships among flow, volume, and pressure. The first trace shows the change in lung volume. The second trace depicts airflow ($\dot{V}$), which is the derivative of volume. Airway resistance stays reasonably constant; therefore, the P_A trace appears to be almost identical in shape to airflow (remember, flow = pressure/resistance). Changes in P_{pl} lead to changes in lung volume, which in turn generate the changes in P_A. Figure 15-2B illustrates the expected changes as an individual breathes more deeply. The waveforms are similar although the excursions are greater. Figure 15-2C demonstrates the pressures generated by a breath that is held at the end of inspiration with the glottis open. At the peak of this steady-state or *static* maneuver, there is no airflow; however, constant inspiratory muscle contraction is needed to keep the lung at its expanded volume above FRC. This constant muscle contraction maintains the P_{pl} near its end inspiratory value. When the glottis is closed and the inspiratory muscles relax, the thoracic cavity decreases in size, and the air in the lung compresses, leading to the increased P_A and the less negative P_{pl} (indicated by the *asterisk* in Figure 15-2D).

Flow = pressure/resistance

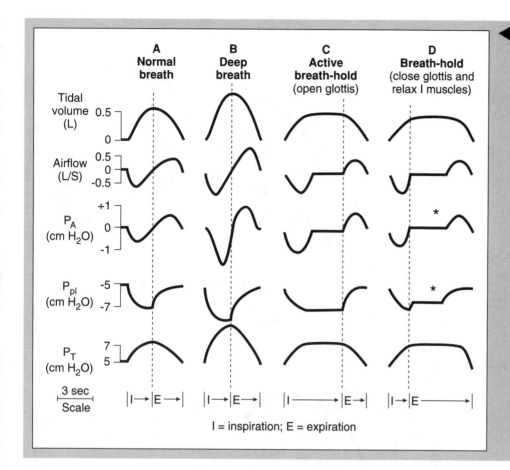

FIGURE 15-2
Pressure, Volume, and Flow Traces. (A) For a normal breath, (B) a deep breath, (C) a breath-hold with an open glottis, and (D) a passive breath-hold at end-inspiratory volume. Inspiration (I) and expiration (E) are indicated below the traces. The asterisk (*) indicates the increase in intrapleural pressure (P_{pl}) and alveolar pressure (P_A) that occurs when the inspiratory muscles relax and the chest size decreases against the end-inspiratory volume still contained in the lung. P_T = transmural pressure.

COMPLIANCE

Compliance is an important concept in both cardiovascular and lung mechanics (see Chapters 3 and 9). Total compliance in the respiratory system depends upon the compliance of both the lung (C_L) and the chest wall (C_{cw}). C_L, in turn, is determined by the elasticity of the lung tissue and by the *surface tension* developed by the air–liquid interface. These properties can be altered in various disease states and by the conformation of the lung. C_{cw} depends upon all the anatomic structures and configuration of the chest.

Compliance = Δ volume/Δ pressure

Lung Compliance

An important property of compliance is that it is not constant but varies with the size of the lung. This dependence on the dynamic state demonstrates *hysteresis*; different curves result from inflating and deflating pressures. C_L is related to the presence of elastin and other structural elements. In restrictive diseases such as *pulmonary fibrosis*, C_L decreases as additional stiff, fibrotic tissue is deposited within the connective tissue of the lung parenchyma. Similarly, pulmonary edema and collapse of lung regions decrease the compliance. In contrast, the loss of lung tissue in diseases such as emphysema actually increases the C_L. Unfortunately, this increase in C_L makes the peripheral airway diameters more dependent on extra-alveolar pressures and may create a *Starling resistor*, thereby creating a significant obstruction or resistance to airflow. Figure 15-3A illustrates the pressure–volume relationship in an excised lung, while panel B presents the calculated C_L plotted against the same pressure abscissa. Generally, Figure 15-3A is called the compliance curve; however, the *slope* of the pressure–volume relationship describes the instantaneous compliance. An average value for C_L is approximately 0.2 L/cm H_2O. The curve of Figure 15-3B shows that this is the compliance on the inflation curve in the normal operating range of P_T (3–7 cm H_2O).

FIGURE 15-3 ▶

Static Lung Compliance Curves. (A) Lung volume (L) is plotted as a function of the transmural pressure (P_T) required to hold that volume. Significant hysteresis is seen between the inflation and deflation curve. Compliance is calculated at two representative regions of the curve. The instantaneous slopes of these curves are compliance. (B) The instantaneous compliance (slopes) of the curves in A are plotted as a function of P_T. An average value for lung compliance is typically given as 0.2 L/cm H_2O. $C_1 = C_1$ over lung volume (1); $C_2 = C_2$ over lung volume (2); ΔP_1 = change in pressure over range (1); ΔP_2 = change in pressure over range (2); ΔV_1 = change in volume over range (1); ΔV_2 = change in volume over range (2).

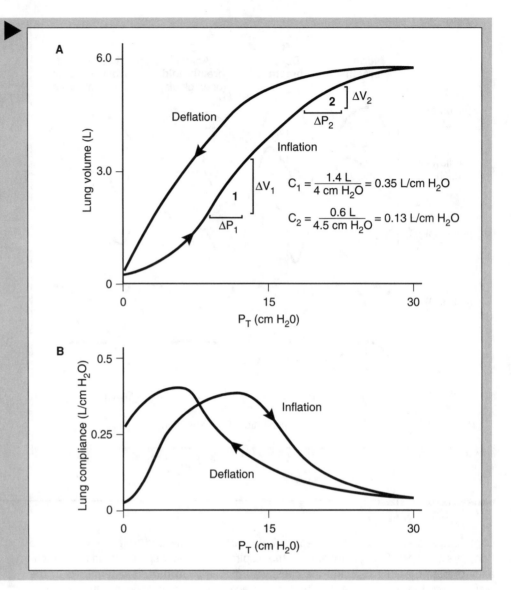

$$C_1 = \frac{1.4 \text{ L}}{4 \text{ cm } H_2O} = 0.35 \text{ L/cm } H_2O$$

$$C_2 = \frac{0.6 \text{ L}}{4.5 \text{ cm } H_2O} = 0.13 \text{ L/cm } H_2O$$

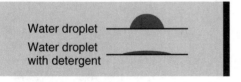

Water droplet ⎯⎯⎯⎯⎯⎯

Water droplet
with detergent

There is considerable variation in the *regional* C_L because of the nonhomogeneous distribution of pressures within the lung. With normal tidal breathing just above FRC, the apices of the lung are relatively distended, and their compliance for any further expansion is low (C_2 in Figure 15-3A). The base of the lung is, however, operating in its maximum compliance range (C_1 in Figure 15-3A). These different compliances result in a greater change in volume for the lower lung regions than for the apices during a normal breath.

Although the curves shown in Figure 15-3 are useful in understanding the mechanical properties of the respiratory system, it is important to realize that most of the actual respiratory movements occur in the middle portions of these curves and not at the extremes. Figure 15-3B shows that the C_L falls off dramatically at the high and low transpulmonary pressures. One can infer that the energy cost of moving a given volume of air is much higher in these low-compliance conditions.

C_L depends upon both the elasticity of the lung tissue and the *surface tension* within the alveoli. Because water molecules at a gas–liquid interface tend to aggregate, a significant force is developed. This surface tension is responsible for the rounded shape of a water droplet placed on a flat surface and its ability to "float" a sewing needle. Surface tension can be minimized by limiting the molecular interactions by adding a detergent. If the excised lung shown in Figure 15-3 is filled with saline instead of air, a new compliance curve is generated (Figure 15-4), indicating that the gas–liquid interaction exerts a strong influence to decrease C_L. If that same lung is rinsed several times to remove the native detergents and then reinflated with air, the C_L decreases considerably.

Surface tension in the lung is minimized by the presence of *surfactant*, an extremely effective detergent agent secreted by the type II alveolar cells of the lung. Surfactant is a mixture of proteins and fatty acids; the major component, dipalmitoyl phosphatidylcholine, constitutes approximately 40%–60% of the secretion. Surfactant is produced relatively late in fetal development. Its deficiency is a major concern in premature births because it leads to a condition known as *hyaline membrane disease, infant respiratory distress syndrome,* or *surfactant deficiency syndrome* (SDS). Synthetic surfactants have been developed that are reasonably effective in treating SDS.

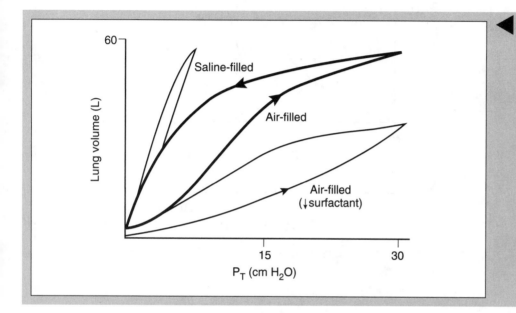

FIGURE 15-4
Static Compliance Curves for Several Different Conditions. *Filling the lung with saline removes the air–liquid interface and therefore eliminates the force of surface tension. Lung compliance is increased greatly in this condition. Repeated rinsing of the lung to decrease the surfactant concentration eliminates the normal effect of surfactant to decrease surface tension, and the lung becomes much less compliant. Restrictive diseases have a similar effect; obstructive diseases usually increase compliance.* $P_T = P_A - P_{pl}$.

Chest Wall Compliance

C_L is most accurately determined by removing the lung from the chest; to measure C_{cw} directly, it is also necessary to remove the lungs and measure the pressure–volume relationship of the empty thoracic cavity. Therefore, it is much simpler to measure the *total compliance* (C_T), which is the compliance of both the chest wall and the lung. The compliance of both components together is less than the compliance of either element alone. C_T can be determined from the static pressure–volume curve of the intact lung, as shown in Figure 15-5. C_L can also be determined from the P_{pl}–volume relationship and then used to calculate the C_{cw}. Similar to the C_L, the C_{cw} depends on the chest wall's previous size and shows significant hysteresis when determined under dynamic conditions. Since C_{cw} is affected by the positions of the diaphragm and chest wall muscles, it may be altered by unusual postures, obesity, pregnancy, or skeletal muscle problems affecting muscle tone.

$1/C_T = 1/C_L + 1/C_{cw}$

The work of breathing is increased in the latter stages of pregnancy as the diaphragm is displaced by high abdominal pressures, and the C_{cw} decreases.

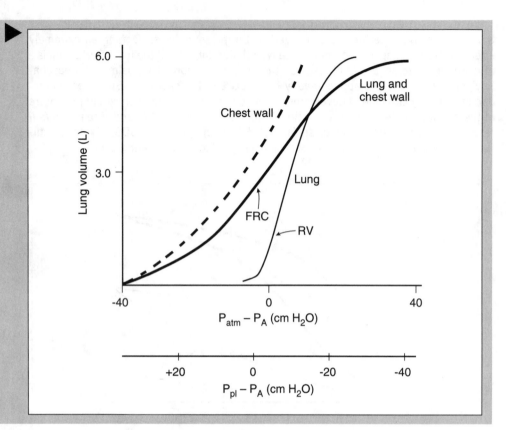

FIGURE 15-5 ▶

Pressure–Volume Curve. *This curve shows compliance of the chest wall and the lung, and the combined compliance of both structures. FRC = functional residual capacity; RV = residual volume; P_A = alveolar pressure; P_{atm} = atmospheric pressure; P_{pl} = pleural pressure.*

FLOW-VOLUME CURVES

Chapters 4 and 9 discuss how the force and velocity of muscle shortening are dependent upon the initial length (or preload) of the muscle. A similar relationship is important for generating expiratory muscle movements and airflow. However, maximal inspiratory flow is limited more by the resistance of the airways than by the maximal effort of the musculature. The peak inspiratory flow rate is about 8 L/sec, and it can be maintained over a wide range of lung volumes (Figure 15-6). Maximal expiratory flow rates are slightly lower and can be generated only at initial lung volumes above 80% of the total lung capacity. At smaller lung volumes, the expiratory flow rate is also limited by airway resistance. The very high $+P_{pl}$ developed during maximal expiratory efforts can lead to significant collapse of the extra-alveolar airways, an increase in airway resistance, and a definite limitation of expiratory flow rate. Although the curves shown in Figure 15-6 demonstrate the maximal flow velocities, such rates are seldom achieved because the energy cost for producing these high flow rates is tremendous.

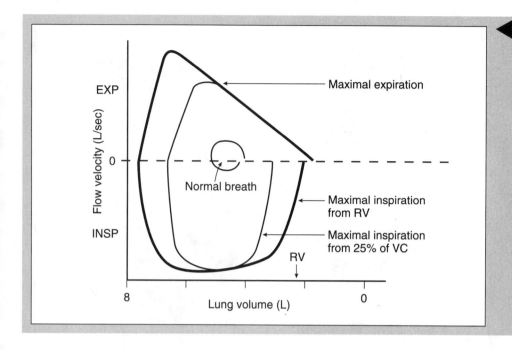

Relationship Between Lung Volume and Maximal Flow Velocities during Inspiration and Expiration. The heavy line shows the results of a forced vital capacity effort. Maximum inspiratory flow rates are similar throughout most of the range; however, the peak expiratory flow rate is very sensitive to lung volume and can be observed only when lung volumes are above 80% of total lung capacity. The typical flow–volume loop for a normal tidal breath is also shown. RV = residual volume; VC = vital capacity.

WORK OF BREATHING

Work done by the respiratory muscles is usually graphed and observed as the area inside a pressure–volume curve, just as for the heart. The respiratory muscles overcome three major types of forces: (1) elastic forces that resist the changes in lung and chest volumes, (2) flow-resistive forces of the airways, and (3) inertial forces that depend on the mass of tissues and gases. In addition to these forces, the respiratory muscles work against forces that act to distort the thoracic cavity such as gravity, a tight belt, a full stomach, and so on.

Figure 15-7 depicts the work of breathing for four separate conditions. In panel A, a breath of 1.0 L is inhaled and exhaled. Elastic work and resistive work are illustrated by the *shaded* and *crosshatched regions*. Resistive work is done in both inspiration and expiration. The resistive work of expiration falls within the stored energy of the elastic work performed during inspiration, so no additional energy expenditure is necessary for this passive expiration. However, in panel B, the same volume of air is moved, but expiration is forced. In this case, the stored energy from the elastic work of inspiration is not sufficient to account for the work of expiration, and additional energy is required to complete the expiratory effort. During forced expiration, resistive work is substantially increased. Panels C and D show the enhanced work required for each breath in restrictive and obstructive diseases. Resistive work is increased in obstructive diseases; in restrictive diseases, elastic work increases markedly to overcome the decreased compliance.

When the body is at rest, the work of breathing accounts for 1%–3% of the total body energy expenditure. However, the cost of ventilation increases rapidly as ventilatory rate and depth increase. As the depth of breathing increases, the resistive component of work may decrease (R_{aw} is inversely related to lung volume), but the elastic work increases as the compliance decreases. As the frequency of breathing increases, both elastic and resistive work tend to increase. The actual pattern of breathing is normally well regulated to minimize the overall work of breathing. As metabolic demands necessitate an increase in alveolar ventilation, both breathing frequency and depth increase in a fashion that keeps the total work as low as possible. This activity is illustrated in Figure 15-8, which shows the work of breathing as a function of respiratory frequency. To achieve a total alveolar ventilation of 30 L/min, a wide range of tidal volumes and frequencies can be used. However, the minimal work to attain this ventilation occurs with a respiratory frequency of about 22 breaths/min. Under normal circumstances, individuals breathe at the frequency that minimizes their total work.

FIGURE 15-7

Pressure–Volume Curves Showing the Work Done to Overcome Elastic and Resistive Forces. (A) Slightly larger than normal breath from functional residual capacity with a passive expiration. (B) An active expiration requires additional work performed beyond the energy of the stored elastic work. (C) In restrictive disease processes such as fibrosis or pulmonary congestion, the total resistive work is about the same; however, the elastic work is greatly increased as extra effort is needed to overcome the decreased compliance. (D) In obstructive diseases, the resistive work is greatly increased. P_{pl} = pleural pressure; E = expiration; I = inspiration.

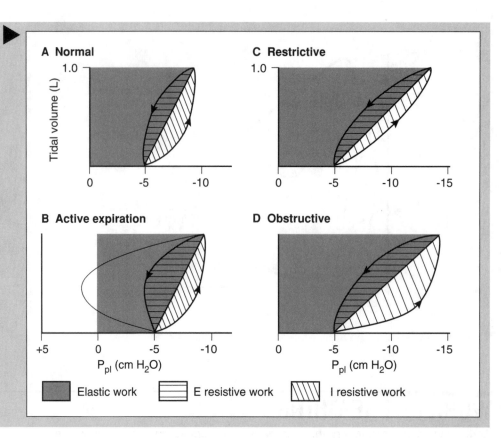

FIGURE 15-8

Respiratory Work as a Function of Respiratory Frequency. Two curves are shown for alveolar ventilation ($\dot{V}_A$) of 6 L/min (resting ventilation) and 30 L/min (ventilation during moderate exercise). As ventilation increases, the work of breathing must obviously increase. Normal breathing patterns match the changes in depth and frequency of breathing to minimize the total work performed (circles on both curves). The two lighter curves show the relative contribution of elastic work and resistive work for the $\dot{V}_A$ of 6 L/min. If an individual breathes very slow, deep breaths, almost all the work is elastic; however with rapid, shallow breathing the elastic work is very small, and the resistive work is large.

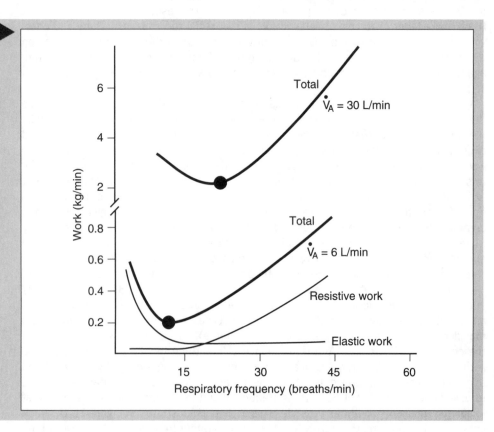

RESOLUTION OF CLINICAL CASE

The spirometry findings for the patient presented indicated an obstructive disease causing a marked increase in airway resistance because there was a substantial decrease in the FEV_1 and the ratio of FEV_1/FVC. The patient's history of smoking and the observation of expiratory flow problems suggested the likelihood of emphysema. As lung tissue is destroyed, the compliance of the lung actually increases. Although this makes the lung easier to inflate and lessens the work of inspiration, the airways tend to collapse as a result of the loss of traction around them. As the airways narrow, there are distinct expiratory flow limitations. Unfortunately, any effort to increase the expiratory P_A by exhaling harder is counterproductive because it exacerbates the collapse of airways. To maintain patency of the airways, the patient increased intra-airway pressures by adding a significant downstream resistance in the form of pursed lips. This allowed him to exhale more completely, although it did add considerably to the work of breathing. His respiratory reserves were small, and the resulting poor ventilatory abilities imposed severe exercise limitations. Patients with emphysema tend to breathe at elevated FRCs because the lung recoil forces are reduced. This increase in chest wall diameter tends to decrease the C_{cw}. In this case, the patient's obesity also hindered chest wall expansion.

The patient's arterial blood gases showed a moderate hypoxia and hypercapnia. His arterial pH remained within the normal range as a result of effective compensation by the kidneys. Because of the loss of functioning alveoli, the surface area for gas exchange decreased dramatically, leading to poor gas exchange (see Chapter 17). However, these levels did not represent a significant threat to his body metabolism, which accounted for the absence of cyanosis and clubbing (a symptom of chronic hypoxia). However, these blood gas levels tend to excite chemoreflexes, leading to this patient's increased resting ventilation, respiratory rate, heart rate, and arterial blood pressure.

REVIEW QUESTIONS

Directions: For each of the following questions, choose the **one best** answer.

1. Which of the following comparisons is correct during inspiratory airflow, where P_{atm} = atmospheric pressure; P_{pl} = pleural pressure; P_A = alveolar pressure; and P_m = mouth pressure?

   (A) $P_{atm} < P_{pl} < P_A < P_m$

   (B) $P_{atm} > P_{pl} < P_A < P_m$

   (C) $P_{atm} < P_{pl} > P_A < P_m$

   (D) $P_{atm} > P_{pl} > P_A < P_m$

   (E) $P_{atm} > P_{pl} < P_A > P_m$

2. Which of the following do **not** affect airway resistance?

   (A) Autonomic nervous system control of bronchiolar smooth muscle

   (B) Changes in lung volume

   (C) Alveolar pressure (P_A)

   (D) Projections of cilia into the lumen

   (E) Excessive secretions of the airways

3. Standing neck-deep in a swimming pool would affect respiratory mechanics by

   (A) decreasing lung compliance

   (B) decreasing the airway resistance

   (C) decreasing the work of breathing

   (D) increasing the functional residual capacity

   (E) increasing the alveolar pressure during inspiration

4. Which of the following would be expected to increase lung compliance?

   (A) Pulmonary congestion

   (B) Fibrosis

   (C) Decreased surfactant

   (D) Emphysema

   (E) Lung edema

ANSWERS AND EXPLANATIONS

1. The answer is B. During inspiration, the lowest, most negative pressure is P_{pl}, which causes expansion of the lungs, thereby making P_A negative and less than P_m. Since P_m is very close to P_{atm}, if P_{atm} were less than P_{pl}, air would move out of the lungs.

2. The answer is D. Autonomic nervous system control of bronchiolar smooth muscle, changes in lung volume, P_A, and excessive secretions of the airways can influence the diameter of the airway lumen, thereby influencing resistance.

3. The answer is A. The weight of the water would compress the chest and lung, creating a less negative pleural pressure and a smaller lung volume. Because of the tethering effect on airways, the airways would also decrease in size and increase airway resistance. The compliance at small lung volumes is low, and the work of breathing would be increased.

4. The answer is D. Emphysema increases lung compliance by destroying lung tissue. Pulmonary congestion, fibrosis, decreased surfactant, and lung edema add structural elements that tend to decrease the ability of the lung to expand. Pulmonary vascular congestion and edema both increase the weight and stiffness of the lung. Similarly, in fibrosis the lungs stiffen. Decreased surfactant allows an increased surface tension, which also makes the lung less elastic.

16

COUPLING OF THE PULMONARY AND CARDIOVASCULAR SYSTEMS

INTRODUCTION OF CLINICAL CASE

A 35-year-old man presented to the emergency room for cough and shortness of breath. A chest radiograph showed a large infiltrate in the left lung. His arterial blood gases at presentation were: partial pressure of arterial oxygen (Pa_{O_2}) = 52 mm Hg and partial pressure of arterial carbon dioxide (Pa_{CO_2}) = 39 mm Hg. His minute volume at this point was 12 L/min.

The patient was placed on 100% oxygen breathing via a face mask. Subsequently, his blood gases were Pa_{O_2} = 60 mm Hg, and Pa_{CO_2} = 30 mm Hg. The physician then asked the patient to lie on his right side. This procedure improved his Pa_{O_2} to 77 mm Hg.

PULMONARY VASCULAR DYNAMICS

Pulmonary Vascular Pressures

Figure 16-1 is a review of the distribution of blood pressure from the right atrium through the heart and into the major arteries. From this figure it can be seen that, in general, pressures in the pulmonary circulation are about one-tenth those found in the systemic arteries. Considering that the same cardiac output (CO) passes through both the pulmonary circulation and the distributing arteries, it can be deduced that pulmonary vascular resistance is roughly one-tenth that of the systemic circulation. This raises the following question: what are the characteristics of the pulmonary circulation that make it a low-resistance system?

FIGURE 16-1 ▶

Distribution of Blood Pressure from the Right Atrium through the Heart and into the Major Distributing Arteries.

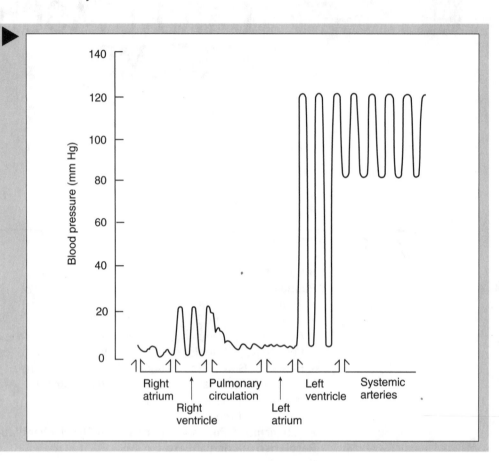

*The reason why **distensive forces** play such a dominant role in the pulmonary circulation is that both the arterial and venous sides of the pulmonary circulation have a high compliance.*

Determinants and Regulation of Pulmonary Vascular Resistance

The pulmonary circulation is markedly different from the systemic circulation in several factors that impact on the control of vascular resistance. First, in the systemic circulation, arterioles are the major sites of vascular resistance; however, essentially all vessels in the pulmonary circulation contribute to vascular resistance. Second, passive forces (e.g., vascular distension caused by gravity) have very little effect on systemic vascular resistance; however, such forces play a very important role in determining and regulating pulmonary vascular resistance. Third, unlike the systemic circulation, pulmonary vessels have a low basal tone, exhibit little or no autoregulation, and their response to sympathetic vasomotor neurons is not well understood in terms of either mechanisms or function.

From a teleologic point of view, it can be argued that the pulmonary circulation has no "need" to be regulated because it must, out of necessity, accept all of the CO. On this point, it can be argued that the high compliant–low resistant pulmonary circulation is well suited to accept wide variations in right ventricular output. According to this line of reasoning, what regulates CO would therefore regulate pulmonary blood flow. Nevertheless, the weight of evidence indicates that pulmonary vascular resistance is regulated by mechanisms that fall into two general categories: (1) active adjustments mediated by constrictor or dilator responses of pulmonary vascular smooth muscle, and (2) passive changes in diameter caused by stress forces, such as pressure. Active adjustments are probably confined to the pulmonary arterioles and small arteries, whereas passive changes involve all components of the pulmonary circulation (i.e., arteries, arterioles, capillaries, venules, veins).

Active Adjustments in Pulmonary Vascular Resistance

One of the more pronounced active regulatory adjustments of the pulmonary circulation is the phenomenon of *hypoxic vasoconstriction*. During situations in which individual alveoli become underventilated to the point where the partial pressure of alveolar oxygen (P_{AO_2}) falls below approximately 70 mm Hg, the nearby small arteries and arterioles vasoconstrict [2]. *Hypoxic vasoconstriction in the pulmonary circulation facilitates the matching of ventilation to perfusion by shifting blood flow from underventilated alveoli to those that are adequately ventilated.* Although this phenomenon has been known for quite some time, the underlying mechanism has yet to be clearly elucidated. Recent evidence suggests that several mechanisms may be involved, including adenosine-elicited vasoconstriction and the release of endothelial-derived constrictor factors [3].

In addition to local hypoxic vasoconstriction, the pulmonary circulation also constricts in response to *systemic hypoxia*, a condition common in situations such as high altitude. The mechanism is probably sympathetic-elicited vasoconstriction secondary to peripheral chemoreceptor stimulation [4]. The functional significance can only be hypothesized, but a tenable possibility is that reduced pulmonary blood flow in the face of reduced alveolar oxygen may optimize gas exchange by increasing the transit time of the pulmonary blood flow–alveolar interface.

> The **vasoconstrictor response** of the pulmonary circulation to low oxygen tension is the exact opposite of the response of systemic arterioles. The mechanisms for this difference are not yet known.

> The pulmonary vascular effects of **systemic hypoxia** may serve a role in altitude adjustment by increasing the transit time of blood flow past the alveoli. This should allow a slightly higher oxygen–hemoglobin association than would otherwise occur.

Passive Adjustments in Pulmonary Vascular Resistance

The relatively low basal tone of the pulmonary circulation and the ability of this circulation to adjust passively to forces such as intravascular pressure are both manifestations of the unique structure of the pulmonary circulation. In Chapter 11, resistance to the flow of blood through a vascular network was shown to be inversely proportional to the fourth power of the radius of the vessels and to the number of vessels in parallel. In this context, part of the reason that the pulmonary circulation has a low resistance is that pulmonary microvessels are generally larger compared to their systemic counterparts. For example, perfused pulmonary capillaries are in the order of 10–15 μ as opposed to a range of 4–8 μ for systemic capillaries. Furthermore, the pulmonary capillary network covers a total surface area of approximately 70 m², which is approximately 40 times the surface area of the human body. This implies that there are an enormous number of pulmonary capillaries in parallel. There is a widespread school of thought that holds that pulmonary capillaries do not interconnect in the manner of a vascular network but rather the capillary *walls* act like pillars separating an upper and lower layer of endothelial cells, much like supporting posts in a parking garage. In this manner, pulmonary capillary flow is thought to occur in a sheet-like, rather than in a stream-like, manner. Thus, at least part of the reason why pulmonary vascular resistance is low is that pulmonary vessels have relatively large diameters, and at least at the capillary level, vascular interconnections are so massive that flow appears to occur as a single sheet between endothelial layers.

Effects of Gravity on Pulmonary Vascular Resistance

A unique factor that contributes to pulmonary vascular resistance is the relative ease with which modest changes in hydrostatic pressure alter pulmonary vascular diameter and, therefore, pulmonary blood flow. The effect of gravitational forces on pulmonary blood flow is illustrated in Figure 16-2, which is a schematic presentation of the relative distribution of pulmonary blood flow in an apex-to-base (top-to-bottom) direction. Such information is usually obtained by isotope clearance techniques in upright subjects during breath holding at end expiration (i.e., with alveolar pressure equal to zero). As described by West and his colleagues, the relationship between pulmonary blood flow and the anatomic position of the lungs is divided into three zones classified in accordance to dynamic relationships between alveolar and intravascular pressures [5].

FIGURE 16-2 ▶

Relative Changes in Pulmonary Blood Flow from the Apex (top) to Base (bottom) of the Lungs across the Different Respiratory Zones. The illustrations indicate that in zone I the pulmonary capillaries are collapsed at both arterial and venous ends. Accordingly, there is very little blood flow in this zone. In zone II, the venous side of the pulmonary capillaries is collapsed. This creates a waterfall effect of pulmonary blood flow, in which flow is governed by the arterial to alveolar pressure gradient. In zone III, both arterial and venous sides of the pulmonary capillaries are open, and pulmonary blood flow is governed by the arteriovenous pressure gradient.

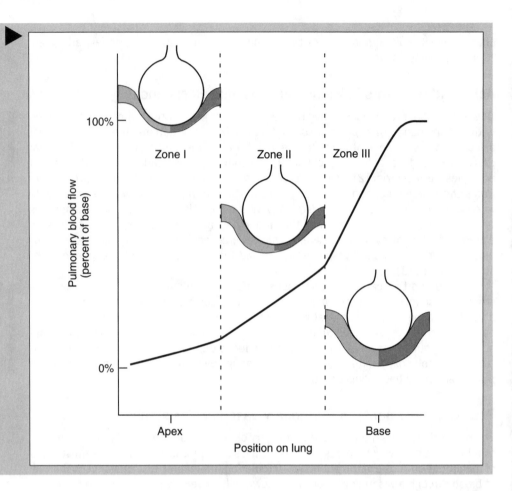

Zone I pertains to the apical regions of the lungs, which are generally above the level of the heart. At this level, pulmonary vascular pressures tend to be subatmospheric and lower than alveolar pressure at both arteriolar and venular ends of the pulmonary capillaries. This situation causes collapse of a large population of pulmonary capillaries in the zone I region, thereby shutting off blood flow in these vessels.

In *zone II*, the vessels tend to reside just above heart level in a manner such that pulmonary arterial pressure is positive, but venous pressure remains subatmospheric. Therefore, the venous ends of the capillaries tend to remain collapsed, and blood flow is determined by the difference between pulmonary arterial pressure and alveolar pressure. Flow in zone II is often compared to that of a waterfall, in which the rate of flow is unaffected by the height of the river below the fall unless it rises to a level equal to the waterfall itself. In a similar manner, as long as pulmonary venous pressure is below alveolar pressure, it has no influence on the rate of pulmonary blood flow.

Zone III is characterized by the fact that pulmonary venous pressure is consistently higher than alveolar pressure. Accordingly, pulmonary blood flow is determined by the usual arteriovenous pressure gradient seen in the systemic circulation.

The general rise in pulmonary blood flow with a descending position in the lungs reflects a decrease in pulmonary vascular resistance. This drop in resistance is associated with a gravitational-related increase in intravascular pressure, which elicits two major effects on the pulmonary circulation: (1) an increase in diameter of the arterioles and (2) the opening (i.e., recruitment) of collapsed capillaries. Toward the lower end of zone III—the very base of the lungs—these effects tend to become limited, thereby resulting in a leveling out of the pulmonary blood flow (i.e., the plateau phase at the far right of Figure 16-2).

The changes in pulmonary vascular pressures caused by gravity are gradual and continuous in going from the apex to the base of the lungs. Therefore, the transitions between zones I, II, and III are also gradual. Furthermore, these zones are classified in accordance to functional, rather than anatomic, criteria. As such, borders between the

In this context, the pulmonary vessels in zone II are behaving very much like a "Starling resistor" as described in Chapter 15.

*The phenomenon of **capillary recruitment** also occurs in the systemic circulation. An example of this is discussed in Chapter 11 in conjunction with adjustments of the skeletal muscle circulation with exercise.*

zones are constantly shifting in response to different physiologic conditions. For example, during forced expiration against an airflow resistance, the alveolar pressure may rise to levels much higher than pulmonary arteriolar pressure, thereby considerably expanding the region of zone I. Other conditions that may expand or contract the zones are discussed below.

INFLUENCE OF THE HEART ON PULMONARY BLOOD FLOW

Because the pulmonary arterial and venous systems are respectively coupled to the right and left cardiac chambers, it is reasonable to anticipate that cardiac dynamics would have a major influence on pulmonary blood flow. Some of the more salient features of pulmonary vascular and cardiac interactions are reviewed in this section.

Influence of the Right Ventricle

Right ventricular stroke volume (SV) is a major determinant of pulmonary arterial pressure. Pulmonary arterial pressure, in turn, plays a major role in the distribution of pulmonary blood flow. The result of these interactions is presented in Figure 16-3 as relative pulmonary blood flow under different conditions. The 100% value represents that at the base of the lungs for the various conditions.

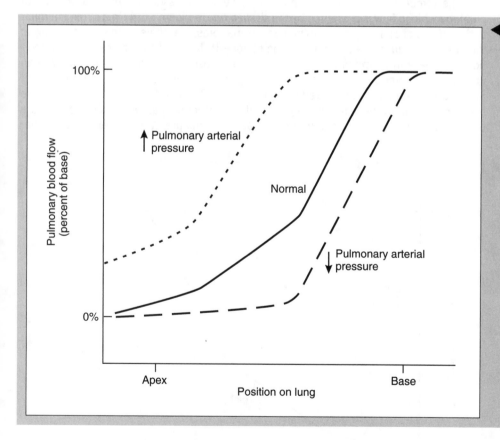

FIGURE 16-3
The effects of an increase (short dashed line) and a decrease (long dashed line) in pulmonary arterial pressure on the distribution of pulmonary blood flow. The solid line represents the normal condition illustrated in Figure 16-2.

The *short dashed line* in Figure 16-3 illustrates the influence of an increase in pulmonary arterial pressure that could occur, for example, with an exercise-induced increase in SV. The point is made in Chapter 20 that adjustments in SV that occur during dynamic exercise are to a large degree elicited by the Frank-Starling mechanism (i.e., an increase in cardiac preload). Thus, it is not the exercise per se that increases pulmonary arterial pressure but rather the increase in diastolic filling. In this context, right heart failure, which is a pathologic condition, can have the same effect on end-diastolic volume and, therefore, on pulmonary arterial pressure as exercise. Thus, the *short dashed line* in

Swimming *elicits the most pronounced increase in SV attributed to the Frank-Starling mechanism (i.e., Starling's law of the heart). This is because the body is in a buoyant horizontal position, and the muscle pump mechanism is operative.*

Figure 16-3 could represent the influence of either a physiologic (e.g., exercise) or a pathologic (e.g., right heart failure) condition on pulmonary blood flow.

As noted in Figure 16-3, one of the effects of an increase in pulmonary arterial pressure is that pulmonary blood flow is positive at the apex of the lung. The reason for this modification is that pulmonary arterial and capillary pressures exceed alveolar pressure at all levels of the lung; therefore, capillary vessels remain open; that is, there is no longer a zone I condition. In proceeding down the lungs, pulmonary blood flow increases. However, this effect plateaus higher up on the lungs compared with the control condition because, with the elevated pulmonary arterial pressure, maximal arteriolar dilation and capillary recruitment occur closer to the level of the heart.

The *long dashed line* in Figure 16-3 illustrates the effects of a decrease in pulmonary arterial pressure that could occur with hemorrhage. Under these conditions, the lungs are perfused over only approximately half of the apex-to-base distance. This is due to alveolar pressure exceeding pulmonary capillary pressure (i.e., zone I conditions) over most of the top portion of the lungs.

Influence of the Left Ventricle

The pulmonary venous system drains into the left ventricle by way of the left atrium and mitral valve. Accordingly, any influence that tends to dam up blood in the left atrium (e.g., mitral stenosis) would affect pulmonary venous pressure and, therefore, the distribution of pulmonary blood flow.

The effect of an increase in pulmonary venous pressure on the distribution of pulmonary blood flow is presented by the *dashed line* in Figure 16-4. In a manner similar to the effects of an increase in pulmonary arterial pressure, there is now positive flow at the apex of the lung (i.e., an elimination of zone I), followed by a more-or-less proportional increase in pulmonary blood flow (i.e., decrease in resistance). Also, as with an increase in arterial pressure, the flow versus position curve tends to level off (plateau) higher up on the lungs, compared with the control. These effects can be attributed to back pressure from the veins dilating the pulmonary venules as well as arterioles and a recruitment, or opening, of capillaries. Because venous pressure now exceeds alveolar

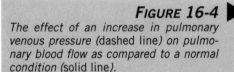

A common pathologic condition that elevates pulmonary venous pressure is **left ventricular failure;** the failing heart is described in Chapter 10.

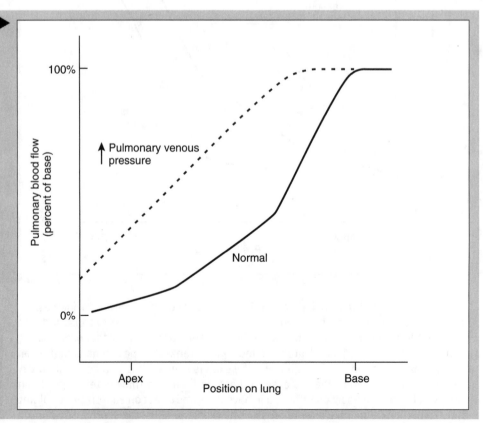

FIGURE 16-4 ▶

The effect of an increase in pulmonary venous pressure (dashed line) on pulmonary blood flow as compared to a normal condition (solid line).

pressure throughout the lungs, there is no longer a waterfall effect. Accordingly, the entire pulmonary circulation is a zone III condition, in which flow is determined by the arteriovenous pressure gradient.

A major disruptive influence of an elevation in pulmonary venous pressure is that pulmonary capillary pressure exceeds plasma oncotic pressure in a considerable portion of the pulmonary circulation. Accordingly, there is a tendency towards pulmonary edema, as seen in congestive heart failure (CHF).

RELATIONSHIP OF PULMONARY PERFUSION TO ALVEOLAR VENTILATION

To achieve maximal gas transport, the ventilation of the alveoli must match the blood flow they receive. Physiologists compare ventilation to pulmonary blood flow by a parameter known as the ventilation-perfusion ratio ($\dot{V}/\dot{Q}$). This ratio is achieved by dividing minute ventilation ($\dot{V}$) by CO ($\dot{Q}$). Because minute ventilation and CO are approximately equal at normal resting conditions, the value for $\dot{V}/\dot{Q}$ at rest is usually given as 1.0. However, it is important to recognize that this represents an average value for the total lung and that $\dot{V}/\dot{Q}$ varies considerably in different regions of the lung, even under rest conditions.

Measurements in humans have shown that in the supine posture there is essentially no difference in ventilation between basal and apical portions of the lungs; whereas, in the upright posture there is a base-to-apex distribution of ventilation similar to that seen in blood flow [6]; that is, there is a higher airflow in the base of the lungs compared to the apex. However, regional differences in ventilation are much lower compared to those of blood flow. This difference in the distribution of ventilation and perfusion is presented schematically in Figure 16-5. Even without quantifying these data, it can be seen that the upper portions of the lung tend to be overventilated ($\dot{V}/\dot{Q} > 1.0$), whereas the lower portions tend to be overperfused ($\dot{V}/\dot{Q} < 1.0$). In the resting state, these differences do

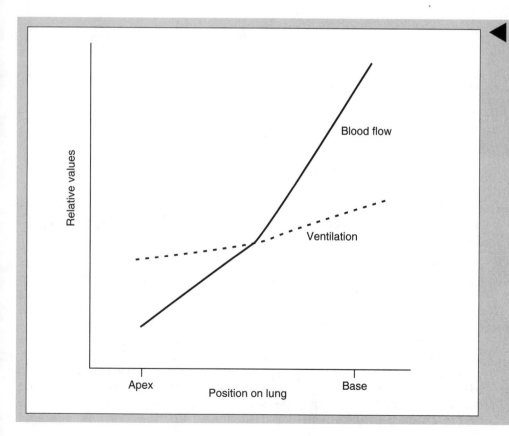

FIGURE 16-5
Relative changes in pulmonary blood flow (solid line) and minute ventilation (dashed line) from the apex to the base of the lungs under normal resting conditions.

not seem to affect the maintenance of adequate blood-gas exchange for the lung as a whole. However, during periods of physical activity, a closer match of ventilation and perfusion becomes necessary. The mechanism by which this is achieved appears to be that during exercise the difference in pulmonary blood flow between the basal and apical portions of the lungs diminishes, as shown in Figure 16-6 [6, 7]. Comparing this figure to Figure 16-5, it can be seen that both ventilation and perfusion are, in general, higher and more closely coupled during exercise compared with the resting state (i.e., the $\dot{V}/\dot{Q}$ ratio becomes more homogeneous among different regions of the lungs). However, it is very important to recognize that minute ventilation increases at a greater rate with increased exercise intensity than does CO [8]. Thus, although ventilation and perfusion become more homogeneous among various regions of the lungs during exercise, the overall $\dot{V}/\dot{Q}$ ratio progressively increases as exercise intensity increases.

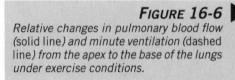

FIGURE 16-6 ▶
Relative changes in pulmonary blood flow (solid line) and minute ventilation (dashed line) from the apex to the base of the lungs under exercise conditions.

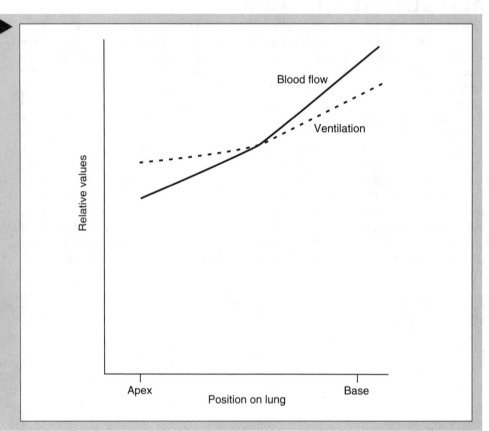

RESOLUTION OF CLINICAL CASE

The patient described at the beginning of the chapter was experiencing severe pneumonia, which was confined to the left lung. His high minute volume of 12 L/min (norm: 6 L/min) with a low Pao_2 and a normal $Paco_2$ suggested a severe $\dot{V}/\dot{Q}$ imbalance, which in this case partly took the form of a *functional* right-to-left shunt; that is, the alveoli in his lungs may have been adequately perfused, but oxygen exchange in the left lung, with the pneumonia infiltrate, was inadequate.

The observation that Pao_2 was only modestly improved by breathing 100% oxygen (from 52 mm Hg to 60 mm Hg) is a clear indication of a functional right-to-left shunt. Because under conditions of 100% oxygen breathing, blood perfusing the alveoli should be saturated with oxygen, the degree to which Pao_2 is less than predicted is a quantitative indicator of the magnitude of the right-to-left shunt [1]. As a rule, the percentage of a right-to-left shunt can be estimated as 1% of the CO for every 20 mm Hg difference between alveolar and arterial Po_2 [1]. At one atmosphere of oxygen pressure (100% oxygen breathing) $PAo_2 = 673$ mm Hg. The Pao_2 of our patient under these conditions was 60 mm Hg. Therefore, his estimated shunt was (673 − 60) mm Hg/20 mm Hg, or approximately 31% of his CO.

With such a large estimated right-to-left shunt in conjunction with the radiographic findings, it could be concluded that his left lung was almost completely dysfunctional. In this context, the objective of having the patient lie on his right side was to improve perfusion of the good lung, because pulmonary perfusion is dependent on gravity. Indeed, this was reasonably successful as indicated by an improvement in the Pao_2 to 77 mm Hg.

A puzzling aspect of this case is why the patient's $Paco_2$ was not elevated. Why was he able to exchange carbon dioxide but not oxygen? This is a normal finding for conditions producing ventilation-perfusion inequalities. The solution to this scenario is found in the *sigmoidal* nature of the oxygen–hemoglobin dissociation curve compared to the *linear* curve for carbon dioxide (see Chapter 17). However, to understand the present case, as the Pao_2 increases above 60 mm Hg, there is a substantial flattening of the oxygen dissociation curve, which prevents much additional oxygen transport despite the increasing partial pressure. Therefore, ventilating with 100% oxygen has only a slight beneficial effect on $\dot{V}/\dot{Q}$ because the extra oxygen in the ventilated areas contributes only a small increase in oxygen content. Fortunately for these patients, a relatively small increase in Pao_2 can be quite beneficial.

In this patient, the oxygenated blood, which perfuses his relatively normal right lung, may have a Pao_2 approaching 673 mm Hg during 100% oxygen breathing. However, when this superoxygenated blood mixes with that from the edematous left lung, the superoxygenated blood gives up oxygen to hemoglobin from the poorly oxygenated blood. With a 31% "functional" shunt, approximately 4 L of blood perfuse functional alveoli and are "supersaturated" during 100% oxygen breathing. This blood would have a Pao_2 in excess of 600 mm Hg, whereas the approximate 2 L of blood perfusing nonfunctional alveoli would end up with a Pao_2 of 26 mm Hg (50% saturation). The resultant 6 L of mixed blood would have a oxygen saturation of approximately 83% and a Pao_2 of approximately 60 mm Hg.

In contrast to oxygen, the portion of CO that is perfusing the well-ventilated portion of the lung efficiently exchanges its carbon dioxide and results in a $Paco_2$ of approximately 35 mm Hg, whereas the portion perfusing the diseased lung would have a $Paco_2$ of approximately 50 mm Hg. However, because the carbon dioxide dissociation curve is almost linear, the resultant $Paco_2$ in the mixed arterial blood is 39 mm Hg.

---

*The **oxygen saturation** (O_2 Sat) of mixed blood from normal and from physiologically shunted regions of the lungs can be calculated as follows:*

- Total Q x mixed O_2 Sat = nonshunted Q x O_2 Sat + shunted Q x O_2 Sat
- 6 L/min x mixed O_2 Sat = 4 L/min x 100% + 2 L/min x 50%
- Mixed O_2 Sat = 83%.

As discussed in Chapter 17, an oxygen saturation of 83% results in a Pao_2 of approximately 60 mm Hg.

REVIEW QUESTIONS

Directions: For each of the following questions, choose the **one best** answer.

1. If the bronchioles to a particular region of lung become constricted or blocked, pulmonary blood flow in the region would decrease because of which one of the following explanations?

    (A) The reduced shear stress on the type I alveolar cells elicits secretion of vasoconstrictor substances

    (B) Bronchiole vasoconstriction passively constricts pulmonary arterioles

    (C) The reduced local Pao_2 elicits constriction of pulmonary arterioles

    (D) Mechanoreceptors in the alveoli trigger a reflex constriction of the pulmonary arterioles

2. The "waterfall" concept applies to which one of the following aspects of pulmonary blood flow?

    (A) Pulmonary blood flow in zone I

    (B) Pulmonary blood flow in zone II

    (C) Pulmonary blood flow in zone III

    (D) Pulmonary capillary blood flow in general

3. A common feature of congestive heart failure (CHF) and dynamic exercise is that they reduce or eliminate which one of the following zones of pulmonary blood flow?

    (A) Zone I

    (B) Zone II

    (C) Zone III

4. Pulmonary perfusion characteristics in a neonate with a patent ductus arteriosus would be expected to show an increase (i.e., expansion) in the extent of

    (A) zone I

    (B) zone II

    (C) zone III

5. Mitral stenosis would be expected to result in an increase in pulmonary

    (A) venous pressure and an expansion of zone I

    (B) venous pressure and an expansion of zone III

    (C) arterial pressure and an expansion of zone I

    (D) arterial pressure and a contraction of zone III

6. During exercise, the ventilation-perfusion ratio ($\dot{V}/\dot{Q}$) is

    (A) greater than 1.0, but there is less variation in $\dot{V}/\dot{Q}$ within the lungs

    (B) approximately 1.0, but there is less variation in $\dot{V}/\dot{Q}$ within the lungs

    (C) less than 1.0, but there is less variation in $\dot{V}/\dot{Q}$ within the lungs

    (D) approximately 1.0, but there is more variation in $\dot{V}/\dot{Q}$ within the lungs

ANSWERS AND EXPLANATIONS

1. The answer is C. The reduced local partial pressure of oxygen (Po_2) elicits constriction of the pulmonary arterioles. This is the phenomenon of hypoxic vasoconstriction, whereby a reduction in oxygen tension within the alveoli causes a local hypoxia that elicits constriction of pulmonary vascular smooth muscle. This is the opposite from the response of systemic vascular smooth muscle, which responds to hypoxia by vasodilation. The mechanisms related to this difference are not known.

2. The answer is B. Zone II is the zone in which blood flow is determined by the difference between pulmonary arterial pressure and alveolar pressure. Pulmonary venous pressure plays no role in determining blood flow in this zone, just as the height of a river below a waterfall plays no role in determining the rate of flow over the falls.

3. The answer is A. Zone I is the zone near the apex (top) of the lungs in which there is little blood flow at rest because the pulmonary capillaries tend to collapse as a result of the intravascular pressure being subatmospheric. In CHF and dynamic exercise, pulmonary arterial pressure increases, thereby elevating pressure in the arterial, and often venous, sides of the pulmonary capillaries. Thus, regions previously characterized as zone I become more like zone II or zone III.

4. The answer is C. In a neonate with a patent ductus arteriosus, pressures in the pulmonary circulation are equivalent to those in the systemic arterial system. Under these conditions, pulmonary blood flow is determined by the difference between pulmonary arterial and venous pressures—a zone III condition—throughout the lungs.

5. The answer is B. Mitral stenosis would cause an increase in left atrial and, therefore, pulmonary venous pressure. If severe enough, it would also result in an elevation of pulmonary arterial pressure. With elevated pulmonary pressures, zone III would expand as explained for the previous question.

6. The answer is A. With exercise, blood flow is more even throughout the lungs, and, as a result, there is less base-to-apex variation in $\dot{V}/\dot{Q}$. However, as exercise intensity progressively increases, minute ventilation ($\dot{V}$) increases to a greater degree than cardiac output ($\dot{Q}$). Therefore, $\dot{V}/\dot{Q}$ becomes greater than 1.0.

REFERENCES

1. Berne RM, Levy MN: *Case Studies in Physiology*. St. Louis, MO: C. V. Mosby, 1994, pp 69–70, 179–181.
2. West JB: *Respiratory Physiology: The Essentials*, 5th ed. Baltimore, MD: Williams and Wilkins, 1995, pp 43–45.
3. Levick JR: *An Introduction to Cardiovascular Physiology*, 2nd ed. Oxford, UK: Butterworth-Heinemann, 1995, pp 249–254.
4. Comroe JH: *Physiology of Respiration*, 2nd ed. Chicago, IL: Year Book, 1974, pp 142–157.
5. West JB, Dollery CT, Naimark A: Distribution of blood flow in isolated lung; relation to vascular and alveolar pressures. *J Appl Physiol* 19:713–724, 1964.
6. Bryan AC, Bentivoglio LG, Beerel F, et al: Factors affecting regional distribution of ventilation and perfusion in the lung. *J Appl Physiol* 19:395–402, 1964.
7. West JB, Dollery CT: Distribution of blood flow and ventilation-perfusion ratio measured by radioactive CO_2. *J Appl Physiol* 15:405–410, 1960.
8. Hlastala MP, Berger AJ: *Physiology of Respiration*. New York, NY: Oxford University Press, 1996, pp 233–256.

17 BLOOD-GAS EXCHANGE

INTRODUCTION OF CLINICAL CASE

On a cold November morning, a woman was found unconscious in her home by her neighbor. Her blood pressure was 110/70 mm Hg, and her breathing was shallow at a rate of 15 breaths/min. She was brought by ambulance to the emergency department. Suspecting carbon monoxide poisoning, the paramedics administered 100% oxygen. The neighbor reported that the woman had complained of excessive, unexplained fatigue and headache the previous day. Blood gas analysis revealed a hematocrit of 35 and a partial pressure of arterial oxygen (Pa_{O_2}) of 650 mm Hg with an oxygen saturation (Sa_{O_2}) of 50%. Further tests revealed that her hemoglobin (Hb) was 50% saturated by carbon monoxide.

BACKGROUND

Previous chapters discuss the ventilatory mechanisms that deliver oxygen to the alveoli and remove carbon dioxide. They also examine the perfusion that transports oxygen from the lungs to the tissues and then returns carbon dioxide to the lungs. Chapter 16 stresses the importance of matching the delivery of oxygen to the alveoli (ventilation) with the delivery of blood (perfusion) so that maximal gas exchange can occur between the air and blood. This chapter further describes the important interactions between these systems and the special adaptations that facilitate gas transport. The mechanisms involved in the movement of gases across the cardiopulmonary interface depend on many of the physical forces that are introduced in Chapter 3.

PARTIAL PRESSURES

*In a mixture of gases, each gas exerts a **partial pressure** proportional to its presence in that mixture (Dalton's law; see Chapter 3). For example, air contains 20.9% oxygen. Therefore, in dry air the P_{O_2} is equal to atmospheric pressure (P_{atm}) times the fraction of oxygen ($F_{O_2} = 0.209$):*

$P_{O_2} = (760\ mm\ Hg)\,(0.209) = 159\ mm\ Hg$

Both oxygen and carbon dioxide are small, soluble compounds that diffuse through water and lipid. Their exchange does not require any specialized transport system across the cell membranes, and their rapid movement depends upon the *partial pressure* gradients underlying passive diffusion. The concentration gradient for gas diffusion is reflected in the difference in partial pressure between any two compartments. Therefore, the body uses several strategies to keep the partial pressure of oxygen (P_{O_2}) as high as possible to promote rapid diffusion of oxygen to its ultimate utilization site—the mitochondria.

Standard atmospheric pressure at sea level is 760 mm Hg, and almost all of this pressure is contributed by oxygen and nitrogen. However, atmospheric pressure is somewhat variable due to weather conditions and temperature. In addition, it decreases with increasing altitude above sea level. The content of air also varies with the addition of water vapor to the oxygen and nitrogen. Therefore, to standardize measurements, gas pressures are usually corrected to body temperature (37°C) and saturated with water vapor. At 37°C, the water pressure is equal to 47 mm Hg. Because inspired air is saturated with water vapor, the water pressure reduces the partial pressures contributed by nitrogen and oxygen.

Oxygen

Because oxygen comprises 20.9% of the air, it accounts for 20.9% of the barometric pressure, or approximately 159 mm Hg (0.209 × 760 mm Hg) when the air is dry. As the air is inspired through the upper airways, it is warmed and humidified. With the addition of water vapor to the inspired air, the P_{O_2} in the trachea decreases to 149 mm Hg (0.209 × [760−47 mm Hg]). As the inspired air mixes with the gas sequestered within the residual capacity of the lung, the P_{O_2} is further reduced to approximately 100 mm Hg in the alveoli. Oxygen diffuses into the thin water layer lining the alveoli until it reaches equilibrium with the oxygen concentration in the alveolar gas. The partial pressure of any gas in a solution equals the partial pressure of that gas in the gas mixture at the air–liquid interface. Therefore, the P_{O_2} in the venous end of the pulmonary capillaries is approximately equal to the partial pressure of alveolar oxygen (P_{AO_2}) [Table 17-1]. There is a large gradient for molecules of oxygen to move into the red blood cells (RBCs) until the Hb is fully saturated with oxygen. Hb within the RBCs binds oxygen with a great affinity, and the bound oxygen no longer contributes to the P_{AO_2}. The P_{O_2} in the RBC and in the arterial blood approaches 100 mm Hg only after the Hb has been almost completely saturated. This binding of oxygen by Hb greatly increases the number of oxygen molecules that can be carried in the blood.

Tissues depend on oxygen to produce adenosine triphosphate (ATP) in the mitochondria. As the oxygen is consumed, the P_{O_2} decreases in the mitochondria and in the cells. This low cellular and tissue P_{O_2} creates a gradient for the movement of oxygen from its higher concentration in the plasma. Consequently, the P_{AO_2} begins to drop as oxygen moves from the plasma to the tissues. The drop in P_{AO_2}, in turn, creates a gradient for

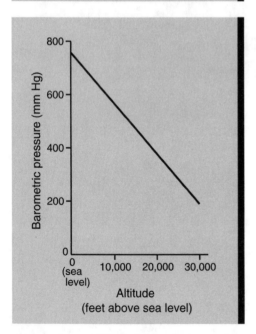

At Sea Level

$P_{atm} = 760\ mm\ Hg$

$P_{O_2\ (inspired)} = (P_{atm} - P_{H_2O})\,(F_{O_2\ (inspired)})$

$P_{IO_2} = (760 - 47\ mm\ Hg)\,(0.209)$

$\quad = 149\ mm\ Hg$

At 5000 Feet (Denver)

$P_{atm} = 620\ mm\ Hg$

$P_{IO_2} = (P_{atm} - P_{H_2O})\,(F_{IO_2})$

$P_{IO_2} = (620 - 47\ mm\ Hg)\,(0.209)$

$\quad = 120\ mm\ Hg$

Partial Pressures (mm Hg)			Content (mL gas/L air* or mL gas/100 mL fluid**)	
Po_2	Pco_2	Location	Co_2	Cco_2
160	0	Atmospheric air	209*	0*
149	0	Inspired humidified air	196	0*
100	40	Expired humidified air (alveolar air)	132	52
95	40	Arterial blood	20**	48**
		Dissolved	0.3	2.5
		Bound to hemoglobin	19.7	2.5
		As HCO_3^-	—	43
40	46	Mixed venous blood	15**	52**
		Dissolved	0.1	2.8
		Bound to hemoglobin	14.9	3.8
		As HCO_3^-	—	45.4
≤40	≥46	Extracellular fluid	0.1**	51**
		Dissolved	0.1	3
		Bound to hemoglobin	...	...
		As HCO_3^-	...	48
≤40[a] May typically be near 0	≥46[a]	Mitochondria	Almost 0[a]	

[a] These values vary greatly and depend on both the metabolic rate and the distance from an oxygenated capillary.

oxygen to move out of the RBCs into the plasma. Because Hb binds oxygen in a reversible fashion, as the Po_2 in the RBC decreases, additional oxygen molecules are released from oxyhemoglobin to blunt the decline in Po_2. Additional features of the binding of Hb and oxygen also contribute to this unloading.

At the cellular level, the Po_2 may decrease to relatively low levels. The lowest levels are observed within the mitochondria, where the oxygen is used by the electron transport chain to generate ATP. With increased metabolism, the tissue Po_2 declines even lower. When inadequate oxygen is delivered, cells must either decrease their activity or switch to *anaerobic metabolism* to generate ATP. Some cells, such as neurons and cardiac myocytes, depend almost exclusively on aerobic metabolism, and these cells must have a continuous supply of oxygen. Anaerobic metabolism results in the production of *lactate* and hydrogen ions (H^+). It also generates an *oxygen debt* that must eventually be repaid.

Carbon Dioxide

The atmosphere contains negligible amounts of carbon dioxide, and the partial pressure of carbon dioxide (Pco_2) in inspired air is close to 0 mm Hg. However, the body tissues are constantly generating carbon dioxide that is returned to the lung. Air in the lung typically has a partial pressure of alveolar carbon dioxide ($Paco_2$) of 35–40 mm Hg. With each inspiration, this value is reduced slightly as the inspired air dilutes the carbon dioxide concentration. However, during expiration, the $Paco_2$, $Paco_2$, and the partial pressure of carbon dioxide in mixed venous blood ($P\bar{v}co_2$) all increase as carbon dioxide is returned to the lungs from the tissues. In the blood, some carbon dioxide is bound by Hb and carried by carbaminohemoglobin. However, *most of the carbon dioxide is combined with water in the presence of carbonic anhydrase to form H^+ and bicarbonate ions (HCO_3^-).* The importance and handling of these ions are further discussed in Chapter 18.

Diffusion of Blood Gases

The major gases present in the alveoli are nitrogen, oxygen, and carbon dioxide. All three gases diffuse readily across the barriers that separate the lung gases from the plasma (Figure 17-1). These barriers include a thin water layer that lines the alveoli, a thin alveolar epithelial cell, an intercellular space containing a basement membrane, and the capillary endothelial cell. Ultimately, most of the blood gases also diffuse into the RBC. As they cross into (or out of) the cell, they must pass through a lipid membrane. The rate

$D_L = \dot{V}$ *of gas/ΔP*

$D_L \propto$ *(area of diffusive surface/thickness of diffusive membrane)(solubility/$\sqrt{MW}$)*

of diffusion depends on the solubility of the gas, the partial pressure gradient for diffusion, and the diffusing capacity of the lung (D_L). Because D_L is defined as the flow of gas for a given pressure gradient, it has units of mL gas/min/mm Hg. It is difficult to measure the diffusing capacity for most gases in vivo because the pressure gradients change alinearly along the length of the pulmonary capillary. However, it is possible to determine the diffusing capacity for carbon monoxide, and this value can be used as an indicator for the diffusing capacity of the lung for oxygen ($D_L O_2$). From the equation in the margin note, the D_L is proportional to the surface area for gas exchange. Because the capillary perfusion of the alveoli is sheetlike, the effective surface area is usually equivalent to the surface area of the alveoli. Therefore, any disease or perturbation that decreases the surface area decreases the D_L. Diffusing capacity is inversely affected by the thickness of the diffusive membrane.

FIGURE 17-1

Barriers to Diffusion between the Alveolar Gases and the Plasma. *Diffusion across the alveolocapillary membrane depends on the concentration gradient established by the partial pressures on either side of the membrane. For carbon dioxide, the partial pressure in blood is higher than the partial pressure in the alveolus, so the net flow is from the capillary into the alveolus. For oxygen, the pressure gradient causes net diffusion from the alveolus to the capillary. The blood gases must diffuse in the air of the alveolus, through the lipid membranes of the alveolar epithelial cell, the capillary endothelium, and the red blood cell (RBC). The diffusing capacity of the lung is proportional to the area for diffusion divided by the thickness of the membrane.*

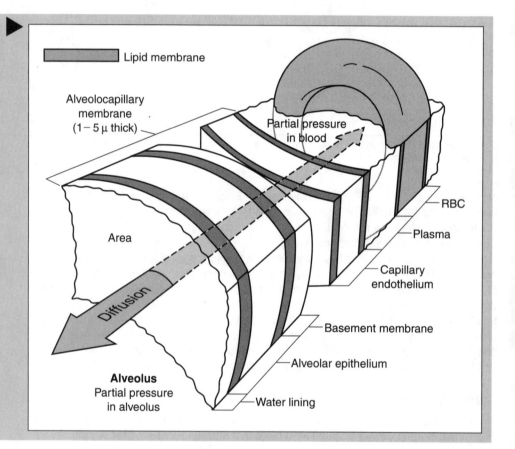

CONTENT

Because of the concentration gradients established by ventilation and perfusion, the gases exhibit a net movement that normally brings their partial pressures in the blood and lungs to near equilibrium, and the alveolar–arterial difference in partial pressure (PA − Pa) is small. Although the partial pressures representing the "free" gases are in equilibrium, their content (C) is not equal because blood contains special mechanisms to bind and transport both oxygen and carbon dioxide. The solubility of a gas also helps to determine the total number of molecules (content) that dissolve in solution at any partial pressure. The partial pressures and contents for both oxygen and carbon dioxide are shown in Table 17-1. The distinction between partial pressure and content is very important because the partial pressure establishes the gradient for diffusion, whereas the content denotes the amount of gas available in a solution (normally expressed as mL gas/100 mL blood). *Because of the characteristics of the transport systems, partial pressure and content are not linearly related.* Sensory transduction mechanisms responsible for maintaining homeostasis of the blood gases are designed to monitor the partial pressure and not the content (see Chapter 19).

At rest, an adult consumes approximately 250 mL O_2/min and produces approximately 200 mL CO_2/min. With a typical cardiac output (CO) of 5 L/min, it can be seen that the average extraction of oxygen from the arterial blood must be approximately 5 mL O_2/100 mL blood. Similarly, the 200 mL of carbon dioxide produced each minute indicates that approximately 4 mL CO_2/100 mL blood must move from the pulmonary capillary into the alveoli. These calculated numbers match the differences observed in content between mixed arterial and venous blood. Table 17-1 presents the contents of the various compartments in the resting state. The content of oxygen in arterial blood (Cao_2) is 20, and the content of oxygen in venous blood (Cvo_2) is 15; therefore, the Cao_2 difference is 5 mL O_2/100 mL blood. Similarly, the normal venous–arterial difference in carbon dioxide content ($C_{v-a}co_2$) is approximately 4 mL CO_2/100 mL blood (see Table 17-1; $Caco_2$ is 48 mL CO_2/100 mL blood, and $Cvco_2$ is 52). With exercise, the delivery of oxygen and the removal of carbon dioxide are augmented by increasing both the amount of blood flow and the amount of gas exchanged (the C_{a-v} difference).

$\dot{V}o_2$/blood flow = O_2 consumed/100 mL blood
= (250 mL O_2/min) / 5000 mL blood/min
= 5 mL O_2/100 mL blood

$\dot{V}co_2$/blood flow = CO_2 produced/100 mL blood
= (200 mL CO_2/min)/5000 mL blood/min
= 4 mL CO_2/100 mL blood

Capillary Transit Time

Although the surface area for gas exchange between the alveoli and the pulmonary capillaries is great, the blood volume of the pulmonary capillaries is relatively small. Because most of the cardiac output passes through these capillaries, the flow velocity must be rapid. In fact, blood normally traverses the pulmonary capillary in approximately 0.75 seconds (Figure 17-2). Thus, the diffusion of oxygen and carbon dioxide must be completed during this *transit time*. Under normal conditions, this does not pose a problem because the exchange of both oxygen and carbon dioxide is complete within 0.25–0.35 seconds. Generally, the diffusion of oxygen is completed slightly quicker than that of carbon dioxide. However, when pathologies such as edema increase the time required for diffusion, the rate of oxygen exchange is usually the most severely affected. With exercise, the pulmonary capillary transit time may decrease to approximately 0.25 seconds. This poses no diffusion limits upon the healthy lung. However, when Pao_2 is low due to disease or high altitude, the exchange of gas across the alveolocapillary membrane may be inadequate to maintain maximal exercise (see Figure 17-2).

Because the Po_2 and Pco_2 normally equilibrate before the blood leaves the pulmonary capillary, there is a substantial period of time when no net diffusion occurs across the alveolocapillary membrane. Diffusion increases if more blood is available; therefore, the movement of oxygen and carbon dioxide is described as *perfusion limited*. This term implies that more gas could be exchanged if there were more perfusion. As the CO —*cardiac output* increases during exercise, there is a decrease in the transit time for blood in the pulmonary capillaries. The decreased transit time reduces the perfusion limitation, and the time spent by the RBCs in the pulmonary capillary may decrease to approximately 0.25 seconds without affecting the Pao_2. However, if the transit time falls below approximately 0.25 seconds, the Po_2 in the pulmonary capillary does not reach equilibrium with the Pao_2, and a *diffusion limitation* occurs because the movement of the gas is limited by the D_L. Diffusion limitations for oxygen can occur in diseases that increase the thickness of the alveolocapillary membrane, such as pulmonary edema. The patient's oxygen transport can be improved by increasing the gradient for diffusion by breathing supplemental oxygen.

FIGURE 17-2 ▶

Transit Time for Diffusion of Oxygen and Carbon Dioxide in the Pulmonary Capillary. At rest, blood normally requires approximately 0.75 seconds to traverse the pulmonary capillary. The top panel shows that the Po_2 in the capillary equilibrates with Pao_2 within 0.25 seconds as blood flows through the first third of the capillary. When the diffusing capacity is reduced (e.g., by any disease that decreases the area for diffusion, such as emphysema, or increases the thickness, such as in pulmonary edema), the required time for equilibrium is increased. When the Pao_2 is abnormally low, the gradient for oxygen diffusion is reduced. Because the same number of molecules are moved (to meet metabolic needs), the reduced gradient mandates a longer diffusion time for equilibrium to be reached. Similar changes for diffusion of carbon dioxide are seen in the lower panel.

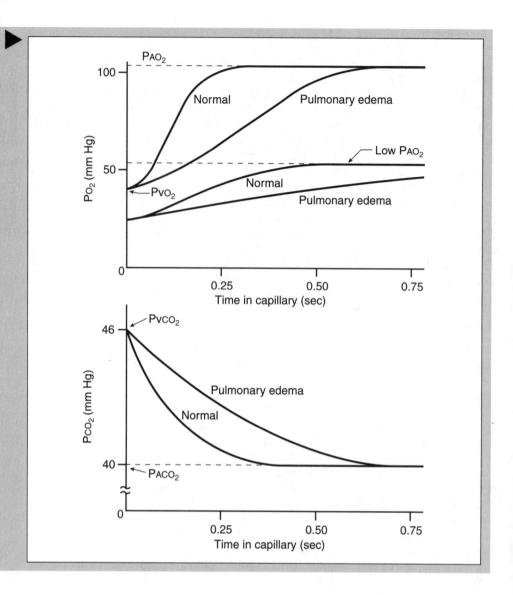

HEMOGLOBIN

RBCs contain Hb, a very important molecule. Each Hb molecule contains four polypeptide subunits, each of which contains a ferrous iron ion (Fe^{2+}) that can bind one molecule of oxygen. This heme group can bind other molecules, including carbon dioxide and carbon monoxide. There are several forms of Hb and its related compounds. In the muscle cells, there is a molecule that resembles a single subunit of Hb known as *myoglobin*. Myoglobin binds a single molecule of oxygen and provides a ready local store of oxygen for the muscle. *Hemoglobin A* (HbA) is the normal adult hemoglobin, and it contains two alpha and two beta polypeptide subunits. *Hemoglobin F* (HbF) is the fetal form of hemoglobin, and it has a greater affinity for oxygen. The enhanced affinity helps to move the bound oxygen from the maternal Hb to the placental Hb. Because of the altered affinity, HbF is 50% saturated at a Po_2 of 20 mm Hg while for HbA this occurs when the Po_2 is 27 (see Figure 17-3). Abnormal variants include *hemoglobin S* (HbS), which causes sickle cell anemia, and *methemoglobin*, which contains ferric iron ions (Fe^{3+}). Most of these variants have a reduced capacity for binding oxygen, and the shape of their dissociation curve differs from HbA.

ie - saturated at lower partial pressures of O_2?

Hemoglobin–Oxygen Dissociation Curve

As each Hb subunit binds oxygen, there is a conformational change that increases the binding affinity for the next molecule of oxygen. This characteristic of Hb and oxygen binding gives rise to the sigmoidal *hemoglobin–oxygen dissociation curve* in Figure 17-3.

This curve is also known by several other names including the *hemoglobin–oxygen equilibrium curve* and the *oxygen saturation curve*. If no oxygen is present, all the Hb exists in a reduced form as *deoxyhemoglobin*. However, in the presence of oxygen, Hb binds oxygen to form *oxyhemoglobin*. Hb is almost completely saturated at a Po_2 of approximately 100 mm Hg. Oxyhemoglobin has a bright red color characteristic of arterial blood. In contrast, deoxyhemoglobin has a dark red color that is typical of venous blood. When the concentration of deoxyhemoglobin is high, vascularized areas of the skin appear blue, or *cyanotic*. Although *cyanosis* is an important clinical symptom usually correlated with hypoxia, it is not necessarily diagnostic by itself. Hypoxia can occur without cyanosis (e.g., anemia), and cyanosis can occur without significant tissue hypoxia (e.g., polycythemia).

It is useful to think of the hemoglobin–oxygen dissociation curve (see Figure 17-3) as representing two domains. A flat, *plateau* range from 70–100 mm Hg is typically encountered within the lung and is important to oxygen loading in the lungs. A steep *dissociation* range from 20–70 mm Hg dominates in the tissues. The *plateau* region of this curve assures that near-maximal oxygen transport into the pulmonary capillary blood occurs even if there is a decline in Pao_2. For example, in Figure 17-3, it can be determined that a 20% decrease in Pao_2 from 100 mm Hg to 80 mm Hg causes approximately a 5% decrease in oxygen saturation (Sao_2). Therefore, at an altitude of 5000 feet, the barometric pressure is decreased approximately 20%, and the Pao_2 is decreased somewhat less. However, there is minimal change in the oxygen content of the arterial blood. Clinically, this means that a patient could have a 20% impairment in ventilation or diffusion with only a very small, clinically insignificant change in oxygen carriage.

Textbook definition of... cyanosis => more than 5g/100ml blood deoxygenated Hb

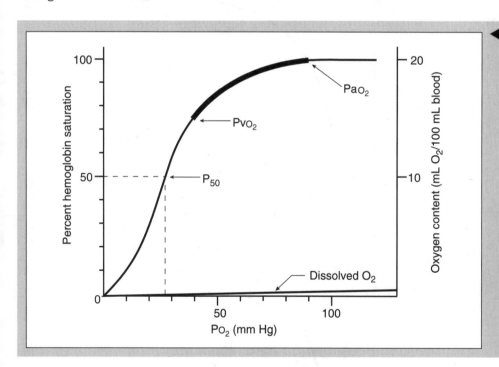

The hemoglobin–oxygen percent saturation curve is a useful measure of the binding characteristics of Hb, and if one knows the Hb concentration of the blood, the *oxygen content* (Co_2) can be easily calculated. In fact, most saturation curves plot both the percent Hb saturation and the oxygen content on the y-axis. One gram of Hb binds 1.34 mL of oxygen. Because a normal value for Hb content is approximately 15 g/100 mL blood, the typical oxygen content is approximately 20 mL O_2/100 mL blood. Some oxygen is dissolved in the plasma, but the total amount of oxygen physically dissolved in blood is very small in comparison to that carried by Hb because the solubility of oxygen is only approximately 3×10^{-5} mL O_2/mL blood/mm Hg. By increasing the Po_2 it is possible to carry a little more oxygen in a dissolved form; however, even with breathing 100% oxygen, the Pao_2 may increase to approximately 600 mm Hg, and the

[Hb] ≅ hematocrit/3 g Hb/100 mL blood

Oxygen dissolved in 100 mL blood = (sol-ubility)(100 mL blood)(Pao$_2$)
= (3 × 10^{-5} mL O$_2$/mL blood/mm Hg)
(100 mL/100 mL)(100 mm Hg)
= 0.3 mL O$_2$/100 mL blood

dissolved oxygen is only approximately 1.8 mL O$_2$/100 mL blood. Therefore, the primary rationale for placing a patient on oxygen is to increase the partial pressure gradient of oxygen between the alveoli and pulmonary capillary, thereby improving the hemoglobin–oxygen saturation. This assists in overcoming a diffusion barrier, but it cannot substantially increase the amount of oxygen dissolved in the blood.

Anemia and Polycythemia

Changes in the number of RBCs affect the amount of Hb available for oxygen transport. The concentration of Hb is decreased in *anemia*. Although the shape of the saturation curve is not affected, the maximal oxygen binding or content is reduced (Figure 17-4). If the concentration of Hb is reduced to half of normal (i.e., 7.5 g/100 mL blood), the maximal oxygen content bound to Hb is 10 mL O$_2$/100 mL blood. The number of RBCs is normally well regulated; however, their number may be decreased by diseases that impair their formation or hasten their destruction. Acute blood loss is another major cause for a reduced hematocrit.

When the hematocrit exceeds 55%, the condition is known as *polycythemia*. Polycythemia is a normal adaptation to altitude and chronic hypoxemia. When the kidney is chronically hypoxic, it produces a hormone known as *erythropoietin* (or *hemopoietin*), which stimulates the production of RBCs. Although this greatly increases the oxygen-carrying capacity of the blood, it has the deleterious side effect of increasing the vis-

hypoxaemia = reduction of the [O₂] in arterial blood.

hypoxia = deficiency of O₂ in the tissues.

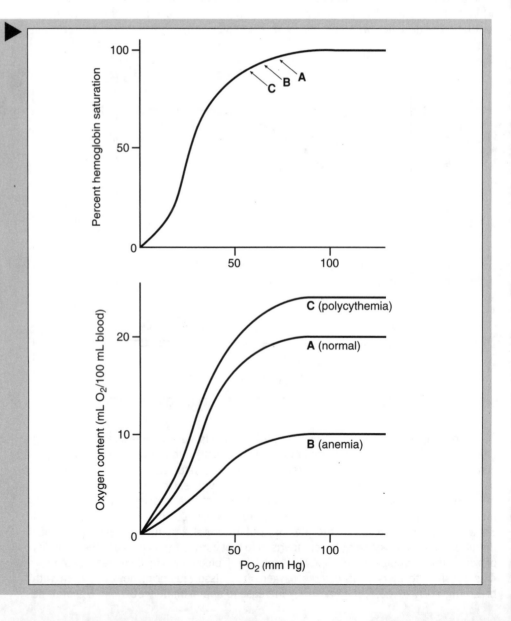

FIGURE 17-4 ▶

Hemoglobin Saturation Curves and Oxygen Content Curves. *The top graph shows that the percent saturation of hemoglobin (Hb) is identical under normal conditions (curve A) and conditions of anemia (curve B) and polycythemia (curve C). Despite the identical shape of the curves, the bottom graph shows that the oxygen content is markedly altered because of the different concentrations of Hb.*

cosity of the blood and, therefore, increasing the resistance to the flow of blood. The increased viscosity ultimately increases the work of the heart.

Carboxyhemoglobin

Hb has a much higher affinity for carbon monoxide than for either oxygen or carbon dioxide. Thus, it preferentially binds carbon monoxide to form *carboxyhemoglobin* (not to be confused with carbaminohemoglobin, which is Hb and carbon dioxide). Because the affinity of Hb for carbon monoxide is more than 200 times greater than that for oxygen, breathing 0.5% concentrations of carbon monoxide can be lethal because all the Hb binding sites become occupied by carbon monoxide rather than by oxygen. In addition to reducing the amount of oxygen that can be transported, the shape of the oxygen dissociation curve is greatly affected by the presence of carboxyhemoglobin. The adjacent margin note shows the change from a normal sigmoidal curve to a hyperbolic curve. With carbon monoxide poisoning, oxygen is unloaded from Hb only at a very low P_{O_2}. Cigarette smoke is a significant source of carbon monoxide, and in heavy smokers, approximately 10% of their Hb may be chronically bound as carboxyhemoglobin. Accidental poisoning usually results from malfunction or improper venting of a fuel-burning device.

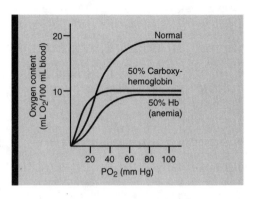

Admixture of Blood

Because of the curvilinear nature of the oxygen saturation curve, the content of oxygen in the blood is not linearly related to the P_{O_2}. Most of the arterial oxygen is bound to Hb, and the total amount bound depends on the P_{O_2} in the plasma. Although the P_{AO_2} in each healthy alveolus usually reaches equilibrium with the P_{aO_2} in the adjacent capillary, differences in the mixed alveolar and arterial values do occur normally.

Approximately 2% of the cardiac output enters the *bronchial circulation*, which perfuses the lung structures. Because this blood is not oxygenated when it returns to the pulmonary vein, it tends to absorb oxygen from the blood that perfused the pulmonary capillaries. In addition to this bronchial blood, the arterial blood in the left ventricle also includes blood from the perfusion of the left heart that enters the ventricle through the *thebesian circulation*. Pathologic conditions, such as mismatching of ventilation–perfusion or regional deficiencies in diffusion, can result in significant alveolar–arterial differences. The P_{O_2} in the mixed arterial blood of the left atrium depends upon the average oxygen content of the blood from the various regions of the lung. The adjacent margin note provides an example of the calculations that predict the mixed P_{aO_2}.

	Pulmonary Circulation	**Bronchial Circulation**
Volume	CO	2% CO
Blood entering	Unoxygenated	Oxygenated
Target	Alveoli and small airways	Major airways
Arterial pressure	15 mm Hg	100 mm Hg
Venous pressure	5 mm Hg	1–2 mm Hg
Resistance	Low	High

Bohr Effect

There is a significant gradient for oxygen to diffuse from the capillary to the mitochondria as the oxygenated, arterial blood perfuses the capillaries in the tissues. Movement of oxygen from the plasma decreases the P_{O_2} of the plasma, which, in turn, results in the release of more oxygen from oxyhemoglobin. Several factors generated by the tissues influence the affinity of Hb for oxygen, thereby changing the equilibrium of the hemoglobin–oxygen dissociation. The accumulation of H^+, carbon dioxide, and 2,3-bisphosphoglycerate (2,3-BPG, sometimes called 2,3-DPG) all shift the curve to the right. An increase in temperature also causes a right shift (Figure 17-5). Shifting of the dissociation equilibrium to the right results in a decreased affinity of Hb for oxygen and a greater release of oxygen for the same drop in P_{O_2}. In exercising tissue, all of these changes increase the availability of oxygen and help to "unload" the oxygen at a higher P_{O_2}. *Keeping the capillary P_{O_2} as high as possible is an important mechanism for increasing the gradient for diffusion of oxygen into the metabolically active tissue.* The hemoglobin–oxygen dissociation relationship normally functions over a series of curves as the capillary blood accumulates H^+ and carbon dioxide from the periphery. In Figure 17-5, line A illustrates the normal relationship in arterial blood, whereas line B shows the curve for venous blood in an exercising muscle. Line C depicts the further right shift that occurs in venous blood in muscle during strenuous exercise. Because both the oxygen utilization and the carbon dioxide production are increased, the oxygen extraction is greatly increased. However, the P_{vO_2} is much higher than it would have been if the curve had not shifted.

Lung 1
$P_{aO_2} = 100$ mm Hg
Blood flow = 2 L/min

Lung 2
$P_{aO_2} = 40$ mm Hg
Blood flow = 2 L/min

(Mixed C_{O_2}) (4 L/min) = (C_{O_2} in lung 1) (2 L/min) + (C_{O_2} in lung 2) (2 L/min)

(Mixed C_{O_2}) (4 L/min) = (20 mL O_2/100 mL blood) (2 L/min) + (15 mL O_2/100 mL blood) (2 L/min)

Mixed C_{O_2} = (400 mL O_2 + 300 mL O_2)/4000 mL blood = 17.5 mL O_2/100 mL blood

From the hemoglobin–oxygen curve, a content of 17.5 mL O_2/100 mL blood occurs at a P_{aO_2} of approximately 55 mm Hg.

Pathway for Oxygen
Air → alveolus → across alveolocapillary membrane → plasma → RBC → bind to Hb → circulation → in tissue, unload from Hb → diffuse to plasma → extracellular fluid → cell → mitochondria

FIGURE 17-5 ▶

Shifts in the Hemoglobin–Dissociation Curve during Exercise. The standard curve (A) is based on a body temperature of 37°C, a pH_a of 7.4, and a $Paco_2$ of 40 mm Hg. The 50% saturation point (P_{50}) for each curve is indicated by the x. A typical Pvo_2 for each condition is indicated by the dot on each line. As the blood traverses the capillary, oxygen is lost from the capillary blood, and carbon dioxide is added. This change in Pco_2 and the resulting decrease in pH both affect the affinity of hemoglobin for oxygen and shift the curve toward line B. With moderate exercise (curve B), there is a right shift of the dissociation curve in the muscle because of the increased [H+] carbon dioxide production, and temperature. The oxygen extraction can increase to provide an arteriovenous oxygen difference of 10 mL O_2/100 mL blood without much change in the Pvo_2. During strenuous exercise, the generation of heat and the accumulation of lactic acid, H+, and carbon dioxide cause a further right shift of the dissociation curve (C). The right shift increases the amount of oxygen released at a given Po_2 and helps to keep the partial pressure high to facilitate diffusion.

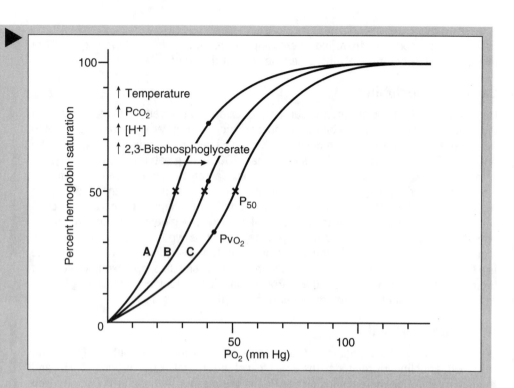

Chloride Shift

In the peripheral tissues, the increased Pco_2 causes an effect known as the *chloride (Cl⁻) shift* (Figure 17-6). As carbon dioxide diffuses into the RBC, the action of the enzyme *carbonic anhydrase* causes the formation of H+ and HCO_3^-. (Although there is very little carbonic anhydrase in the plasma, some H+ and HCO_3^- is generated directly in the plasma by the endothelial cell.) Most of the H+ remains inside the RBC where it is buffered by Hb; however, the HCO_3^- diffuses out of the cell down its concentration gradient using a membrane transport molecule that cotransports Cl⁻. This movement of Cl⁻ into the RBC helps maintain the electrical equilibrium and creates an osmotic gradient for water to enter the RBC, which swells in size. This Cl⁻ shift is reversed in the lung as the carbon dioxide leaves the plasma for the alveoli. As Cl⁻ and water both leave the RBC, it returns to its normal size. This shift in Cl⁻ content and cell size happens routinely with each pass through the systemic and pulmonary circulation.

Haldane Effect

As the venous blood with its reduced Hb returns to the lung, it encounters an environment with a high Po_2 and a lower Pco_2. This results in a decreased affinity of Hb for carbon dioxide that aids in the release of carbon dioxide from the *carbaminohemoglobin* and the subsequent binding of oxygen. Therefore, the *Haldane effect* facilitates the unloading of carbon dioxide and the loading of oxygen in the lung. Its action is the opposite of the Bohr effect that predominates in the peripheral tissues.

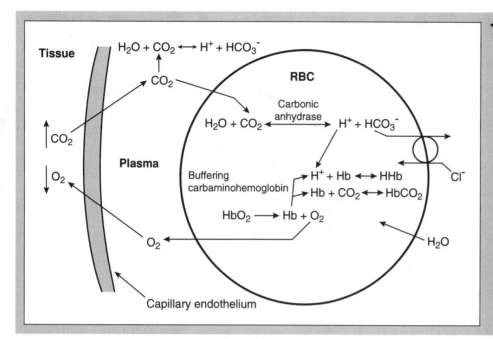

FIGURE 17-6
Movements of Carbon Dioxide and Oxygen in the Peripheral Capillaries. As the tissues produce carbon dioxide and consume oxygen, gradients are created that drive the movement of these molecules. As carbon dioxide enters the plasma, some is converted to H^+ and HCO_3^-, but most passes into the red blood cell (RBC), where it is acted on by carbonic anhydrase. Some of the HCO_3^- leaves the RBC in exchange for Cl^-. As the tonicity of the RBC increases, water moves into the cell to keep the cell isotonic. This results in a slight swelling of the cell described as the chloride shift. As oxyhemoglobin (HbO_2) is reduced, it binds and buffers excess H^+ and carbon dioxide.

TRANSPORT OF CARBON DIOXIDE

Carbon dioxide is transported from the tissues to the lungs in several forms that have already been mentioned (dissolved, as carbaminohemoglobin, and as HCO_3^-). Most of the carbon dioxide is converted to H^+ and HCO_3^- through the action of carbonic anhydrase, and approximately 90% of the carbon dioxide in the blood exists in the RBCs and plasma as HCO_3^-. Dissolved carbon dioxide and carbon dioxide that is bound to Hb to form carbaminohemoglobin each account for approximately 5% of the total carbon dioxide. Table 17-1 shows the approximate values for these contents. Although nearly 90% of the carbon dioxide exists as HCO_3^-, the venous-to-arterial differences in carbon dioxide content suggest that both carbaminohemoglobin and dissolved carbon dioxide transport more carbon dioxide from the tissues to the lung than might be expected.

The carriage of carbon dioxide by Hb is affected by the concentration of oxyhemoglobin. With a Po_2 of 100 mm Hg, most of the Hb is bound to oxygen; however, as the Po_2 drops, the formation of carbaminohemoglobin is increased. This binding characteristic is responsible for the different carbon dioxide dissociation curves of Figure 17-7. Within the normal physiologic range, these carbon dioxide dissociation curves are almost linear, whereas the oxygen dissociation curves are sigmoidal. As blood moves through the systemic capillaries, oxygen leaves the capillary, and the Po_2 decreases. The "physiologic" carbon dioxide dissociation curve is therefore described by the *arrow*, which moves from the $Paco_2$ on the oxyhemoglobin curve to the $Pvco_2$ on the 75% saturation curve. During the increased oxygen desaturation that occurs in exercise, the physiologic curve moves even farther toward the appropriate saturation line.

FIGURE 17-7 ▶
Carbon Dioxide Dissociation Curve at Different Levels of Oxygen Saturation. *The carriage of carbon dioxide in the blood varies as a function of Pco_2 and Po_2. Because of the influence of oxyhemoglobin (HbO_2) on the binding of carbaminohemoglobin, the carbon dioxide dissociation curve is affected by the degree of oxygen saturation. The normal arterial (a) and venous (v) points are indicated, and the arrow connecting them describes the normal physiologic binding curve that occurs in the systemic and pulmonary capillaries.*

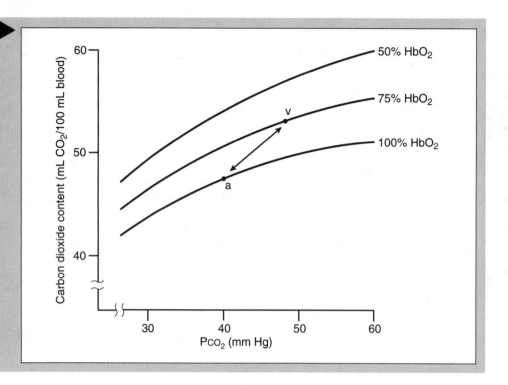

HYPOXIA, HYPOXEMIA, AND HYPERCAPNIA

Hypoxia and *hypoxemia* are often used interchangeably to describe conditions of low oxygen. Hypoxemia specifically suggests a low oxygen condition in the blood, whereas hypoxia suggests a low alveolar oxygen concentration. Both hypoxia and hypoxemia result from deficiencies in the transport of oxygen from the atmosphere to the tissues. Four clinically relevant types of hypoxia are recognized: *hypoxic hypoxia, anemic hypoxia, stagnant hypoxia,* and *histotoxic hypoxia.* They are distinguished by the site of the respiratory defect and can be characterized as seen in Table 17-2.

TABLE 17-2 ▶
Partial Pressures and Content of Oxygen Correlated with Different Types of Hypoxia

	P_{AO_2}	Pa_{O_2}	Ca_{O_2}	Pv_{O_2}	Cv_{O_2}
Hypoxic hypoxia					
High altitude	Low	Low	Low	Low	Low
CNS depression	Low	Low	Low	Low	Low
Respiratory muscle weakness	Low	Low	Low	Low	Low
Abnormal lung mechanics	Low	Low	Low	Low	Low
Diffusion impairment	Normal	Low	Low	Low	Low
Anatomic shunt	Normal	Low	Low	Low	Low
Ventilation–perfusion mismatch	Normal	Low	Low	Low	Low
Anemic hypoxia					
Anemia	Normal	Normal	Low	Low	Low
Carboxyhemoglobin	Normal	Normal	Low	Low	Low
Stagnant hypoxia	Normal	Normal	Normal	Low	Low
Histotoxic hypoxia	Normal	Normal	Normal	High	High

Note: The descriptors high, normal, and low are used to compare the values to normal values for a healthy individual. P_{AO_2} = partial pressure alveolar oxygen; Pa_{O_2} = partial pressure arterial oxygen; Ca_{O_2} = content arterial oxygen; Pv_{O_2} = partial pressure oxygen in mixed venous blood; Cv_{O_2} = content of oxygen in mixed venous blood.

Hypoxic Hypoxia

Hypoxic hypoxia is associated with inadequate delivery of oxygen into the pulmonary capillary. Therefore, any condition that decreases the Pa_{O_2} or impairs the diffusion of oxygen across the alveolocapillary membrane can cause this type of hypoxia. Significant hypoxias are often averted by the feedback mechanisms of the peripheral and central chemoreceptors (see Chapter 19). When the Pa_{O_2} declines below approximately 60 mm Hg, the peripheral chemoreceptors are stimulated, and they initiate a reflex increase in ventilation. Therefore, severe hypoxic hypoxias occur only after normal mechanisms for maintaining oxygen transport are significantly compromised.

Some common pathologies that lead to alveolar hypoventilation include depression of the central nervous system (CNS), respiratory muscle weakness, and impaired lung mechanics. The Pa_{O_2} can also be reduced in healthy individuals by breathing low P_{O_2} gas mixtures. This occurs naturally when breathing at high altitude or in closed areas from which the oxygen has been depleted. Alveolar hypoventilation caused by a disease process is often accompanied by an increased Pa_{CO_2} or *hypercapnia*.

Central Nervous System (CNS) Depression. CNS depression can result from many causes, including anesthesia, drug overdoses, brainstem trauma, and stroke. All of these conditions can decrease the descending central drive to breathe and reduce the ventilatory effort, which in turn leads to a decrease in the Pa_{O_2}. Spinal cord injuries or phrenic nerve injury can also reduce the efficacy of the respiratory pump and lead to a low Pa_{O_2} and an elevated Pa_{CO_2}.

Respiratory Muscle Weakness. Some muscle wasting diseases can affect the respiratory pump muscles and decrease the contractile ability of the chest wall muscles. Similarly, muscle control pathologies, such as myasthenia gravis, can also impair normal function of the respiratory pump. Although there may be a significant central drive to breathe, the musculature is physically incapable of generating normal levels of inspiratory and expiratory force.

Abnormal Lung Mechanics. Normally, the elastic and resistive work of breathing is minimized so that the total work of breathing is very small. However, the respiratory pump may be unable to overcome the airway resistance completely when the airways are significantly obstructed in chronic obstructive pulmonary diseases (COPD) such as emphysema, bronchitis, and asthma. Similarly, diseases that decrease lung compliance may make the elastic work of breathing so great that alveolar ventilation is reduced.

Diffusion Impairment. Even if the alveolar ventilation is normal, hypoxic hypoxemia may occur if there is a significant barrier to the diffusion of oxygen. Loss of alveoli decreases the surface area for diffusion and may further limit the uptake of oxygen in the lung. Abnormal diffusion can also result from an increased thickness of the alveolocapillary membrane associated with fibrosis or pulmonary edema. Because carbon dioxide is more soluble than oxygen, it is not uncommon to see diffusion impairments causing hypoxemia without an accompanying hypercapnia. Oxygen therapy with higher inspired concentrations of oxygen are beneficial in treating this type of hypoxia.

Anatomic Shunts. Right-to-left anatomic shunts are discussed in Chapter 16. In a shunt, the unoxygenated pulmonary artery blood is returned directly to the left heart without exchanging any gas with the alveoli. With an anatomic shunt, hypoxemia may result despite a normal Pa_{O_2}.

Ventilation–Perfusion Mismatching. The matching of ventilation and perfusion in the lung is essential for adequate gas exchange. If ventilation and perfusion are not distributed appropriately, there can be areas where either ventilation or perfusion is wasted because there is little gas exchange in those areas. The lack of adequate gas exchange leads to a *physiologic shunt*. These ventilation–perfusion inequalities are discussed in detail in Chapter 16. Again, they often result in hypoxemias without concomitant hypercapnia.

Anemic Hypoxia

This category of hypoxia includes abnormalities related to inadequate Hb binding and carriage of oxygen. The normal [Hb] is approximately 15 g/100 mL blood; if this value is decreased, the oxygen content of the blood is decreased. In anemia, there is a decrease in the number of RBCs and an accompanying decline in [Hb]. The reduced hematocrit can result from decreased production of RBCs, increased destruction of RBCs, or loss through hemorrhage. Although the shape of the oxygen dissociation curve is not affected by a loss of Hb, the oxygen content is severely limited. This can result in a very low P_{O_2} in the tissues. Clinically, anemia is characterized by excessive fatigue and a very limited ability to increase the oxygen consumption. Because the Pa_{O_2} is usually normal, there is very little increased drive to breathe because the peripheral chemoreceptors sense the Pa_{O_2}, not the blood content. Although hyperventilation could increase the Pa_{O_2}, it would not result in any significant increase in oxygen delivery to the tissues.

Abnormal variants of Hb that fail to bind sufficient oxygen (e.g., sickle cell anemia) can also produce a hypoxia that is classified as an anemic hypoxia. Carbon monoxide poisoning is another related pathology because again the tissue hypoxemia is due to inadequate carriage of oxygen by Hb.

Stagnant Hypoxia

Hypoxia in the tissues can also be caused by inadequate systemic blood perfusion. In this situation, the Pa_{O_2} is normal, and there is normal diffusion and Hb binding of oxygen; however, the delivery of the RBCs to the tissue is inadequate to meet metabolic needs. With poor perfusion, almost all the oxygen content can be removed from the blood, and the arteriovenous difference may be comparatively large. The tissue becomes severely hypoxic when the oxygen extraction is nearly complete, and the Pa_{O_2} decreases substantially below normal. This type of hypoxia is called by several names, including *stagnant hypoxia, hypoperfusion hypoxia*, and *circulatory hypoxia*. Stagnant hypoxias may occur either locally or throughout the body. They can be caused by low blood pressure caused by reduced CO or by regional vasoconstriction that limits perfusion. Hemorrhage can reduce blood flow, especially through the bowel or kidneys, and results in significant damage due to this type of hypoxemia.

Histotoxic Hypoxia

The final form of hypoxemia relates to a failure of the cells to use the oxygen that is delivered to them. A typical example of histotoxic hypoxia is *cyanide poisoning*. Cyanide blocks the action of mitochondrial enzymes in the electron transport chain and prevents oxygen from being used. Although the local P_{O_2} is greatly elevated from normal and may even approach the Pa_{O_2}, the cell behaves in the same way as if no oxygen were present.

RESOLUTION OF CLINICAL CASE

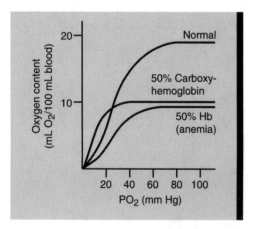

Carbon monoxide poisoning is most frequently associated with breathing the exhaust of heating appliances that generate carbon monoxide as a by-product of combustion. The reported symptoms of fatigue and headache are consistent with a tissue hypoxia caused by the inadequate delivery of oxygen to the tissues, especially the brain. The patient's comatose condition results from partial failure of her neurons caused by *anemic hypoxia*. Although her hemoglobin is 50% saturated with oxygen, the carboxyhemoglobin alters the normal dissociation curve so that oxygen is unloaded only at a very low P_{O_2}. This low P_{O_2} decreases the gradient for diffusion, and it is likely that the mitochondria that are distant from a capillary are exposed to a P_{O_2} that is almost 0.

Despite the patient's severe tissue hypoxia, her Pa_{O_2} remained normal, so there was no increased drive to breathe from the peripheral chemoreceptors. Her shallow, slow breathing was primarily caused by the CNS depression resulting from hypoxia. This hypoventilation may have resulted in a slight increase in Pa_{CO_2} and Pa_{CO_2}. The increased Pa_{CO_2} would stimulate both central and peripheral chemoreflexes to limit any further CNS suppression of breathing.

Breathing 100% oxygen increases the dissolved oxygen slightly, which may have some slight benefit for this seriously compromised patient. However, the increased oxygen delivery can provide only approximately 40% of the normal resting requirements (approximately 1.8 mL O_2/100 mL blood can be dissolved at 600 mm Hg). The major benefit of the 100% oxygen is to provide a gradient to increase the oxygen binding by Hb and speed the removal of carbon monoxide from the carboxyhemoglobin.

Because her hematocrit is slightly below normal, her ability to transport oxygen is further compromised. A hematocrit of 35 in a woman probably does not represent any pathology, but it does warrant subsequent monitoring.

After 6 hours of breathing 100% oxygen, the patient's oxygen–hemoglobin saturation increased to 80%. She resumed breathing room air and was kept overnight for observation. The next day, she appeared healthy and was released. Her faulty furnace was repaired, and she purchased a carbon monoxide detector.

REVIEW QUESTIONS

Directions: For each of the following questions, choose the **one best** answer.

1. Which of the following statements best describes the effect of carbon monoxide?
    (A) Carbon monoxide poisoning stimulates the peripheral chemoreceptors and increases the respiratory rate
    (B) Carbon monoxide changes the shape of the sigmoidal oxygen dissociation curve
    (C) The binding of carbon monoxide to hemoglobin (Hb) creates carbamino-hemoglobin
    (D) The Pao_2 is decreased by carbon monoxide poisoning
    (E) Carbon monoxide binds irreversibly to Hb

2. During exercise, the delivery of oxygen to the tissues is facilitated by which one of the following actions?
    (A) An increased pulmonary capillary transit time
    (B) Peripheral vasoconstriction
    (C) The production of carbon dioxide and H^+ by the muscle
    (D) An increase in pH from 7.35 to 7.45
    (E) The formation of methemoglobin

3. The content in 100 mL of blood is greatest for which one of the following substances?
    (A) Dissolved oxygen
    (B) Oxygen bound to oxyhemoglobin
    (C) Dissolved carbon dioxide
    (D) Carbon dioxide in the form of bicarbonate (HCO_3^-)
    (E) Carbon dioxide bound to carbaminohemoglobin

4. Which one of the following is the essential enzyme for transport of carbon dioxide?
    (A) Hemoglobin reductase
    (B) Bicarbonase
    (C) Carbonic anhydrase
    (D) Erythropoietin
    (E) Carbaminohemoglobin

5. Which one of the following actions would increase the rate of diffusion of oxygen from the alveolus?
    (A) Increasing the capillary blood perfusion rate
    (B) Decreasing the surface area
    (C) Increasing the thickness of the alveolocapillary membrane
    (D) Decreasing the Pao_2–Pvo_2 gradient
    (E) Decreasing the pH_a

6. In a patient with a normal hematocrit, the ventilation of one lung is compromised by severe emphysema and airway collapse. This results in a ventilation–perfusion mismatch such that one lung receives 1 L/min of inspired air with a perfusion of 2 L of blood/min. The P_{AO_2} in this lung is 40 mm Hg. The other lung has a P_{AO_2} of 100 mm Hg and a perfusion of 3 L blood/min. Using the graph below, what is the mixed arterial P_{O_2}?

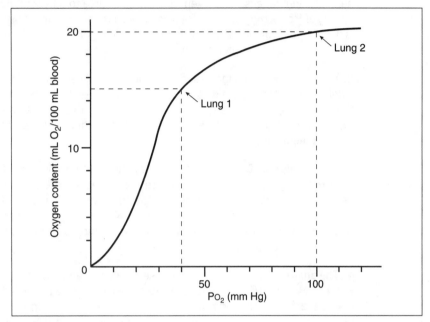

   (A) 30 mm Hg
   (B) 50 mm Hg
   (C) 60 mm Hg
   (D) 70 mm Hg
   (E) 90 mm Hg

7. Acute hemorrhage causes a reduction of Hb content to 60% of the normal value in an otherwise healthy individual. If the alveolar ventilation and oxygen consumption rates remain the same as before hemorrhage, which one of the following conditions is likely to occur after the hemorrhage during rest?

   (A) Normal P_{aO_2}, normal P_{vO_2}
   (B) Low P_{aO_2}, normal P_{vO_2}
   (C) Low P_{aO_2}, low P_{vO_2}
   (D) Normal P_{aO_2}, low P_{vO_2}
   (E) High P_{aO_2}, normal P_{vO_2}

8. The oxygen capacity of arterial blood can be reduced to 10 mL O_2/100 mL blood by either a 50% poisoning with carbon monoxide or by a 50% loss in Hb. Which one of the following statements describes the comparative effect of these conditions?

   (A) Both conditions result in a similar decrease in tissue P_{O_2}
   (B) Carbon monoxide poisoning is most severe because there is less oxygen in the blood
   (C) Carbon monoxide poisoning is most severe because the gradient for oxygen diffusion from the plasma to the tissues is lower
   (D) A 50% anemic condition is most severe because the maximal oxygen available for exchange is 10 mL O_2/100 mL blood
   (E) A 50% anemic condition is most severe because the deoxyhemoglobin cannot form as much carbaminohemoglobin

ANSWERS AND EXPLANATIONS

1. The answer is B. When carbon monoxide binds to Hb, the formation of carboxyhemoglobin changes the oxygen dissociation curve to a hyperbolic shape. Although the affinity of Hb for oxygen at low Pa_{O_2} is increased, the amount of oxygen that can be bound is decreased. Typically, the Pa_{O_2} is the same or slightly elevated, so there is no increase in peripheral chemoreceptor activity.

2. The answer is C. The increased concentrations of carbon dioxide during exercise cause a right shift in the oxygen dissociation curve that results in the unloading of oxygen from the oxyhemoglobin. These molecules also cause a peripheral vasodilation to increase systemic capillary blood flow. With increased cardiac output, the pulmonary capillary transit time decreases.

3. The answer is D. Table 17-1 shows the content for each form of gas carriage. Approximately 43 mL of carbon dioxide are carried as HCO_3^-, in the arterial blood. It is useful to rank order these answers and give their values in mL gas/100 mL blood: carbon dioxide in the form of HCO_3^- (43) > oxygen bound to oxyhemoglobin (20) > dissolved carbon dioxide and carbon dioxide bound to carbaminohemoglobin (2.5) > dissolved oxygen (0.3).

4. The answer is C. Carbonic anhydrase catalyzes the conversion of carbon dioxide and water to H^+ and HCO_3^-. Because most carbon dioxide is carried as HCO_3^-, carbonic anhydrase is very important. Carbaminohemoglobin is a polypeptide formed by the binding of carbon dioxide to hemoglobin. Erythropoietin is a renal hormone that stimulates RBC production.

5. The answer is A. Normally, the diffusion of oxygen is perfusion limited, and Hb is almost completely saturated most of the time that the blood is in the pulmonary capillary. By increasing the perfusion, more oxygen can diffuse. Decreasing the surface area, increasing the thickness of the alveolocapillary membrane, and decreasing the PA_{O_2}–Pv_{O_2} gradient would all decrease oxygen diffusion because $D_L{O_2} = (A/T)\ (D_{O_2})\ (PA_{O_2} - Pv_{O_2})$. Decreasing the pH_a would shift the oxygen dissociation curve to the right and decrease the affinity of Hb for oxygen slightly. However, it would probably not affect the overall diffusion.

6. The answer is D. The curve is used to convert the Pa_{O_2} to a content; the contents are then averaged.

(Ca_{O_2})(total blood flow) = $(C_{O_2}$ lung 1)(lung 1 blood flow) + $(C_{O_2}$ lung 2)(lung 2 blood flow)
(Ca_{O_2}) (5 mL/min) = (15 mL/100 mL blood)(2 L/min) + (20 mL O_2/100 mL blood)(3 L/min)
(Ca_{O_2}) = (30 mL O_2/100 mL blood + 60 mL O_2/100 mL blood)/5 = 18 mL O_2/100 mL blood

Again using the oxygen dissociation curve, this content occurs at a 90% Hb saturation and a Pa_{O_2} of approximately 70 mm Hg.

7. The answer is D. The Pa_{O_2} in a healthy individual without any significant shunting is determined by the PA_{O_2}. Therefore, although the oxygen content is low from the patient's blood loss, the Hb is fully saturated, so the Pa_{O_2} is normal. Because the metabolism is normal, approximately 5 mL O_2/100 mL blood is extracted from the saturated blood. The Ca_{O_2} is approximately 12 mL O_2/100 mL blood (60% of the normal 20 mL O_2/100 mL blood). Therefore, the Cv_{O_2} would be 7 mL O_2/100 mL blood. For this anemic individual, this Cv_{O_2} would correspond to a Pv_{O_2} of approximately 30 mm Hg.

8. The answer is C. With either a 50% depletion of Hb or a 50% saturation of Hb with carbon monoxide, the maximal oxygen content is the same at approximately 10 mL O_2/100 mL blood. However, the Po_2 at which the Hb unloads its oxygen is much lower in carbon monoxide poisoning because carbon monoxide changes the shape of the hemoglobin–oxygen binding curve. This results in oxygen being released from the Hb at a much lower Po_2. The lower plasma Po_2 decreases the gradient for oxygen O_2 to diffuse.

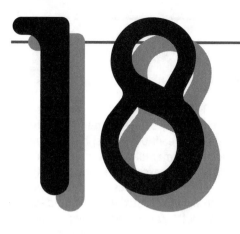

18

ROLE OF THE CARDIOPULMONARY SYSTEM IN ACID-BASE BALANCE

CHAPTER OUTLINE

INTRODUCTION OF CLINICAL CASE

A known diabetic is brought to the emergency room in a comatose state. She is breathing on her own approximately 15 times per minute. Arterial blood-gas analysis reveals a pH of 7.25, partial pressure of arterial oxygen (Pao$_2$) of 85 mm Hg, partial pressure of arterial carbon dioxide (Paco$_2$) of 31 mm Hg, and a bicarbonate ion concentration ([HCO$_3^-$]) of 15 mEq/L. Additional blood work indicates poor control of glucose levels and a significant ketoacidosis.

[handwritten margin note: Intercellular => between cells. Intracellular = situated or occurring inside cells. Extracellular = situated or occurring outside cells.]

INTRODUCTION TO ACID-BASE BALANCE

Most of the numerous biochemical reactions that occur within a human organism are very sensitive to the hydrogen ion concentration ([H$^+$]) within the extracellular and intracellular fluids. The activity of the enzymes that catalyze these reactions are greatly influenced by the pH of the environment. With this in mind, it is axiomatic that homeostasis of [H$^+$] is an essential element of total body homeostasis. The [H$^+$] in most body fluids is approximately 40 nM/L. This value is miniscule when compared to other ions, such as extracellular calcium concentration [Ca^{2+}] (2 mM/L or 2,000,000 nM/L). Despite the low concentration, small changes in [H$^+$] have profound effects on chemical reactions. Because of the very low concentration, it is common to express [H$^+$] in terms of pH, where pH = −log[H+]. Although [H+] and pH are used interchangeably, the student must remember that an increase in [H+] results in a decreased pH.

Although a small amount (approximately 100 mEq [millimoles]) of H+ is ingested in the foods we eat, the major source of H+ in the human body comes from the more than 10,000 mEq of H+ produced per day through metabolic reactions. Thus, humans must constantly deal with a heavy acid (i.e., H+) load. Fundamentally, this is achieved by chemically buffering the excess acid, converting it to an excretable form, and then eliminating it from the body. The sum of all physiologic processes by which acid is neutralized and eliminated is what is meant by the term *acid–base balance* or *acid–base homeostasis*. The objective of this chapter is to review the role of the cardiopulmonary system in acid–base balance. In so doing, the text focuses on cardiovascular and pulmonary physiology. Related topics, such as the biologic sources of acid and acid–base chemistry, are covered very superficially. For those interested in the fundamental framework of acid–base chemistry in biology, the classic monograph of Davenport is recommended [1].

ACID–BASE RELATIONSHIPS

A minor portion of the daily acid load comes from the anaerobic catabolism of glucose to lactic acid. However, the preponderance (essentially all) of metabolic acid production results from the aerobic combustion of glucose and fatty acids to carbon dioxide and water. Obviously, this reaction by itself does not produce H+. As described in Chapter 17 on blood-gas transport, *aerobically generated H+ comes from the conversion of carbon dioxide and water to H+ and HCO_3^- by the enzyme carbonic anhydrase in red blood cells* (RBCs). These reactions are expressed in the following equation, which forms the basis of acid–base balance in humans:

$$CO_2 + H_2O \longleftrightarrow H_2CO_3 \longleftrightarrow H^+ + HCO_3^- \qquad (1)$$

The relationship between these compounds is determined by the Henderson-Hasselbalch equation, where pK represents the negative logarithm of the dissociation constant:

$$pH = pK + \log ([HCO_3^-]/[CO_2]) \qquad (2)$$

or

$$pH = 6.1 + \log \{[HCO_3^-]/0.03(P_{CO_2})\} \qquad (3)$$

Sometimes this relationship is described simply by the Henderson equation, where:

$$[H^+] = K ([HCO_3^-]/[CO_2]) \qquad (4)$$

Because the $[HCO_3^-]$ is controlled by relatively slow processes of the kidneys, and the carbon dioxide is controlled rapidly via the lungs, this equation may be conceptually simplified to:

$$[H^+] = kidneys/lungs \qquad (5)$$

As indicated previously, the reaction that converts carbon dioxide to H+ and HCO_3^- generates approximately 10,000 mEq of H+ per day. If the H+ produced in this manner were not immediately buffered, it would be impossible to carry out any level of metabolic activity compatible with life without generating a lethal acidosis. However, for the most part, the H+ generated within RBCs do not leave the RBC. Instead, they are buffered within the RBC by binding to hemoglobin, and in the process, oxygen dissociates from the hemoglobin molecule. Thus, the role of the circulatory system in acid–base balance is to provide an adequate number of RBCs containing the enzyme carbonic anhydrase and an appropriate hemoglobin content in those cells. In short, *carbonic anhydrase catalyzes the conversion of carbon dioxide and water to HCO_3^- and H+, then hemoglobin helps to buffer the latter.*

The relationship between carbon dioxide and the HCO_3^- and H+ is reversible, as indicated by the *double arrows* in equation 1. Therefore, the relationship is driven by the chemical *law of mass action*. If the H+ and HCO_3^- were not affected by any other buffers or reactions, the relationship between these compounds could be graphed as in Figure 18-1. This relationship is often described as the *hemoglobin buffer line* because it reflects the buffering capacity of hemoglobin for the H^+ produced from carbon dioxide. As the concentration of carbon dioxide changes, there is a commensurate change in $[H^+]$ and $[HCO_3^-]$ and a corresponding shift along this line. At the tissue level, where P_{CO_2} is comparatively high, the reaction favors the generation of HCO_3^- and H^+, and the point on this line shifts to the left (i.e., high $[HCO_3^-]$ and low, acidic pH). However, within the oxygen-rich and carbon dioxide–poor environment of the alveoli, the high oxygen concentration helps to dissociate H^+ from the hemoglobin. Subsequently the H^+ combine with HCO_3^- to form carbonic acid (H_2CO_3), and, with the help of carbonic anhydrase, the H_2CO_3 is converted to carbon dioxide and water, which are then exhaled. This change of events causes a right shift along the line of Figure 18-1A. The normal physiologic operating range is relatively narrow, as indicated by the *heavy line*. If the concentration of hemoglobin falls, the ability to buffer the H^+ falls. Thus, the line indicating anemia shows a greater change in pH for any given change in $[HCO_3^-]$.

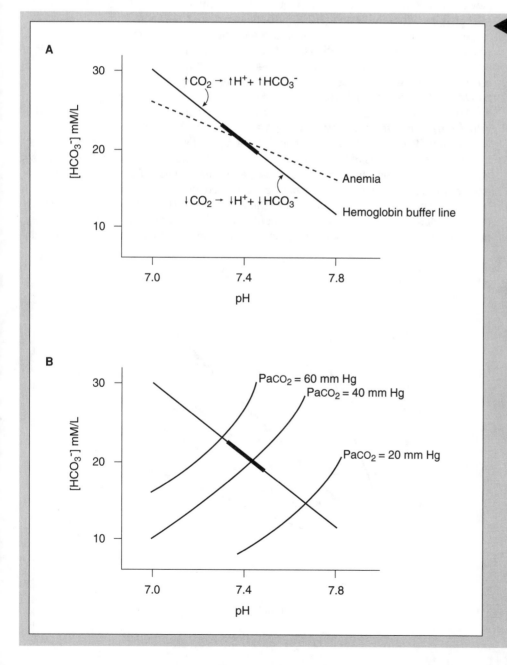

FIGURE 18-1
Relationships among $Paco_2$, H^+, and HCO_3^-. (A) Hemoglobin buffer line shows the relationship between pH and $[HCO_3^-]$ in the blood. The thick portion of the line depicts the normal physiologic range of this relationship. With anemia (dashed line), the reduced hemoglobin concentration decreases the buffering capability of the blood so that $[H^+]$ changes more for any given change in $[HCO_3^-]$. (B) Addition of $Paco_2$ isobars demonstrates the relationship between pH and $[HCO_3^-]$ at several levels of constant $Paco_2$.

FUNDAMENTAL CATEGORIES OF ACID-BASE DISTURBANCES

Because three variables ($Paco_2$, pH, and [HCO_3^-]) interact in equations 1–3, the relationships are complex and depend on which factor is changed. Ventilatory problems produce an initial change in the concentration of carbon dioxide, whereas metabolic abnormalities can alter either [H^+] or [HCO_3^-]. The concentrations for these ions are usually given in either milliequivalents/L (mEq/L) or millimoles/L (mM/L). Because both ions have only a single charge, these units can be used interchangeably for both [H^+] and [HCO_3^-].

A primary change in any one variable results in modification of the others. Several experimental manipulations illustrate these relationships. For example, if the $Paco_2$ is held constant (by adjusting the concentration of carbon dioxide in the inhaled air) while [HCO_3^-] levels are altered (by infusing either H^+ or HCO_3^-), the *isobars* showing this new relationship can be added to Figure 18-1B. Each isobar indicates the multiple relationships between pH and [HCO_3^-] that can occur at the same Pco_2.

The complex relationship between these variables is demonstrated in Figure 18-2, which shows the multiple solutions for the Henderson-Hasselbalch equation. There is a unique point on this graph for any physiologic combination of these three variables. The *dashed lines* show the intersection point for normal resting values for arterial blood (i.e., a $Paco_2$ of 40 mm Hg, a [HCO_3^-] of 24 mEq/L, and a pH of 7.4). The $Paco_2$, [HCO_3^-], and [H^+] all increase as the blood moves through the capillaries into the veins and the values move along the *short arrow* through a succession of isobars.

To simplify the understanding of acid–base regulation, it is useful to recognize that the two main categories of abnormal pH status are *acidosis* and *alkalosis*. Both of these pathologic conditions can be caused either by abnormal values of $Paco_2$ resulting from a *respiratory* (pulmonary) disturbance or by abnormal concentrations of [H^+] and [HCO_3^-] resulting from *metabolic* disturbances at the tissue level. The relationships shift along the hemoglobin buffer line in primary acid–base disturbances caused by pulmonary problems. In contrast, metabolic disturbances result in a shift along the carbon dioxide

Acidosis and *alkalosis* are associated with mechanisms that decrease and increase pH, respectively. These terms are used without any absolute reference to the arterial pH. *Acidemia* refers to an arterial blood pH_a lower than 7.36, and *alkalemia* is used when the pH_a is greater than 7.44. It is possible for an alkalosis to occur simultaneously with acidemia.

FIGURE 18-2
Relationships among pH, Pco_2, and [HCO_3^-]. *The complex interactions among these three variables show that if any single parameter changes, there must be a resulting change in at least one other variable. The normal physiologic values in arterial blood are indicated by the dotted lines. As blood moves through metabolizing tissue, the Pco_2, [HCO_3^-], and pH all increase as indicated by the arrow originating from this point. The asterisk at the end of the arrow represents the values associated with venous blood.*

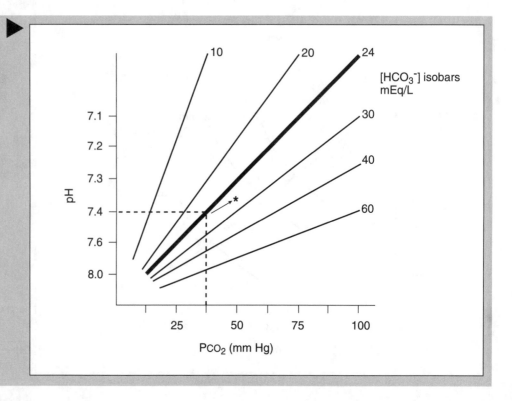

isobars. Therefore, there are four major categories of acid–base disturbance: metabolic acidosis, metabolic alkalosis, respiratory acidosis, and respiratory alkalosis. These categories are depicted in the Davenport diagrams of Figure 18-3. Figure 18-3A is a plot of plasma [HCO$_3^-$] versus plasma pH, with only one point on the graph. This *central point* shows the normal values of these variables when the blood is in optimal acid–base balance. Drawing a horizontal and a vertical line through this point divides the graph into four quadrants, each of which represents a different type of acid–base disturbance.

It is essential to recognize that the cardiopulmonary system is regulated by several different sensors responsive to both [H$^+$] and Paco$_2$. Increases in either stimuli increase ventilation, thereby providing a negative feedback important for homeostasis. Sometimes the [H$^+$] and the Paco$_2$ change in opposite directions because of the mass action effect on the carbon dioxide–bicarbonate reaction. This provides contradictory signals to the respiratory controller. These sensors and their reflexes are described in detail in

In **respiratory acidosis**, there is an increase in Paco$_2$ typically leading to a decrease in pH$_a$. In **respiratory alkalosis**, there is an decrease in Paco$_2$ typically leading to an increase in pH$_a$. In **metabolic acidosis**, there is a decrease in [HCO$_3^-$]$_a$ typically leading to a decrease in pH$_a$. In **metabolic alkalosis**, there is an increase in [HCO$_3^-$]$_a$ typically leading to an increase in pH$_a$. Each of these **primary** processes can be homeostatically counterbalanced by a secondary **compensatory** process.

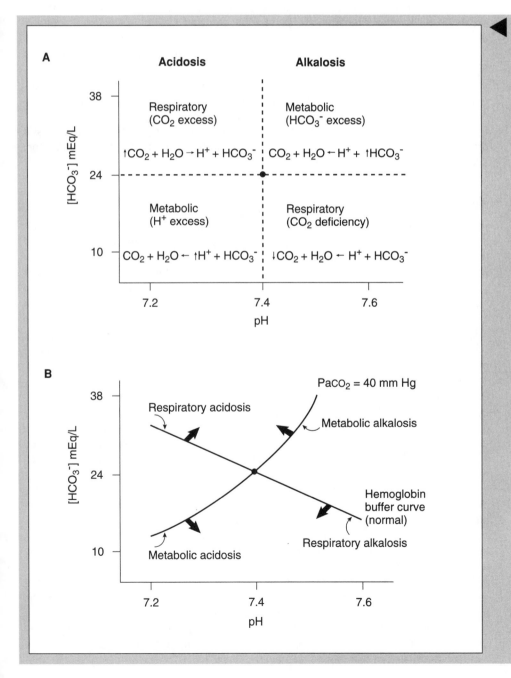

FIGURE 18-3
Davenport Diagrams Depicting the Major Acid–Base Problems and Their Compensation. (A) A simple graph showing the normal set point for plasma and the four major acid–base disturbances. For each perturbation, the primary change is indicated along with the resulting change in the carbon dioxide–bicarbonate reaction. Note that the direction of the reaction can change. An increase in any parameter results in a decrease of the other variable on that same side of the reaction and an increase in both variables on the other side of the equation. (B) Addition of the hemoglobin buffer line and the 40 mm Hg Paco$_2$ isobar to the axes of part A. The intersection of these two lines occurs at the normal resting values for arterial blood. Primary acid–base disturbances cause a shift along one of the four line segments originating from this point. For example, in metabolic acidosis, one could predict a [HCO$_3^-$] of 20 mM/L and a pH of 7.3. These primary disturbances are usually offset by compensatory mechanisms indicated by the heavy arrows.

Chapter 19. However, at this time it is important to know that the respiratory chemo-reflexes normally limit perturbations of these parameters within very narrow ranges. Relatively small changes in these variables can have a major impact on numerous body functions.

Alkalotic Conditions

The *upper right* quadrant of Figure 18-3A depicts the situation of metabolic alkalosis, in which pH is higher than normal (i.e., a low [H+]), and plasma [HCO_3^-] is elevated. The chemical reaction given in that quadrant demonstrates that the elevated [HCO_3^-] shifts the reaction to the left, resulting in a lower [H+] and a higher $Paco_2$. One of the more common causes of this condition is the excessive loss of gastric acid that can occur with chronic vomiting. It is not the loss of gastric acid per se that elicits metabolic alkalosis but rather the secretion of base (HCO_3^-) into the circulatory system by the gastric parietal cells as they secrete H+ into the gastric lumen, which is then emptied by vomiting. Other common causes for metabolic alkalosis include a loss of potassium (K+), excessive ingestion of bicarbonate (antacids), elevated steroid levels, or the use of diuretics.

The condition of respiratory alkalosis is represented by the lower right quadrant of Figure 18-3A. This situation is commonly initiated by hyperventilation, which elicits a net loss of carbon dioxide and, therefore, a shift of the carbon dioxide–bicarbonate reaction (equation 1) to the left, resulting in a loss of both HCO_3^- and H+. Hyperventilation can be induced by anxiety, fever, overventilation, and some drugs (e.g., aspirin). Conditions that cause severe hypoxia provide a strong drive to breathe and a dramatic drop in $Paco_2$; thus, asthma and breathing at high altitudes can both result in respiratory alkalosis.

Acidotic Conditions

In contrast, respiratory acidosis results from hypoventilation and a corresponding increase in plasma carbon dioxide. The high concentration of carbon dioxide "pushes" the carbon dioxide–bicarbonate reaction (equation 1) to the right, resulting in an elevation in both H+ and HCO_3^-. This condition is depicted in the *upper left* quadrant of Figure 18-3A. Respiratory acidosis can result from depression of the central respiratory control mechanisms (see Chapter 19) or from any pathology that impedes adequate air movement. Additional factors eliciting respiratory acidosis include weakness of the respiratory muscles, decreased chest wall and lung compliance, severe airway obstruction, and diseases causing decreased gas diffusion (e.g., pulmonary edema, pneumonia).

Finally, metabolic acidosis, the most common type of acid–base disturbance, is represented in the *lower left* quadrant of Figure 18-3A. This condition could be elicited by any type of situation in which there is a net increase in [H+] (or a decrease in [HCO_3^-]) in the body *unrelated to the respiratory system*. The increase in [H+] could result from either an increased production or a decreased excretion of H+. Conditions associated with metabolic acidosis include high-intensity exercise, renal failure, untreated diabetes mellitus, excessive loss of HCO_3^- from the lower gastrointestinal tract (via diarrhea), and excess acid ingestion. The excess acid pushes equation 1 to the left, resulting in a depletion of bicarbonate base and subsequent compensatory elimination of carbon dioxide from the lungs.

The use of the four major categories of acid–base balance disturbances can be misleading, because multiple disturbances often can exist simultaneously. The coexistence of these mixed disorders can further complicate the diagnosis and interpretation of acid–base status. When multiple problems exist, the acid–base balance is typically more severely disordered. A common example of a mixed disorder is a patient who has respiratory acidosis caused by severe chronic obstructive pulmonary disease (COPD) and metabolic acidosis caused by marked hypoxemia and lactic acidosis. The respiratory disease results in carbon dioxide retention and a concomitant acid accumulation. The lactic acidosis also contributes to an elevated [H+].

FUNDAMENTAL MECHANISMS OF ACID-BASE HOMEOSTASIS

The initial position that any acid–base disturbance occupies in a diagram like Figure 18-3A (i.e., H^+–HCO_3^- combination) depends on the values of many contributing variables such as hemoglobin content of the blood, affinity of hemoglobin for oxygen, body temperature, and the Pco_2 in the blood. However, the patterns of changes produced by the initial insult and the nature of the compensatory adjustments are similar within any particular type of acid–base disturbance, regardless of the values of auxiliary variables. The hemoglobin buffer line (see Figure 18-1) is included in the Davenport diagram of Figure 18-3B. The four primary acid–base insults lie on the four line segments that meet at the normal arterial blood values (a pH of 7.4, a $Paco_2$ of 40 mm Hg, and a $[HCO_3^-]$ of approximately 24 mEq/L). The stronger the perturbation, the farther the relationship shifts along the appropriate line. When these disturbances occur, homeostatic mechanisms usually attempt to restore normal pH balance through *compensatory* mechanisms. These secondary compensations are indicated by the *heavy arrows* in Figure 18-3B. When the primary insult is metabolic, changes in the blood values initiate chemoreflexes that enable the respiratory system to compensate. Conversely, when the primary perturbation is respiratory-related, the body uses metabolic homeostatic mechanisms to compensate. A primary respiratory acidosis results in a metabolic compensation that returns the pH toward normal. This compensation is sometimes described as a compensatory metabolic alkalosis; however, because the pH is never alkalotic, this seems to be a misnomer. It is probably better to think simply in terms of respiratory and renal compensation.

> *Compensatory mechanisms are never complete because they depend on a negative feedback cycle. If the entire disturbance were removed, the stimuli for compensation would be lost.*

Compensation for Acidotic Conditions

The acid–base insults and their normal compensatory patterns are qualitatively depicted in Figure 18-4 for the two classes of acidosis, metabolic and respiratory. The x-axis in both the upper and lower portions of the figure represents the normal $[H^+]$, $[HCO_3^-]$, and $Paco_2$ at a pH of 7.4 (i.e., a $[H^+]$ of 40 nM/L). The y-axis demonstrates the qualitative change with each intervention. In the condition of metabolic acidosis (see Figure 18-4, *upper left panel*), as the H^+ becomes elevated, the HCO_3^- buffers the excess acid, forming H_2CO_3. The H_2CO_3 is converted to carbon dioxide and water, which are then given off in the expired air. In this manner, there is a simultaneous increase in $[H^+]$ and a decrease in $[HCO_3^-]$. The elevated H^+ level then stimulates respiration (see Chapter 19), resulting in a partial compensation of $[H^+]$ via the lowering of carbon dioxide (*upper right panel*). As the carbon dioxide level is lowered by hyperpnea, $[H^+]$ and $[HCO_3^-]$ subsequently decline. As can be seen in Figure 18-4, this *respiratory compensation* occurs at the expense of a further small depletion of HCO_3^-.

Respiratory compensation for metabolic acidosis is not capable of completely returning pH to its resting level of 7.4 (i.e., $[H^+] = 40$ nM/L). A further and more complete compensation is carried out by the kidneys. Renal perfusion must be adequate for the kidneys to carry out their acid–base function. The H^+ of acidosis serves as a metabolic vasodilator for the afferent arteriole and partial inhibitor of sympathetic vasoconstriction. Then, renal perfusion is matched to the level of acidosis. The mechanisms by which the renal system compensates for a nonrenal metabolic acidosis include reabsorbing nearly 100% of the HCO_3^- from the glomerular filtrate back into the blood.

In respiratory acidosis (*lower portion* of Figure 18-4), the hypoventilation of the lungs results in an increase in $Paco_2$ and a simultaneous increase in both H^+ and HCO_3^-. In this condition, the lungs are the problem; therefore, they cannot be part of the solution. Accordingly, physiologic compensation for respiratory acidosis falls entirely on the renal system. The kidney compensates by reabsorbing essentially all of the filtered HCO_3^- back into the circulatory system and by excreting H^+ in the urine as a fixed acid. These processes are coupled through the carbon dioxide–bicarbonate reaction (equation 1) as shown in Figure 18-5. The high concentration of carbon dioxide in uncorrected

FIGURE 18-4 ▶

Changes in [H+], [HCO₃⁻], and Paco₂ As- sociated with Metabolic (top) and Respira- tory (bottom) Acidosis and Their Com- pensatory Responses. The x-axis depicts the resting values for [H⁺] (40 nM/L), [HCO₃⁻] (24 mM/L), and Paco₂ (40 mm Hg). The y-axis shows qualitative changes in each parameter. In each set of bar graphs, the initial change is indicated by the heavy arrow. The resulting changes based on mass action are indicated by the lighter arrows. In the top panels, the in- creased H⁺ in metabolic acidosis causes a decrease in HCO₃⁻ and an increase in car- bon dioxide. The respiratory compensation in the next panel is a hyperpnea caused by the chemoreflex initiated by the elevated acid and Paco₂. Subsequent to hyper- pnea, the Paco₂ decreases and then shifts the equation toward carbon dioxide, re- sulting in a decrease in both H⁺ and HCO₃⁻. In the lower panels (respiratory acidosis), hypoventilation results in an in- crease in Paco₂ and concomitant in- creases in H⁺ and HCO₃⁻. Renal com- pensation conserves HCO₃⁻ and excretes H⁺.

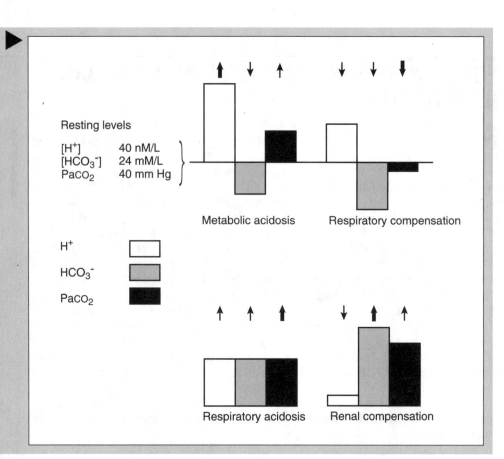

FIGURE 18-5 ▶

Schematic Drawing for Renal Reabsorp- tion of HCO₃⁻ and Excretion of Fixed Acid by the Renal Tubular Cell. Carbonic an- hydrase is essential for this renal function.

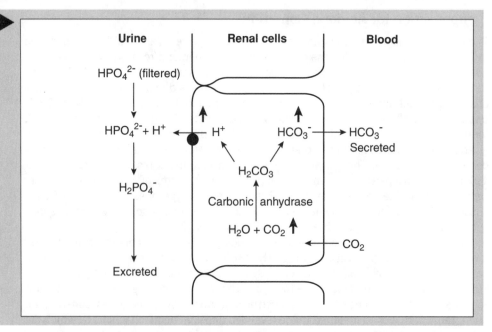

respiratory acidosis favors the diffusion of carbon dioxide into renal tubular cells, where carbonic anhydrase converts it to H_2CO_3. The HCO_3^- then dissociates into H^+ and HCO_3^-, with the former being excreted into the urine and the latter secreted into the blood. Once in the urine, the H^+ is buffered by the secreted phosphate ion. This allows the H^+ to be excreted in the urine as *fixed* acid (i.e., bound to a base).

Compensation for Alkalotic Conditions

Figure 18-6 presents the conditions of alkalosis. During metabolic alkalosis, an increase in HCO_3^- results in a decline in H^+ and an increase in carbon dioxide. The reduced

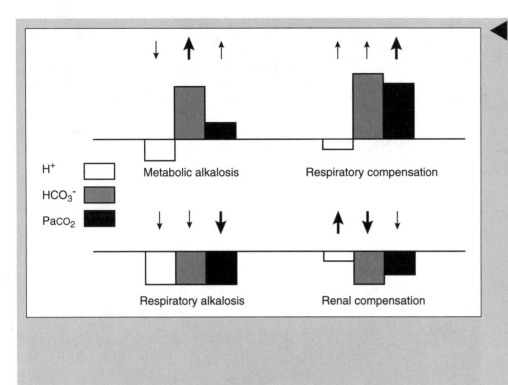

FIGURE 18-6
Changes in [H+], [HCO₃⁻], and Paco₂ Associated with Metabolic (top) and Respiratory (bottom) Alkalosis and Their Compensatory Responses. The x-axis depicts the resting values for [H+] (40 nM/L), [HCO₃⁻] (24 mM/L), and Paco₂ (40 mm Hg). The y-axis shows qualitative changes in each parameter. In each set of bar graphs, the initial change is indicated by the heavy arrow. The resulting changes based on mass action are indicated by the lighter arrows. In the top panels, the increased HCO₃⁻ in metabolic alkalosis causes a decrease in H+ and an increase in carbon dioxide. The respiratory compensation in the next panel is a hypoventilation caused by the chemoreflex initiated by the decreased pH. Subsequent to hypoventilation, the Paco₂ increases and then shifts the equation toward H+ and HCO₃⁻, resulting in an increase in both ions. In the lower panels (respiratory alkalosis), hyperventilation results in a decrease in Paco₂ and concomitant decreases in [H+] and [HCO₃⁻]. Renal compensation conserves H+ and excretes HCO₃⁻ to correct the pH.

plasma H+ decreases respiratory drive, resulting in respiratory compensation by hypoventilation, which partially restores H+ but further elevates HCO₃⁻ and Paco₂.

The hyperventilation of respiratory alkalosis results in hypocapnia and a simultaneous depletion of both acid and HCO₃⁻. Again, because the lungs are the problem, the kidneys carry the burden of compensation by reducing acid excretion while increasing the excretion of base (i.e., the same role they play in compensating for metabolic alkalosis of nonrenal origin).

It is evident from Figures 18-4 and 18-6 that the physiologic mechanisms for correcting acid–base disturbances are incomplete. Although compensatory mechanisms can adjust and correct much of the H+ disturbance, the compensation never returns the blood to the predisturbance level. Intuitively, one recognizes that in a regulated feedback system there always must be some deviation from normal to maintain the feedback effect.

Additional buffers and homeostatic mechanisms further complicate the issue of acid–base balance. Physiologically, some perturbations can cause an acidosis or alkalosis resulting from both respiratory *and* metabolic mechanisms. However, understanding the reaction relating carbon dioxide to H+ and HCO₃⁻ and the consequences of mass action allow the derivation of the basic responses.

RESOLUTION OF CLINICAL CASE

The patient's comatose state is related to her poor regulation of glucose. Because of her poorly controlled diabetic condition, she has been converting fats to ketones. Metabolism of the ketone bodies has produced a metabolic acidosis, which can be diagnosed from her arterial pH of 7.25 coupled with a low [HCO₃⁻]. Figure 18-3A can be used to confirm this diagnosis. The acidotic state stimulates the chemoreceptors, and the normal respiratory compensation for this insult is a hyperventilation to decrease Paco₂ and raise the pH. The compensation is obviously incomplete because pH is still significantly lower than normal. Because the Pao₂ is lower than normal despite the hyperventilation, this patient may also have some pulmonary edema or shunt that is limiting oxygen transport. However, the major immediate concern is to correct the blood glucose levels and the pH by slow intravenous infusion of insulin and HCO_3^-. The kidney can excrete both K^+ and H^+. These ions are typically excreted interchangeably, depending on which is in excess. Therefore, K^+ levels are often inversely related to H^+ levels, so it is important to monitor both values closely.

REVIEW QUESTIONS

Directions: For each of the following questions, choose the **one best** answer.

1. A $Paco_2$ of 50 mm Hg with a pH of 7.3 would be classified as which one of the following conditions?

    (A) A primary respiratory alkalosis

    (B) A primary metabolic alkalosis

    (C) A primary respiratory acidosis

    (D) A primary metabolic acidosis

    (E) Normal ventilation during exercise

2. A $Paco_2$ of 30 mm Hg with a $[HCO_3^-]$ of 20 would be classified as which one of the following conditions?

    (A) A primary respiratory alkalosis

    (B) A primary metabolic alkalosis

    (C) A primary respiratory acidosis

    (D) A primary metabolic acidosis

    (E) Normal ventilation during exercise

3. A $Paco_2$ of 38 mm Hg with a $[HCO_3^-]$ of 23 would be classified as which one of the following conditions?

    (A) A primary respiratory alkalosis

    (B) A primary metabolic alkalosis

    (C) A primary respiratory acidosis

    (D) A primary metabolic acidosis

    (E) Normal ventilation during exercise

4. A comatose patient who has overdosed on drugs would most likely be suffering from

    (A) a primary respiratory alkalosis

    (B) a primary metabolic alkalosis

    (C) a primary respiratory acidosis

    (D) a primary metabolic acidosis

5. The acid–base balance in a patient with a $[HCO_3^-]$ of 30 and a pH of 7.43 would most likely be associated with

    (A) a primary respiratory alkalosis with renal compensation

    (B) a primary metabolic alkalosis with respiratory compensation

    (C) a primary respiratory acidosis with respiratory compensation

    (D) a primary metabolic acidosis with respiratory compensation

    (E) normal ventilation during exercise

ANSWERS AND EXPLANATIONS

1. The answer is C. A pH lower than 7.4 indicates an acidemic condition, and the higher-than-normal Pa_{CO_2} indicates that the primary disturbance is respiratory.

2. The answer is A. This condition is harder to diagnose because the pH is not directly given. Using Figure 18-3 and the carbon dioxide isobars from Figure 18-1, it is apparent that this point lies in the lower right quadrant along the respiratory alkalosis line.

3. The answer is E. The Pa_{CO_2} is normal or just slightly below normal, and the $[HCO_3^-]$ is also near normal. During exercise, there is often a slight hyperventilation that results in a decreased Pa_{CO_2}, although all three variables stay within normal ranges.

4. The answer is C. Many narcotics and anesthetics suppress the respiratory drive to breathe, resulting in hypoventilation and an increase in the Pa_{CO_2}.

5. The answer is B. Because the pH is within the normal range, it appears that compensation is near complete. The pH is on the high side of the normal range, suggesting that the initial problem was an alkalosis. The high $[HCO_3^-]$ is consistent with a metabolic alkalosis and respiratory compensation.

REFERENCES

1. Davenport HW: *The ABC of Acid–Base Chemistry*, 6th ed. Chicago, IL: University of Chicago Press, 1974.
2. Stewart PA: *How to Understand Acid–Base.* New York, NY: Elsevier, 1981.

19

CONTROL OF THE PULMONARY SYSTEM

INTRODUCTION OF CLINICAL CASE

A 45-year-old overweight man has minor injuries from a recent car accident. His major concerns relate to his continued symptoms of narcolepsy. It appears that he fell asleep while driving during the late afternoon and ran off the road. He complained of excessive tiredness and "dozing off" throughout the day despite sleeping 8–10 hours every night. Although he does drink alcohol, he claimed that he did not have anything to drink prior to the accident. In fact, he now seldom drinks because he noticed that he often felt bad the day after having only one or two drinks. Upon questioning, the physician learned that his wife sleeps in a separate room because of his excessive snoring.

BACKGROUND

Unlike the myogenic nature of the cardiac cycle, the respiratory cycle is generated exclusively by the central nervous system (CNS). The fundamental mechanisms that produce the breathing movements are only partially understood. Breathing is typically an involuntary act, although considerable voluntary control can be exerted. However, the voluntary control is limited by homeostatic mechanisms that eventually restore involuntary control. If a person actively hyperventilates or hypoventilates by holding one's

If an angry, headstrong child threatens to hold his breath, he may become hypoxic enough to pass out. However, as soon as consciousness is lost, involuntary breathing resumes. He will suffer a transient memory loss and probably will not remember what angered him.

breath, dizziness or loss of consciousness occurs within a few minutes. At that point, the intrinsic involuntary control mechanisms restore normal function.

The basic mechanisms for this involuntary control include a large number of afferent and efferent systems, extensive brainstem circuitry, and many related neural inputs related to behavior. For the present purpose, it is reasonable to think of the respiratory control system as an interconnected network of positive and negative feedback and feedforward systems. These systems are considered individually in this chapter to simplify the discussion. However, the reader should remember that the actual function of the respiratory control system involves a complex, dynamic integration of many of these feedback loops. The mechanisms and neurons involved in respiratory control overlap extensively with those participating in cardiovascular regulation. In fact, many of the sensors provide important inputs to both systems. Similarly, many individual brainstem neurons respond to both cardiovascular and respiratory stimuli. Thus, in reality it is difficult to separate cardiovascular and respiratory control.

MODELS OF RESPIRATORY CONTROL

Continuous alveolar ventilation ($\dot{V}_A$) is essential to maintain adequate blood–gas homeostasis for metabolism (see Chapters 17 and 18). Remember from Chapter 14 that $\dot{V}_A$ depends upon the depth and rate of breathing. Both rate and depth can be determined by a *central pattern generator* within the CNS, although sensory inputs from the lungs and periphery may modify the basic rhythm and patterns of breathing. In a quiet, relaxed state, breathing tends to be fairly consistent and rhythmic. Generation of this fundamental breathing pattern is often portrayed as a simple *feed-forward* system (Figure 19-1A). However, this model neglects the important feedback nature of respiratory control. A more complete picture is provided by Figure 19-1B, which includes sensors in a controlled cycle diagram. During resting ventilation, the most important of these sensors are those that monitor partial pressure of oxygen in arterial blood (Pa_{O_2}), partial pressure of carbon dioxide in arterial blood (Pa_{CO_2}), and pH. For such a loop to maintain homeostasis, at some point the interaction must be inhibitory in nature, otherwise the loop would continue to move in one direction. The point of inhibition varies, depending on the controlled variable. A partial list of the many different respiratory-related sensors includes peripheral and central chemoreceptors, bronchopulmonary receptors, mechanoreceptors of the lung and chest wall, proprioceptors, nociceptors, and baroreceptors.

FIGURE 19-1 ▶

Block Diagrams of Respiratory Function. (A) Simple diagram depicts the feed-forward chain of command. (B) The addition of sensors to this circuit allows feedback to regulate various parameters. If all the connections were excitatory, this positive-feedback cycle would result in a continuous increase in ventilation. Inhibition limits the unrestrained increase. This inhibition is usually exerted at either of the dark arrows. Sensory input can inhibit the controller (e.g., baroreceptors), or increases in ventilation can decrease the activity of the sensors (e.g., peripheral chemoreceptors).

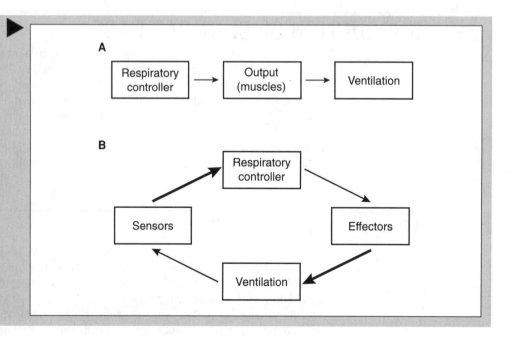

These sensors are discussed on the following pages. The respiratory effectors were discussed in Chapter 14 and include the laryngeal and pharyngeal muscles, airway smooth muscle, the diaphragm, and the intercostal, abdominal, and accessory muscles.

A more complicated version of the respiratory control system is seen in Figure 19-2. This feedback system again depends primarily on the chemosensors for blood gases; however, it does indicate some additional inputs that can influence the respiratory cycle. In particular, cortical inputs, temperature, and mechanoreceptors are but a few of the many inputs that influence the respiratory controller either directly or indirectly.

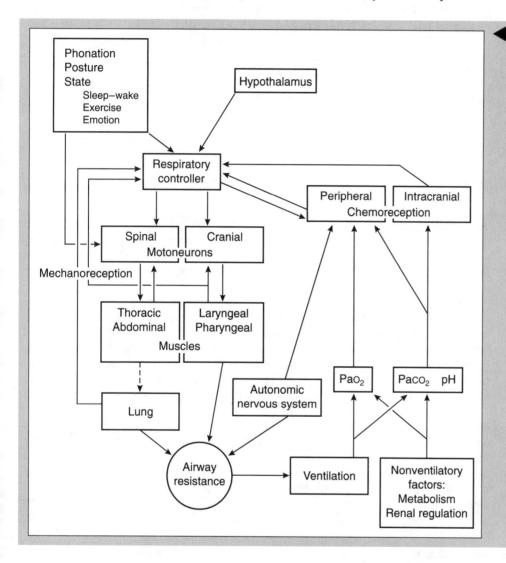

FIGURE 19-2
Schematic Drawing for Neural Control of Ventilation. The output of the controller activates spinal and cranial motoneurons innervating the muscle pumps and airways. Mechanical coupling of the pumps to the lungs results in ventilation. Nonventilatory factors interact with ventilatory processes to determine blood gases (i.e., Pao_2, $Paco_2$) and pH. These variables influence the activity of the chemosensors that provide a major positive input to the respiratory controller. (Source: *Reprinted with permission from Feldman JL:* Handbook of Physiology. *Bethesda, MD: American Physiological Society, 1986, p 464.*)

Respiratory Controller

Thus far, the respiratory controller has been treated as a "black box," with no attention given to its anatomic location or physiologic mechanisms. Although scientists still disagree on the particular brainstem nuclei and neuronal mechanisms for respiratory rhythm generation, there is a consensus that the fundamental respiratory controller resides in the medulla of the brainstem. Brain transection experiments from the 1920s indicate that the basic respiratory cycle is maintained despite removal of the forebrain, midbrain, and cerebellum (Figure 19-3). In fact, there is little change in the breathing patterns of an anesthetized mammal until sequential transections remove the rostral pons. After midpontine transection (at the level of B in Figure 19-3), there is an increase in inspiratory duration, a slowing of respiratory frequency, and an increase in tidal volume. This observation prompted the hypothesis that there was a *pneumotaxic center* in the rostral pons that helped to increase the respiratory rate. Subsequent research has

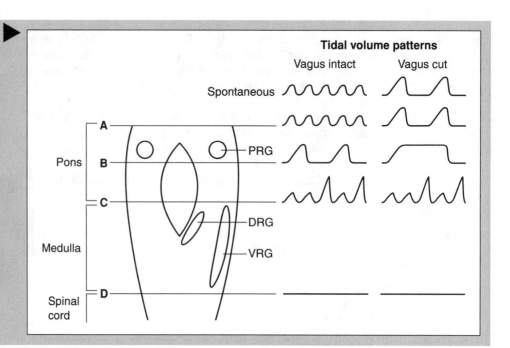

FIGURE 19-3

Respiratory Effects of Brainstem Transections. Transection rostral to the pons (A) has little effect on the spontaneous respiratory rhythm. A midpontine transection (B) eliminates the neurons associated with the pontine respiratory group (PRG) and removes a tonic excitation, resulting in a slowed frequency and increased depth of breathing. Elimination of vagal input from the lung stretch receptors results in apneusis. Transection at the pontomedullary junction (C) results in the irregular breathing pattern of gasping. Removal of vagal afferents has little effect after this transection. Transection of the spinal cord (D) eliminates all descending drive to the spinal motoneurons, and therefore, spinal respiratory movements cease. However, the respiratory rhythm persists in muscles innervated by cranial nerves. DRG = dorsal respiratory group; VRG = ventral respiratory group.

demonstrated that neurons in the region of the nucleus parabrachialis do indeed provide a tonic excitatory effect on respiratory rate. Neurons of this *pontine respiratory group* can show respiratory periodicities under certain conditions. Activation of these neurons can alter respiratory timing. Therefore, respiratory rate slows when this region is damaged.

Because the lung volume receptors also provide an important input that tends to increase respiratory frequency, elimination of these afferents similarly slows respiratory frequency and increases the depth of ventilation. When both the pontine regions and the vagal inputs are eliminated, the loss of both of these excitatory drives greatly depresses the mechanisms that terminate inspiration. This often produces an inspiratory breath-hold, or *apneusis*. Although many texts describe an *apneustic center* in the caudal pons, no anatomically distinct region has been found. Arguing against such a "center" is the finding that wakefulness or increasing other respiratory drives can restore a more normal pattern of breathing. Transection of the brainstem below this level at the pontomedullary border produces a gasping pattern of breathing. This finding indicates that the fundamental *respiratory rhythm generator* is likely to reside within the medulla. Respiratory-related neurons are found in several specific areas of the medulla (Figure 19-4). These "respiratory" areas are in proximity to cardiovascular control areas, and numerous neuronal interactions between these areas have been observed. Therefore, it is often hard to dissociate the mechanisms of cardiovascular control from respiratory control.

Dorsal Respiratory Group (DRG). The DRG is anatomically located in the ventrolateral subnucleus of the nucleus tractus solitarius, which is a major relay for all types of visceral afferent information, including baroreceptors, chemoreceptors, and vagal mechanoreceptors. Within the DRG, almost all of the neurons are inspiratory-modulated, and most of them are premotor neurons projecting to inspiratory motoneurons in the spinal cord. Just medial to the DRG are the motor nucleus of the vagus that innervates the airway smooth muscle and the hypoglossal nucleus that innervates the tongue. Both of these nuclei may have a strong respiratory-related activity.

Ventral Respiratory Group (VRG). The VRG is a much longer column of neurons located in the region of the nucleus ambiguus and nucleus retroambigualis extending rostrally to the region of the facial nucleus. The caudal portions of the VRG contain primarily expiratory-modulated neurons. Many of these are motoneurons projecting to respiratory-related skeletal and smooth muscle through the ninth and tenth cranial nerves, whereas others are premotor neurons that innervate the expiratory-related motoneurons in the spinal cord. The intermediate regions of the VRG contain primarily inspiratory-modulated neurons that are a mixture of premotor and motor neurons. In addition, many of the

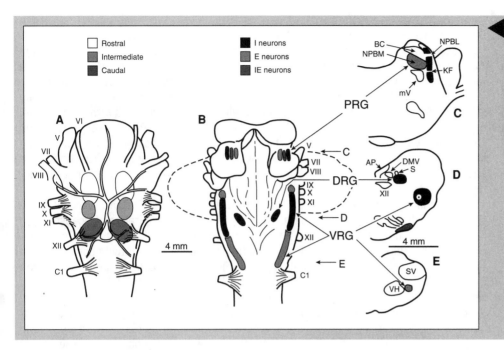

FIGURE 19-4
Brainstem Areas Implicated in Respiratory Control in the Cat. *Ventral view (A), dorsal view (B), and cross-sectional views at three levels (C, D, E) of the brainstem are shown. Ventral medullary areas are implicated in central chemoreception. Other areas of interest include the pontine respiratory group (PRG), dorsal respiratory group (DRG), and ventral respiratory group (VRG). Cross-sections illustrate the approximate location of these areas. Cranial nerves are indicated by the Roman numerals. (Source: Reprinted with permission from Feldman JL:* Handbook of Physiology. *Bethesda, MD: American Physiological Society, 1986, p 475.)*

neurons are interneurons that communicate with other brainstem neurons. The far rostral extent of the VRG contains both inspiratory- and expiratory-modulated neurons.

Ventral Medullary Surface. A fourth important respiratory-related region of the medulla is found very superficially on the ventrolateral surface. This region has historically been associated with the central chemoreceptive region, and there is some evidence that cells in or near this region may also be important in respiratory rhythmogenesis. Once again, this area overlaps extensively with nuclei implicated in cardiovascular control.

The actual mechanism by which the fundamental respiratory rhythm is generated is unknown. Various theories have been proposed based on network properties and pacemaker properties of respiratory neurons. In fact, some investigators have proposed a hybrid system using both pacemaker neurons and network interactions. Regardless of the fundamental mechanism, it is well established that the controller receives considerable afferent information to accomplish its normal function in the behaving animal. The respiratory controller must produce the appropriate spatial and temporal pattern of outputs to optimize its performance and adjust to the various demands that are placed upon the respiratory system.

The timing and coordination of respiratory muscle activation is very important. If the thoracic musculature is recruited to produce deeper breaths and more negative P_A but the upper airways muscles are not activated, the upper airways can be "sucked" closed during inspiration.

RESPIRATORY-RELATED SENSORS

Multiple variables are constantly monitored, and this information is used to adjust ventilation and muscle contraction within a breath and on a breath-to-breath basis. The central controller is responsible for integrating the vast amount of information from these various inputs to achieve the proper output. Sensors are distributed throughout the viscera to transduce the many variables. These sensors may be located within specialized neurons or supporting cells, or they may be associated with a specific structure designed to transduce the variable being controlled. Each receptor can be characterized by its specific stimulus (i.e., to what it responds best) and its ability to adapt, accommodate, or fatigue. The two major classes of these receptors are *chemoreceptors*, which respond best to chemical stimuli, and *mechanoreceptors*, which respond to mechanical stimuli such as stretch and deformation. Many receptors are multimodal and respond to both chemical and mechanical inputs.

Lung Receptors

A variety of mechanoreceptors and chemoreceptors are found within the lung and airways. All of these sensory receptors send their information to the brainstem through

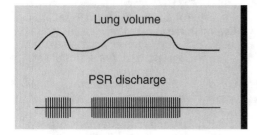

the vagus nerve. The largest and fastest conducting afferent vagal fibers innervate the *pulmonary stretch receptors* (PSRs). These receptors are sometimes called *slowly adapting receptors* because they show very little adaptation to a maintained stimulus. The receptor structures are believed to be free nerve endings in the smooth muscle of the larger airways and bronchioles. The PSRs adapt to a distending stimulus of the lung very slowly. Because of their minimal adaptation, their activity is correlated with lung volume, or more accurately, with the distending pressure on the lung (P_T). These receptors do show some dynamic response, so that at the same volume the discharge is greater during inflation than deflation. Reflexes associated with these afferents are known as the *Breuer-Hering reflexes* (after the student [Breuer], who did the initial work, and his professor [Hering], who got most of the credit).

Neuronal activity from the PSRs is transmitted to the brainstem, where it influences respiratory timing and promotes the termination of inspiration. Because these receptors are normally activated as the lung inflates, PSR discharge frequency increases as inhalation progresses (Figure 19-5). Eventually their activity contributes to the end of inspiration. If tidal volume (V_T) is artificially controlled, the amplitude of the inflation is inversely related to the duration of inspiration (Figure 19-5B). Therefore, with increased activation of the PSRs during inspiration, inspiratory duration is shortened, the respiratory period is shortened, and respiratory frequency is increased. Normally during expiration, PSR activity decreases as the lung deflates. However, if lung inflation is maintained during expiration, the continued discharge of these slowly adapting afferents *prolongs* expiration and *decreases* the respiratory frequency. Therefore, both the intensity of PSR activity and the timing of activation are important. Breathing at an elevated lung volume can result in both a decreased inspiratory duration (increased PSR activity during inspiration) and an increased expiratory duration (increased PSR activity during expiration).

Although the PSR reflexes are very strong in many animal species, in normal adult humans, the PSRs show little reflex activity until lung volumes greater than 1.0 L above

FIGURE 19-5 ▶

Characteristics of Pulmonary Stretch Receptor (PSR) Discharge. (A) The top trace shows three consecutive breaths of increasing depth. The lower trace depicts the discharge frequency of PSRs in response to these breaths. Although these receptors are slowly adapting, they do show a small sensitivity to the rate of change, which accounts for the decline to 0 during late expiration. (B) The relationship between the depth of inflation and the inspiratory duration is attributed to the Breuer-Hering inspiratory reflex. With very large, rapid breaths (e.g., carbon dioxide during rebreathing), the inspiratory duration is very short because of activation of the PSRs. FRC = functional residual capacity.

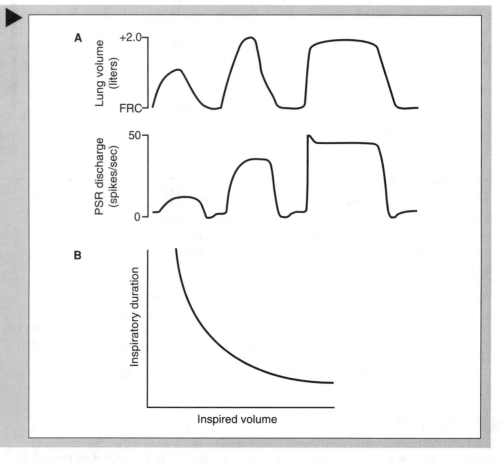

functional residual capacity (FRC) are attained. There is, however, evidence that PSR activity may be altered by any of the factors that affect lung compliance or activity of the airway smooth muscle. Therefore, the PSRs may become more important in various lung pathologies. There also may be a developmental role for these afferent fibers because the Breuer-Hering reflex is believed to be stronger in the neonate than the adult.

The *irritant receptors* or *rapidly adapting receptors* (RARs) comprise a second group of important lung receptors. They account for 25%–50% of the myelinated afferent fibers from the lung. These receptors are free nerve endings localized within the mucosal lining of the trachea and larger airways. Although they respond to stretch and deformation with a rapidly adapting discharge, these afferent fibers also exhibit a strong, longer lasting response to many chemical irritants. The afferent fibers associated with these receptors are small myelinated axons with conduction velocities of 10–20 m/sec. The reflex actions of these receptors in the large airways induce cough, bronchoconstriction, laryngeal constriction, increased airway mucus secretion, and hypertension. *Hyperpnea* is also sometimes associated with activation of similar receptors found deep within the lung tissue. Inhaled irritants that activate the irritant receptors and elicit numerous reflex effects include smoke, nicotine, ammonia, sulfur dioxide, and carbon dust. Endogenous compounds such as histamine and substance P also can activate these receptors and elicit profound reflexes.

Most lung afferent fibers are slowly conducting, nonmyelinated *C-fibers*. These afferents are subclassified as *bronchial* or *pulmonary*, depending on their associated circulation. The pulmonary receptors are located in the lung parenchyma and are most accessible to stimulants injected into the pulmonary circulation. In contrast, the bronchial receptors are most easily activated by substances in the lung blood flow that comes from the left ventricle and perfuses the bronchial arteries. The bronchial and pulmonary C-fiber receptors respond to both mechanical and chemical stimulation. Some of these receptors may sense the deformation of lung parenchyma associated with pulmonary edema. The natural stimuli and the role of C-fibers during normal breathing (eupnea) are not known; however, stimulation of these receptors can produce apnea followed by rapid, shallow breathing and an increase in laryngeal and bronchial resistance. Resistance changes are associated with both smooth muscle activation and enhanced mucus secretion. Bradycardia, vasodilation, and respiratory-related sensations have also been produced by activation of these receptors.

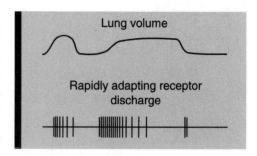

The root -pnea *refers to breathing.* **Hyperpnea** *and* **tachypnea** *refer to rapid breathing;* **apnea** *is an absence of breathing;* **hypopnea** *and* **bradypnea** *refer to slow breathing.* **Eupnea** *is normal breathing.*

Muscle Receptors

Although the mechanoreceptors in lung tissue play an important role in sensing lung perturbations, they are not the only respiratory-related mechanoreceptors. The striated skeletal muscles that comprise the respiratory pump are innervated with numerous proprioceptors, including muscle spindles and Golgi tendon organs. These proprioceptors are very important in spinal reflexes associated with load compensation and postural adjustments. In addition, they can influence the central control of respiratory depth and timing. The diaphragm is unusual for a striated muscle in that it has very few proprioceptors. However, proprioceptive reflexes have been observed even in the diaphragm.

The major effect of these receptors is an inhibition of inspiratory-related activity. Excitation of the intercostal muscle afferent fibers results in a premature termination of inspiratory activity and a shortening of inspiratory duration. These afferent fibers may be involved in the breathlessness associated with a blow to the thoracic cavity. It has also been suggested that these afferent fibers contribute to the perception of *dyspnea*.

Muscle Chemoreceptors. The pump muscles are richly innervated with free nerve endings that are sensitive to chemical stimuli. Most of the substances that activate these receptors are associated with the metabolic wastes or by-products of strenuous muscle activity. Examples of these stimulants include lactic acid, prostaglandins, arachidonic acid, low pH, and high potassium levels. Excitation of these afferent fibers elicits both local and central reflexes affecting respiratory function. It is believed that these afferent fibers play an important role in limiting fatigue of the respiratory muscles. Many of these receptors function as pain receptors or *nociceptors*. Although pain can have a profound effect on the control of respiration, it does not elicit a consistent response. In general, somatic pain tends to cause

Dyspnea *is a sensation of abnormal, labored breathing.*

*Hyperpnea is an increase in breathing frequency; it is not necessarily associated with excessive ventilation. **Hyperventilation** is an excess ventilation resulting in a decreased Paco₂.*

a hyperpnea, whereas visceral pain can cause hypopnea or apnea. Pain can cause a person either to take a very large, deep breath or to hold his or her breath. Other times pain causes a marked hyperpnea and probably *hyperventilation* (e.g., childbirth).

Airway Receptors

The larynx, pharynx, and larger airways are richly innervated by sensory structures that respond to mechanical, chemical, and temperature-related stimuli. The afferent fibers project to the brainstem through the cranial nerves. These receptors are very sensitive to a variety of stimuli, and they have been implicated in the reflex control of airway diameter, bronchial secretions, respiratory timing, respiratory sensations, and cough. Many of the respiratory-related reflexes associated with these receptors are very pronounced.

The mechanical receptors in the upper airways are stimulated by several distending forces including flow, pressure, touch, and mechanical activation of the smooth muscle. Chemical receptors in the airway epithelia detect both osmotic and chemical stimuli. Introduction of distilled water provides a strong osmotic stimulus to activate these receptors. Although the air is usually warmed and humidified in the mouth and nose, the passage of cool air through the pharynx and larynx can activate the "cold" receptors located there. This variety of receptors within the airways contributes to the complicated responses observed physiologically.

Baroreceptors

The arterial baroreceptors and the associated cardiovascular reflexes are described in Chapter 13. These mechanoreceptors are located in the aortic arch and at the carotid sinus. They are designed to sense the pressure within the major arteries, and their discharge frequency increases as the transmural pressure increases. Although they have a profound effect on cardiovascular regulation by influencing both vascular tone and heart rate, they have only modest effects on respiratory control. With increases in arterial baroreceptor activity, there is a decrease in respiratory rate and depth. Strong activation can result in apnea and bronchodilation.

Peripheral Chemoreceptors

The peripheral chemoreceptors are located within the aortic bodies of the aortic arch and the carotid bodies near the bifurcation of the carotid artery. They are innervated by the aortic nerve and carotid sinus nerve, respectively. Therefore, the chemoreceptive structures and fibers are in proximity to the baroreceptors. Although the chemosensors can detect increases in Paco₂, decreases in pH, and decreases in Pao₂, the responses to oxygen are usually the most important physiologically. These sensors are ideally situated to measure the Po₂ in the arterial blood perfusing the brain. The information sensed by these receptors is relayed to interneurons in the brainstem medulla, including neurons in the region of the nucleus tractus solitarius. Processing of this information results in changes in both autonomic outflow and respiratory control. The general response to a decreased delivery of oxygen is to increase both ventilatory and circulatory activity to enhance oxygen transport. The reflexes evoked by these receptors are relatively quick (occurring within seconds), which enables these sensors to influence ventilation and cardiac output on a breath-to-breath basis.

Both the aortic and carotid body receptors influence cardiovascular control and increase the cardiac output when they are activated. For respiratory control, the carotid bodies are much more important than the aortic bodies. The transduction processes in these chemoreceptors depend on sensory cells in both bodies that are very active metabolically. Because they consume oxygen so rapidly, they depend on a substantial pressure gradient for maintaining an adequate rate of diffusion for oxygen. If the Pao₂ falls below 60–80 mm Hg, although the total content of oxygen remains high, the diffusion of oxygen becomes inadequate to meet the metabolic demands, and there is an increase in the discharge rate of the chemoreceptive fibers (Figure 19-6). Because of the rapid uptake of oxygen by these cells, the actual oxygen content of the blood is not a reliable stimulus. To deliver adequate oxygen, both the Pao₂ and the blood flow must remain high. Under normal circumstances, the blood flow rate to these tissues is approx-

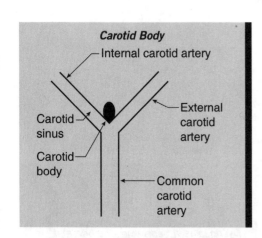

Carotid Body

- Internal carotid artery
- External carotid artery
- Carotid sinus
- Carotid body
- Common carotid artery

*Although the oxygen content of the blood may be significantly decreased by **carbon monoxide poisoning** or **anemia**, neither of these conditions has a marked effect on the carotid chemoreceptors because the Pao₂ is not reduced. In contrast, with **polycythemia**, the oxygen content may be greatly elevated, but the increased viscosity of the blood may reduce blood flow through the chemoreceptors and cause a small drop in the Pao₂ that results in an increased peripheral chemoreceptor activation.*

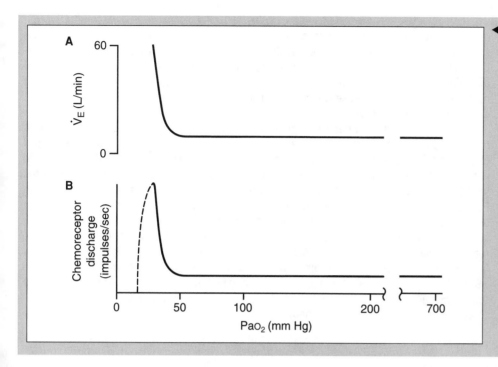

FIGURE 19-6
Ventilatory Reflex and Chemoreceptor Discharge in Response to Hypoxia. Both of these response curves are hyperbolic with a very steep slope. The threshold for a rapid increase in chemoreceptor activity and ventilation occurs at a Pa_{O_2} below 60–70 mm Hg. Breathing 100% oxygen has little effect on the normal responses. When arterial P_{O_2} falls below approximately 30 mm Hg, the chemoreceptors begin to fail, and death is imminent.

imately 20 mL/g tissue/min. Therefore, although the oxygen consumption in the carotid body is comparatively large, the high-flow rate keeps the arteriovenous oxygen difference very small.

> *The average blood flow to the chemoreceptive tissues is approximately 40 times greater than the blood flow in most tissues. For example, a 70-kg man during exercise may have an elevated cardiac output of 35 L/min. The average blood flow rate for the body is calculated at 0.5 mL/g tissue/min (35,000 mL/min/70,000 g).*

Despite the major importance of Pa_{O_2} on these chemoreceptors, it is worth noting that their activity is modulated by Pa_{CO_2} (Figure 19-7). Physiologically, a decrease in oxygen is often accompanied by an increase in carbon dioxide levels; this enhances the sensitivity of these receptors. This effect of Pa_{CO_2} on the Pa_{O_2} response is *multiplicative* in that the response to both stimuli is greater than the added responses of the two stimuli applied independently. Therefore, the normal response to hypoventilation is much stronger than that predicted by the response to either hypoxia or hypercapnia alone.

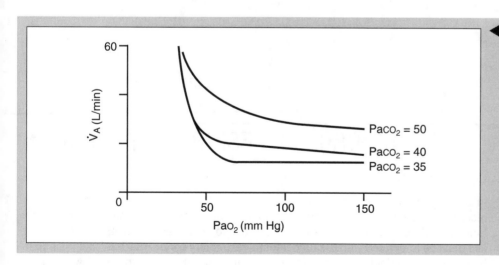

FIGURE 19-7
Sensitivity of Peripheral Chemoreceptor Reflexes to Carbon Dioxide. The three curves show an increasing gain in the chemoreflex with progressive hypercapnia. As Pa_{CO_2} increases, there is a slight increase in ventilation at the normal Pa_{O_2} of 100 mm Hg. However, with moderate hypoxia, these increases are augmented. A similar enhancement of the hypoxic responses is seen with a decrease in pH. V_A = alveolar ventilation.

Central Chemoreceptors

In contrast to the peripheral chemoreceptors, the central chemoreceptor structures have not been positively identified. Although various studies have indicated that Pa_{CO_2} (or some related variable) is sensed near the ventrolateral surface of the medulla, no definitive structure, transduction mechanism, or neuronal cell type has been identified as the sensor. This has led to considerable confusion in our understanding of central chemoreception. Evidence suggests that the final stimuli that are sensed could be the concentration of hydrogen ion [H^+], bicarbonate [HCO_3^-] and carbon dioxide in the extracellular fluid, blood, cerebrospinal fluid, or intracellular fluid compartments. These substances are closely interrelated in the blood and tissues through the action of carbonic anhydrase (see Chapter 18). Because the *blood–brain barrier* provides a significant diffusion barrier for the movement of ions, carbon dioxide is generally believed to be the most likely stimulus because it is more soluble than the related ions and can pass more easily into brain tissues.

Despite the lack of understanding regarding the specific sensor and stimuli, it is well recognized that both $Paco_2$ and pH are normally tightly regulated. Although the central chemoreceptors assist in maintaining the steady-state levels of pH and $Paco_2$, they do not appear to play a major role in the response to sudden changes, requiring 1–2 minutes to initiate a reflex response to an acute experimental change. The relationships between $Paco_2$ and ventilation depend on the integration of both central and peripheral chemoreceptors. The threshold and slope of these carbon dioxide–response curves during several states are shown in Figure 19-8. The reflexes associated with the central chemoreceptors can be altered by chronic pathologic conditions, normal physiologic states (sleep or wakefulness), and certain drugs, including anesthetics and opiates (see Figure 19-8). These factors can influence both the slope or sensitivity of the response as well as the threshold. Severe depression of the chemoreceptor reflexes can lead to life-threatening hypoventilation or apnea.

> *Narcotic overdoses* often present with significant hypoventilation because of depressed central and peripheral chemoreceptor function. Administering 100% oxygen to these patients removes the peripheral chemoreceptor drive and can lead to complete cessation of breathing. Therefore, treatment of these patients begins with artificial ventilation.

FIGURE 19-8 ▶

Ventilatory Responses to $Paco_2$ during Different States. *Within the normal physiologic range of 35–45 mm Hg, the response curve to hypercapnia during wakefulness is linear with a steep slope (approximately 2–3 L/mm Hg). The sensitivity of the reflex is enhanced by conditions that cause a prolonged decrease in the $Paco_2$ (e.g., metabolic acidosis, respiratory alkalosis), whereas the sensitivity is decreased by long-lasting hypercapnic conditions. Sleep and drug-induced suppression of the central chemoreceptors also depresses the carbon dioxide–response curve. $\dot{V}_A$ = alveolar ventilation.*

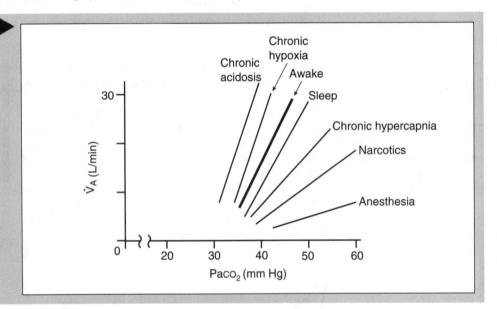

CONTROL OF RESPIRATORY FUNCTION

Cortical Control

In addition to the specific reflexes that are described above, the respiratory system receives numerous inputs from the CNS that help to control and coordinate respiratory function with behavioral tasks. The mechanical and respiratory demands of these behaviors must be integrated with the fundamental respiratory control mechanisms to perform both functions effectively. For example, during speech or singing, airflow must be controlled to permit appropriate vibration of the vocal cords during expiration. When a lecturer speaks rapidly in long sentences without any pause, he or she is transiently hypoventilating because of the long expiration. The next breath is generally a very rapid inspiration with a greater-than-normal tidal volume to provide adequate air for the next sentence. This adjustment is made without much conscious effort. However, the coordination of these behaviors is very noticeable in patients with injured spinal cords (e.g., actor Christopher Reeves), who must coordinate their speech with a preset ventilator-assisted breathing pattern.

Similarly, respiratory patterns must be integrated with digestive behaviors such as swallowing, belching, and vomiting. It is essential that the glottis be closed during these activities to prevent aspiration of ingested food or stomach chyme into the trachea and lungs. Complex brainstem interactions between the respiratory and digestive nuclei, especially in the region of the nucleus tractus solitarius, normally prevent simultaneous activation of these two systems. However, decoupling of the integration can occur with brainstem trauma or with conditions such as polio and Alzheimer's disease.

There are many important cortically controlled interactions between the postural, mechanical, and respiratory demands of the skeletal muscles. Changes in the breathing pattern during weightlifting, swimming, and running are all obvious integrative mechanisms that enhance the function of both systems. Many animals as well as humans tend to *entrain* their respiratory movements to both external and internal stimuli. External entrainment can occur with auditory or vibratory stimuli (e.g., a change in respiratory frequency in response to a fast, driving rhythm from a song on the radio). Internal stimuli from mechanoreceptors can also entrain respiratory frequency. Many athletes find that their respiratory frequency relates to a movement cycle in a regular manner. For example, runners may routinely inspire or exhale when their foot strikes the ground. It is difficult to determine if entrainment is due to involuntary or reflexive control.

Vegetative Control

In addition to the voluntary control exerted by the CNS, the respiratory controller is also influenced by other regulators related to involuntary, vegetative function. *Body temperature* is a very important determinant of respiratory frequency. This is readily apparent by the increased ventilation observed during fever. The effect of body temperature on respiration is exerted by both direct and indirect effects. With increased body temperature, there is normally an increase in metabolic rate leading to enhanced oxygen consumption and carbon dioxide production. These may act as stimuli on the peripheral and central chemoreceptors to increase ventilatory rate and depth. Certain hormones, such as progesterone, have also been shown to influence respiration.

Pathologies of Respiratory Control

Failures of the respiratory control system are fortunately rare because they are often life-threatening. Although the cause of *sudden infant death syndrome (SIDS)* is unknown, a failure of the respiratory rhythm generator has been proposed because hypoxia and apneic periods are frequent occurrences in the children at risk for this syndrome. However, other data suggest that cardiovascular mechanisms and alterations in autonomic control may be the causative factors. In all likelihood, this syndrome probably encompasses malfunction of both the cardiovascular and respiratory systems (remember that central cardiopulmonary control mechanisms are closely intertwined).

Sleep apneas are an important clinical problem. During sleep, there is a marked decrease in the rate and depth of breathing because of a decline in respiratory drives. Even healthy individuals occasionally have a long apneic period that results in significant blood oxygen desaturation. However, when the frequency or duration of apneas increases, it can result in significant disruption of sleep. Sleep apneas are often classified as *obstructive, central,* or *mixed,* depending on the features that attend the apneic episode. With pure *central apneas,* there are no respiratory-related efforts during the apnea, suggesting a failure of the respiratory rhythm generating circuitry. In contrast, during *obstructive apneas,* there is no airflow despite the persistence of respiratory movements. These apneas result from the collapse of the upper airways, usually related to decreased activity of the striated pharyngeal and laryngeal muscles. These apneas are correlated with obesity and snoring and are most prevalent in obese men older than 40 years of age who sleep on their backs. Fat deposition within the pharynx probably leads to a narrowing of the pharynx and obstruction by the tongue. The narrowing, in turn, leads to the development of more negative inspiratory airway pressures, which "suck" the airways closed. As the apnea progresses, the hypoxia and hypercapnia lead to greater respiratory efforts of the diaphragm. Eventually, the muscle effort causes a transient arousal, which leads to reopening of the pharyngeal airway.

*The collapse of the pharyngeal airway is another physiologic example of the important concept of **transmural pressure**. The airways close because the extraluminal pressure exceeds the pressure inside the distensible airway.*

The apneic periods may last for 1 minute or longer and result in significant hypoxia. In severely affected patients, there may be 30–40 apneic episodes per hour. Obviously, if each apnea terminates with a partial arousal, these patients may be sleep-deprived, leading to daytime somnolence and narcolepsy. Treatment for this condition with continuous positive airway pressure (CPAP) during the night is usually successful almost immediately. The positive pressure helps maintain patency of the airway, preventing any subsequent apneic periods. The biggest problem is patient compliance because the mask can be annoying.

In patients with *Ondine's curse*, a lesion of the spinal cord or brainstem eliminates the neuronal pathways for normal, involuntary breathing. However, pathways related to voluntary control still exist, enabling the patient to breathe voluntarily. This obviously requires cortical, conscious control and can maintain adequate ventilation as long as the patient is awake. Unfortunately, during sleep the patient becomes apneic. Unlike the sleep apneas discussed above, there may be little stimulus for arousal, and life-threatening hypoxia may ensue. These patients can be managed by providing artificial ventilation during sleep.

Abnormal breathing patterns such as apneusis, Biot breathing, and Cheyne-Stokes breathing are shown in Figure 19-9. In *Biot breathing* (also known as cluster breathing or periodic breathing), normal breaths of uniform amplitude occur within clusters that are separated by abnormally long expiratory durations. The number of breaths within the clusters and the duration of the long expirations tend to be fairly regular in pattern and rhythm.

FIGURE 19-9 ▶

Abnormal Respiratory Patterns Associated with Periodic Breathing, Cheyne-Stokes Breathing, and Apneusis. Apneusis denotes an abnormally long inspiration. Apnea (a long breath-hold during expiration) can be observed in both periodic and Cheyne-Stokes breathing. The absence of airflow associated with either apnea, hypoventilation, or apneusis can lead to significant declines in Pao$_2$ and smaller declines in arterial oxygen saturation. The large changes in Pao$_2$ suggest an important role for peripheral chemoreceptors in these pathologies. FRC = functional residual capacity.

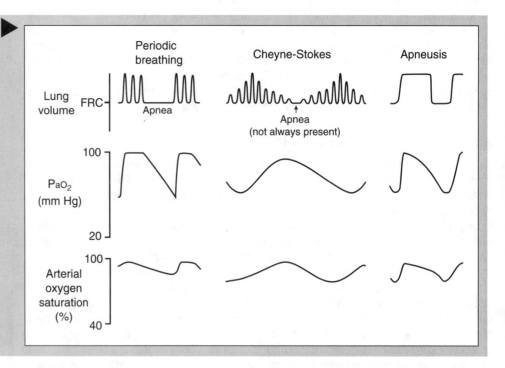

Cheyne-Stokes breathing refers to a waxing and waning pattern of V_T. It can be observed during sleep at high altitude, after brainstem injury, or in infants. This pattern is believed to be associated with pathologic delays in the cardiovascular-to-respiratory sensor coupling or with an abnormal gain of the peripheral chemoreceptors. Experimentally, Cheyne-Stokes breathing can be created by increasing the circulation time from the lung to the peripheral chemoreceptors. The V_T tends to be small during the time when well-oxygenated blood is flowing through the carotid body; however, the small V_T can result in inadequate gas exchange in the lung. Subsequently, as the poorly oxygenated blood reaches the chemoreceptors, it stimulates the sensors and results in a marked increase in breathing, which restores the lung oxygenation to normal (or greater-than-normal) levels. This cycle of alternating hypoventilation and hyperventilation can continue indefinitely.

ARTIFICIAL VENTILATION

Artificial ventilation is an important clinical tool to ensure adequate ventilation. Ventilators are designed to deliver either a constant pressure or a constant volume. Usually these two variables are closely correlated. In some disease states, however, it is preferable to use one parameter over the other. For example, in lungs with low compliance, a fixed volume may generate large pressures that could damage alveolar walls. In contrast, a fixed-pressure ventilator may result in inadequate airflow in a patient with high airway resistance.

Although artificial ventilation is often essential, it can create several problems that must be closely monitored. Most importantly, the arterial blood hydrogen tension (pH_a) and the $Paco_2$ are typically tightly controlled through the feedback provided by the chemoreceptors. However, artificial ventilation can result in hyperventilation with a concomitant decrease in $Paco_2$ and alkalosis. Alternatively, hypoventilation causes the serious problems of hypoxia, hypercapnia, and acidosis. Therefore, the arterial blood gases, or at least the end-tidal gases, must be monitored to maintain appropriate ventilation. If the patient is not paralyzed, there is a tendency for the patient to "fight" the ventilator by establishing his or her own rhythm. However, if the ventilator frequency and volume are near normal, the patient often entrains to the ventilator through the reflexes initiated by mechanoreceptors in the lungs and skeletal muscles. The pulmonary stretch receptors and the Breuer-Hering reflex are especially important in terminating the endogenous inspiratory effort.

RESOLUTION OF CLINICAL CASE

Because of the history of snoring, the patient's wife was questioned further. She described his snoring as a "snorting" often accompanied by excessive movement and thrashing around. The physician suspected a marked obstructive apnea and asked the patient to come to the sleep clinic. Monitoring indicated approximately 20 apneic episodes per hour during sleep. The apneic episodes were obstructive in origin because strong respiratory efforts persist during the apnea. The patient seldom entered rapid eye movement (REM) sleep and was therefore sleep-deprived.

Alcohol consumption and many drugs can decrease the tone in the musculature of the upper airways, thereby contributing to the collapse of the upper airways. Therefore, obstructive apneas are often exaggerated with use of these substances. The worsening of this patient's obstructive symptoms caused further sleep deprivation. This sleep disorder, in turn, caused him to feel "bad."

The patient was instructed in the use of CPAP during the night, and his sleep improved dramatically. The small positive pressure applied to the airways kept them patent, and he did not experience any hypoxic periods during sleep. However, he felt so good after 1 week of CPAP that he considered himself healed and neglected further use of the CPAP mask. Subsequently, his symptoms of daytime somnolence returned. He was counseled to use CPAP routinely.

REVIEW QUESTIONS

Directions: For each of the following questions, choose the **one best** answer.

1. Which one of the following statements best describes respiratory control mechanisms?

    (A) Breathing is normally considered an autonomic motor program

    (B) The pattern of breathing is carefully controlled by several different feedback systems

    (C) Most of the respiratory "effectors" are controlled by the autonomic nervous system

    (D) The respiratory rhythm generator is located within the cortex

    (E) The dorsal respiratory group (DRG) contains mostly motor neurons

2. Which one of the following statements best describes the central chemoreceptors?

    (A) The central chemoreceptor is located in the cerebellum

    (B) A lack of oxygen excites the central chemoreceptors

    (C) The response curve for the central chemoreceptor reflex is increased with sleep and anesthesia

    (D) The central chemoreceptors are not activated by resting levels of H^+ and carbon dioxide

    (E) Many believe that carbon dioxide is the primary stimulus because it is readily soluble, whereas H^+ does not easily cross membranes

3. Which of the following structures is the most important *medullary* structure for *integrating* respiratory-related afferent information?

    (A) Nucleus ambiguus

    (B) Pontine respiratory group

    (C) Swallowing center

    (D) Ventrolateral surface of the medulla

    (E) Nucleus of the tractus solitarius

4. The peripheral chemoreceptors would produce the greatest increase in ventilation in response to which one of the following?

    (A) Breathing 16% oxygen

    (B) Anemia that decreased the hematocrit to 30%

    (C) Moderate poisoning with carbon monoxide

    (D) A Pao_2 of 70 mm Hg

    (E) A 0.2 unit decrease in pH

5. Which of the following statements best describes obstructive sleep apnea?

    (A) Arterial desaturation occurs infrequently

    (B) The upper airways are prone to collapse

    (C) Sleep abnormalities are uncommon

    (D) The lungs are hyperinflated during apneas

    (E) Pleural pressures are less negative than normal

Directions: The group of questions below consists of lettered choices followed by several numbered items. For each numbered item, select the appropriate lettered option with which it is most closely associated. Each lettered option may be used once, more than once, or not at all.

Questions 6–8

Match the respiratory function listed below with the receptor most likely to be associated with it.

    (A) Peripheral chemoreceptors

    (B) Striated muscle pain fibers

    (C) Pulmonary stretch receptors

    (D) Central chemoreceptors

    (E) Pulmonary chemoreceptors

    (F) Pulmonary C-fibers

    (G) Irritant receptors

6. This receptor is most important in maintaining the respiratory drive in a patient suffering from a drug overdose

7. In a patient with pulmonary edema, arterial blood gases were Pa_{O_2} of 70 mm Hg and Pa_{CO_2} of 40 mm Hg. This patient's increased minute ventilation most likely would be elicited by this receptor

8. This receptor would be expected to elicit the greatest effect on respiratory timing in a patient breathing on continuous positive airway pressure (CPAP)

ANSWERS AND EXPLANATIONS

1. The answer is B. Most of the respiratory pump involves striated muscle innervated by the somatic nervous system. Only the smooth muscle of the lung and cardiovascular system are controlled by the autonomic nervous system. The respiratory output is controlled by the rhythm generator in the brainstem. This controller integrates multiple inputs to determine the appropriate output. The DRG contains mostly premotor neurons that send this information to the muscle pumps.

2. The answer is E. Hypoxia actually *inhibits* the central chemoreceptors that are located at or near the ventral medullary surface of the brainstem. The central chemoreceptors are active at normal blood gases and contribute to the drive for resting ventilation. The gain of these receptors is suppressed during sleep, anesthesia, or chronic hypercapnia.

3. The answer is E. The nucleus tractus solitarius is an important sensory relay that receives afferent information from many receptors, including the peripheral chemoreceptors, baroreceptors, and lung afferents. Although the central chemoreceptors are associated with the ventrolateral medullary surface, there are not many other afferents integrated there. The swallowing center and the nucleus ambiguus also receive afferent information, but it is minimal compared to the nucleus tractus solitarius. The pontine respiratory group is another important integrative center; however, it is located in the pons and not the medulla.

4. The answer is E. Although the primary stimulus for the peripheral chemoreceptors is hypoxia, it is important to note that the threshold for hypoxic activation is a Pa_{O_2} of approximately 60. Therefore, options A (breathing 16% oxygen) and D (a $Pao_2 = 70$ mm Hg) are false. Both options B (anemia that decreased hematocrit to 30%) and C (moderate carbon monoxide poisoning) would decrease the oxygen content; however, they have little effect on the Pao_2, which is the major stimulus. Peripheral chemoreceptor activity is increased by increases in H^+ or $Paco_2$. Therefore, a large change in pH from 7.4 to 7.2 would stimulate the peripheral chemoreceptors.

5. The answer is B. The major problem for most patients with obstructive sleep apnea is the collapse of the upper airways during inspiration that leads to very high airway resistance and low airflow (i.e., little or no change in lung volume, despite stronger than normal inspiratory efforts). The reduced ventilation leads to a low Pao_2 and reduced saturation of hemoglobin with oxygen. The periods of obstruction occur frequently during sleep.

6–8. The answers are: 6-A, 7-F, 8-C. Anesthesia suppresses both mechanoreceptor and chemoreceptor reflexes. The central chemoreceptors are severely depressed, and the major stimulus for breathing in drug overdose is hypoxia sensed by the peripheral chemoreceptors. None of the mechanoreceptors is typically involved in maintaining the tonic respiratory drive.

Although severe pulmonary edema can cause hypoxia and sometimes hypercapnia, the blood gases in this patient would not be significant stimuli for the peripheral or central chemoreceptors. Edema does cause deformation of the lung parenchyma, which excites pulmonary C-fibers. Activation of these receptors results in rapid, shallow breathing with an increase in minute ventilation.

CPAP would elevate the resting lung volume (i.e., functional residual capacity) and the end-tidal lung volume. This would increase the activity of the pulmonary stretch receptors, which influence both inspiratory and expiratory timing.

REFERENCES

1. Dempsey JA, Pack AI (eds): *Regulation of Breathing*, 2nd ed. New York, NY: Marcel Dekker, 1995.
2. Feldman JL: Neurophysiology of breathing in mammals. In *Handbook of Physiology*, section 1, *The Nervous System*, vol 4. Edited by Bloom FE. Bethesda, MD: American Physiological Society, 1986, pp 463–524.

20 THE INTEGRATED RESPONSE TO EXERCISE

CHAPTER OUTLINE

INTRODUCTION OF CLINICAL CASE

This is a continuation of the claudication case presented in Chapters 3 and 11. Additional tests performed on this patient at the clinic included maximum walking distance and calf muscle blood flow response to exercise in the affected limb. The walking tolerance test included walking on a treadmill until the onset of leg pain. Healthy individuals do not normally experience ischemic pain while walking, even after several miles. However, the patient in this case could walk fewer than 100 yards before experiencing leg pain.

Immediately after performing mild exercise on a foot ergometer (similar to a stationary bicycle), the patient's leg muscle blood flow increased from a resting level of 5 mL/min/100 g to a peak of 15 mL/min/100 g of muscle tissue. The peak postexercise response for healthy individuals performing mild exercise is in the range of 40–80 mL/min/100 g.

Illustration of typical leg muscle blood flow responses before and after rhythmic exercise in a normal subject (solid dots) and in a patient with sclerotic vascular disease, such as claudication (open squares). Note that the blunted postexercise response of the patient is similar to the blunted reactive hyperemia response shown in Chapter 11, Figure 11-11 for an atherosclerotic patient.

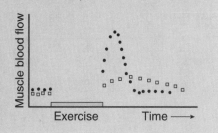

For therapy, the patient was placed on an exercise program consisting of movements, such as marking time to music and walking, for 30 minutes three times a week for 5 months. Repeated testing at the end of the 5-month period showed that his walking tolerance (distance to pain) had increased to 400 yards, whereas postexercise blood flow had increased to only 18 mL/min/100 g. However, the patient "felt better," and his episodes of ischemic pain (claudication) became less frequent.

ENERGETICS OF EXERCISE

"Pooh," I said one day when we were out walking with Piglet to nowhere in particular. "Exercise is the thing. You want to be fit. You want to tone up your muscles and stride through the Forest like a Bear of Great Strength." "I do?" he said. "Well, don't you?" He wondered. "I haven't given it much thought."[1] But hopefully you will after reading this chapter.

Nature of Energy Production

Adenosine triphosphate (ATP)—the molecule that provides most of the high-energy phosphate used in physiologic processes—is the fuel that drives exercise. Aerobic and anaerobic metabolism are the two general processes used to produce ATP from adenosine diphosphate (ADP). As their names imply, aerobic metabolism is the collection of biochemical events that require oxygen to synthesize ATP, whereas anaerobic metabolism produces ATP in the absence of oxygen. Glucose is a common metabolic substrate used in both aerobic and anaerobic processes. Aerobic metabolism provides more ATP per molecule of glucose compared to anaerobic metabolism. However, anaerobic production of ATP occurs relatively fast, such that *per unit time* anaerobic metabolism generates the most ATP. Accordingly, physical activities that require a rapid production of ATP, such as a sprint, rely on anaerobic metabolism for the necessary ATP production. Activities calling for a slow and long-lasting source of ATP, such as walking, utilize aerobic metabolism.

Sources of ATP Production

The various sources of ATP in skeletal and cardiac muscle are illustrated in Figure 20-1. The *bottom* of the figure depicts the fact that actin (A) and myosin (M) bonding, and therefore muscle contraction, occur in a cyclic manner as long as ATP is available. The most readily available source of ATP is the ATP stored within the cytoplasm of muscle cells. However, this source is quite small and can supply ATP for only approximately 1 or 2 seconds during high-intensity exercise.

The next most readily available source of high-energy molecules is creatine phosphate (CP). As shown in Figure 20-1, CP gives up its high-energy phosphate to ADP to make additional ATP for muscle contraction. Although there is approximately four times as much stored CP in muscle tissue compared to ATP, CP is still a relatively small source of high-energy phosphate and can supply ATP for only a few seconds before becoming depleted.

Because the pool of stored high-energy phosphate is relatively small, muscle cells must continuously produce high-energy phosphate molecules to sustain physical activity for any length of time. The most rapid source of ATP production from a metabolic substrate comes from the anaerobic conversion of glucose to pyruvate, which is shown in the *upper left* corner of Figure 20-1. This process, called *glycolysis*, can rapidly produce two ATP molecules per molecule of glucose.

The slowest, but the most enduring, production of ATP comes from the aerobic consumption of acetyl coenzyme A (acetyl CoA) in the Krebs (citric acid) cycle. As noted in Figure 20-1, acetyl CoA comes from either the glycolytic production of pyruvate from glucose or from the breakdown of fat stores to free fatty acids. In this context, note that

[1] Reprinted with permission from Mordden E: *Pooh's Workout Book.* New York, NY: E. P. Dutton, 1984, p 1.

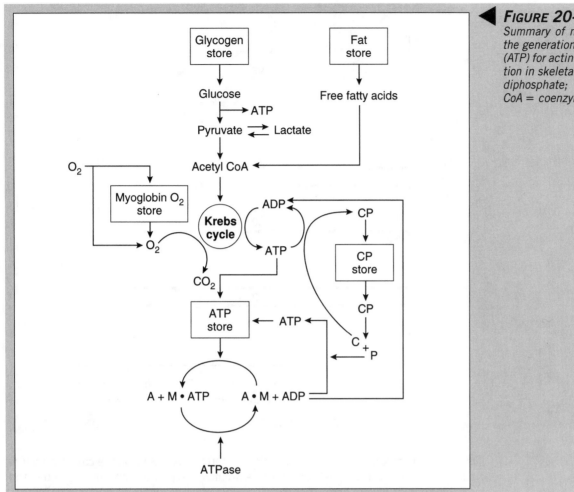

FIGURE 20-1
Summary of metabolic steps involved in the generation of adenosine triphosphate (ATP) for actin (A) and myosin (M) interaction in skeletal muscle. ADP = adenosine diphosphate; CP = creatine phosphate; CoA = coenzyme A.

pyruvate can be converted either to acetyl CoA or to lactate. The direction in which the reaction proceeds depends on the availability of oxygen. If oxygen is present, then the conversion to acetyl CoA via the Krebs cycle is favored. Myoglobin, the muscle pigment that gives red meat its color, assists in the transfer of oxygen to the Krebs cycle by storing a limited amount of oxygen within muscle cells.

In the absence of sufficient oxygen in skeletal muscle, pyruvate is converted to lactate. The lactate produced by skeletal muscle cells diffuses into the blood, which carries it to the heart and liver, where it can be converted back to pyruvate. In this manner, the heart, which has a lower capacity for glycolysis compared to skeletal muscle, is provided with additional substrate for its ATP production.

Although stored glycogen does provide substrate for ATP production, most ATP produced by aerobic means (approximately 80%) comes from fat stored in the liver, adipose tissue, and muscle. In healthy individuals, fat comprises 5%–25% of body weight, and the combustion of fat to carbon dioxide and water represents the primary source of aerobic energy.

Note that fat can be used for the production of ATP only by anaerobic means. Think about the implications of this with regard to the use of exercise for weight reduction.

Energy Utilization of Exercise

Physical activities are rarely, if ever, completely aerobic or anaerobic. Rather, physical work tends to be an admixture, with aerobic energy being dominant in low-level, long-duration activities (e.g., walking), whereas anaerobic energy is dominant in high-level, short-duration activities (e.g., sprinting, lifting heavy objects). The approximate division of anaerobic and aerobic energy utilization with increasing exercise intensity during running is given in Figure 20-2, which is a plot of running speed against the duration at which an average, healthy, conditioned individual can maintain a given speed. The two columns in the center of the graph give the percent distribution of anaerobic and aerobic energy for each of the running speeds. As can be seen, 98% of the energy cost of a sprint

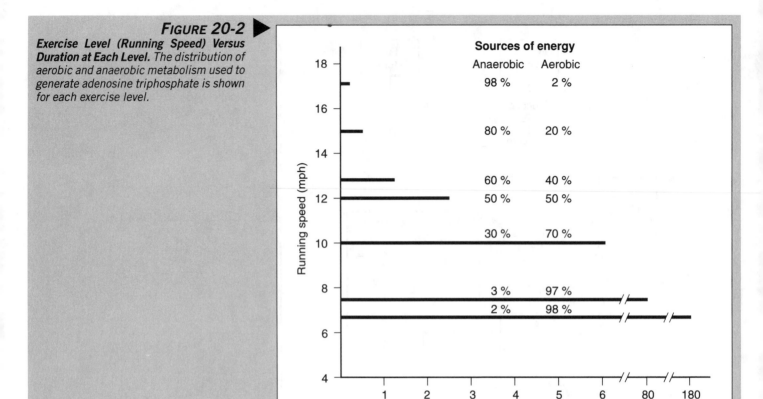

FIGURE 20-2

Exercise Level (Running Speed) Versus Duration at Each Level. The distribution of aerobic and anaerobic metabolism used to generate adenosine triphosphate is shown for each exercise level.

at 17 mph is met by anaerobic metabolism, whereas the reverse is the case for a jog at approximately 6.5 mph. Between these extremes there is a blend of anaerobic and aerobic sources of energy production.

In terms of energy utilization, there is nothing unique about running. Charts similar to those depicted in Figure 20-2 could be constructed for any exercise that can be performed over a wide range of intensities, such as swimming or bicycling. Therefore, in a general context, Figure 20-2 shows that the energetics of exercise involves a combination of aerobic and anaerobic metabolism, with the percentage of distribution being determined by exercise intensity.

If high-intensity exercise is primarily anaerobic, then why does a person breathe so hard after a bout of high-intensity activity? The reason for this is that *anaerobic energy must ultimately be repaid by aerobic means*. This principle is illustrated in Figure 20-3. This figure shows the oxygen cost (*dashed lines*) and oxygen consumption (*solid lines*) versus time for increasing levels of exercise intensity (speed). The oxygen consumption can be directly measured by continual collection of expired air from the subject. By contrast, oxygen cost is a calculated parameter derived by knowing the caloric expenditure of the exercise and the caloric equivalent of the subject's diet. For example, an exercise performed at an intensity of 9.6 kcal/min by a subject whose diet produces 4.8 kcal energy/L consumed oxygen has a cost of 2.0 L oxygen/min (9.6/4.8).

The *shaded area* in Figure 20-3 between oxygen cost and oxygen consumption represents the *oxygen deficit*. This is the energy produced by anaerobic means during exercise. This anaerobic energy production results in a partial depletion of ATP and CP stores, as well as an accumulation of lactate (see Figure 20-1). By contrast, the period indicated by the *clear area* under the solid curve represents production of ATP by aerobic means. ATP production by aerobic means continues after exercise, as indicated by elevated oxygen consumption, until ATP and CP stores are renewed and lactate is cleared by converting it to carbon dioxide and water (in the heart and liver) or by using it to resynthesize glucose (in the liver). The postexercise phase of elevated oxygen consumption is referred to as the *oxygen debt* and provides the oxygen used to pay back the oxygen deficit.

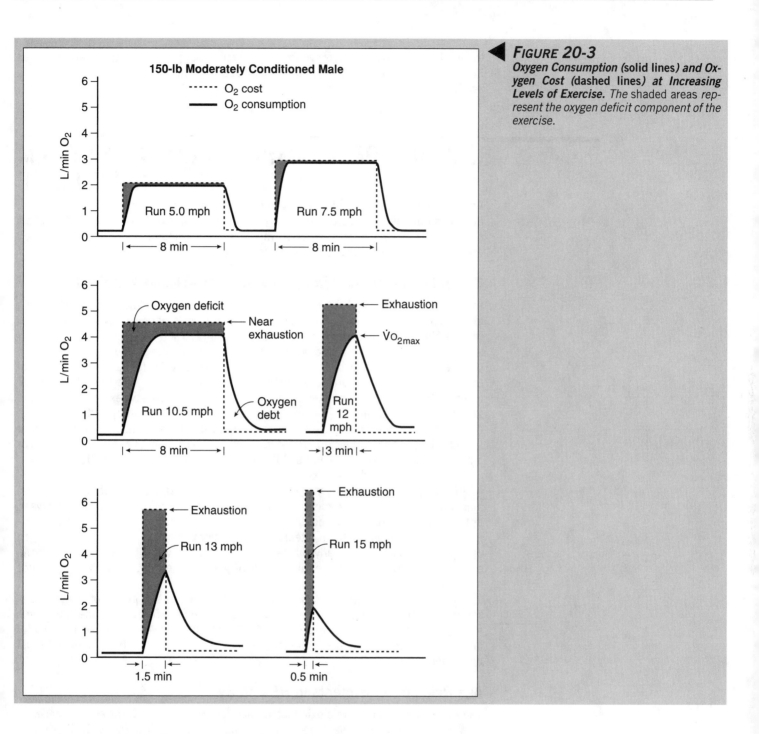

◄ FIGURE 20-3
Oxygen Consumption (solid lines) and Oxygen Cost (dashed lines) at Increasing Levels of Exercise. The shaded areas represent the oxygen deficit component of the exercise.

As can be seen in Figure 20-3, by increasing intensity, the point of exhaustion comes sooner, as was depicted in Figure 20-2. It is not clear what causes the exhaustion, but a likely hypothesis is that intracellular acidosis disrupts muscle contractions. This consideration points to the importance of the lungs in maintaining acid–base balance during physical activity.

Also noted in Figure 20-3 is that oxygen consumption only goes so high—to a level referred to as the *maximal oxygen consumption* ($\dot{V}o_{2max}$), which in this individual is approximately 4.0 L oxygen/min. With high-intensity exercise, exhaustion occurs before $\dot{V}o_{2max}$ is even reached.

Physiologists have debated for decades as to the determinants of $\dot{V}o_{2max}$. Ventilatory limitations of the lungs, limited ability of the heart to pump blood, limited dilatory reserve of arterioles, limited muscle capillary density, and limited muscle oxidative enzymes have all been implicated as causal factors in limiting oxygen consumption. However, because these factors are interactive, all of them probably play a role in limiting the intake and utilization of oxygen during exercise. Support for multiple causes comes from the observation that the aforementioned determinants of Vo_{2max} are all improved by aerobic exercise conditioning.

RESPONSE OF THE CARDIOPULMONARY SYSTEM TO EXERCISE

As indicated above, the limits of oxygen consumption during muscle work are, in part, due to limitations of the cardiopulmonary system to provide oxygenated blood to muscle tissue. This section explores the adjustments of the cardiopulmonary system to graded exercise and identifies possible limiting factors of oxygen consumption.

General Response of Cardiopulmonary Variables to Muscle Work

In Chapter 11, Figure 11-14 describes the distribution of cardiac output (CO) during exercise at increasing levels of intensity. However, it does not give any indication as to whether the cardiopulmonary system is becoming limited at high levels of exercise or, if it is, what components of the cardiopulmonary system are limiting. Figures 20-4 and 20-5 provide information on these issues. These charts respectively illustrate the responses of cardiac and respiratory parameters to acute bouts of exercise. Note the relative increments in heart rate (HR) and stroke volume (SV) from light-to-heavy exercise (see Figure 20-4) as compared with relative increments in respiratory frequency and tidal volume (V_T) from moderate-to-heavy exercise (see Figure 20-5). These comparisons suggest that for both the heart and lungs, increases in pump volume become limited before those of pump frequency; that is, the limits of the increase in CO and ventilation depend on the upper limits of HR and respiratory frequency, respectively.

Figure 20-6 provides further information on *steady-state* levels of cardiac performance as a function of exercise intensity expressed as a percent of maximal oxygen uptake. Again, SV reaches a "ceiling" at relatively low exercise intensity, whereas maximal HR is not reached until an intensity level of approximately 80% of maximal oxygen uptake is reached. This clearly indicates that HR is the variable that determines the extent to which CO can increase with increasing levels of exercise. Then what determines maximal HR?

Theoretically, maximal HR is determined by the refractory period of a myocardial action potential. Because this period is approximately 0.25 seconds, the theoretical maximum for HR would be approximately 240 beats/min. However, it is very unusual for heart rates to be this high. Accordingly, factors other than the refractory period must determine maximal HR.

Age-Related Adjustments in HR and SV

The exact anatomic or physiologic factors that determine maximal HR are not presently known; however, they do seem to depend on age. On this point, Figure 20-7 presents steady-state data from a study by Rodeheffer and colleagues showing HR and CO as a function of work intensity during bicycle exercise in young (25–44 years) and old (65–80 years) healthy male subjects [1]. Note that in the elderly, resting HR, the HR response to exercise, and maximal HR are all lower compared to the younger subjects. Because the response of CO to submaximal exercise is virtually identical in these two groups, the reduction in HR in elderly individuals must be offset by corresponding elevations in SV. This is shown in Figure 20-8, which presents SV, end-diastolic volume (EDV), and end-systolic volume (ESV) as functions of work load and CO for the same groups of subjects shown in Figure 20-7. Note that at any given CO or work load, SV is higher in older individuals and that this is manifested by an increase in EDV (i.e., the Frank-Starling mechanism, or Starling's law of the heart).

Until recently, it was thought that resting CO and the CO response to exercise declined with age. However, the study of Rodeheller and colleagues showed that this is true only for those individuals in which aging was attended by coronary heart disease (CHD) [1]. Healthy individuals with no evidence of subclinical CHD maintain CO with advancing age.

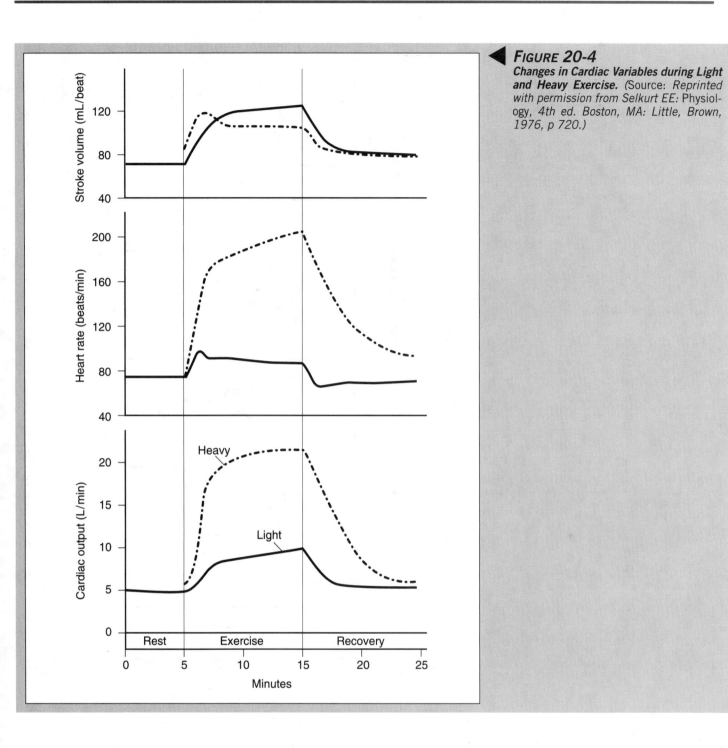

FIGURE 20-4
Changes in Cardiac Variables during Light and Heavy Exercise. (Source: *Reprinted with permission from Selkurt EE:* Physiology, *4th ed. Boston, MA: Little, Brown, 1976, p 720.)*

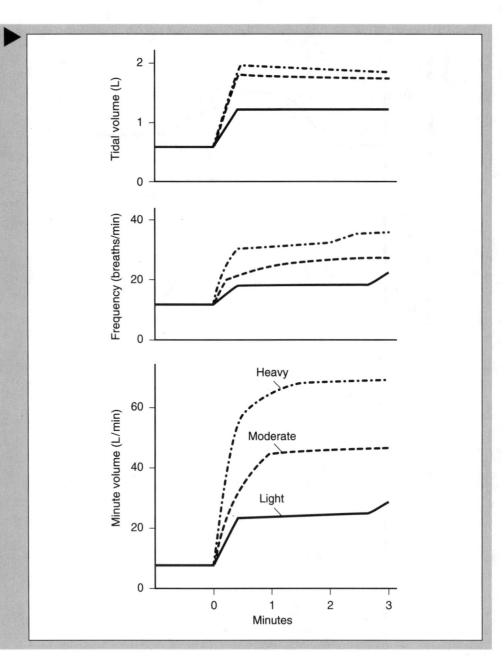

FIGURE 20-5

Changes in Respiratory Variables during Light, Moderate, and Heavy Exercise. (Source: *Reprinted with permission from Stegemann J:* Exercise Physiology: Physiologic Basis of Work and Sport. *Chicago, IL: Year Book, 1981, p 165.*)

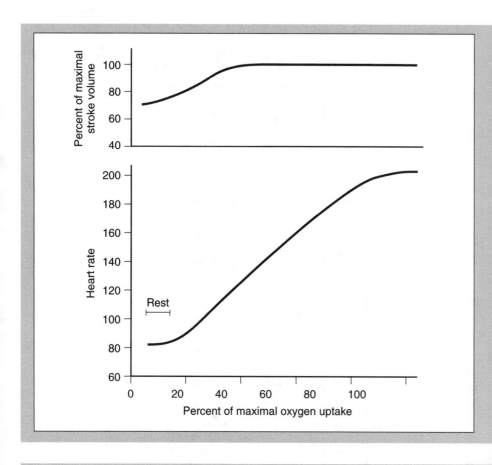

◀ **FIGURE 20-6**
Stroke Volume and Heart Rate as a Function of Exercise Intensity Expressed as a Percentage of Maximal Oxygen Uptake. (Source: *Reprinted with permission from Astrand PO, Rodahl K:* Textbook of Work Physiology. *New York, NY: McGraw-Hill, 1977, p 188.)*

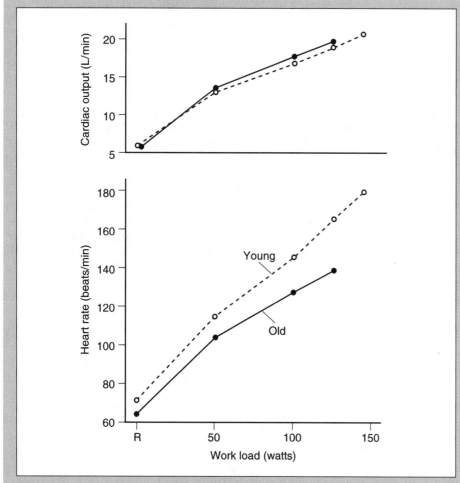

◀ **FIGURE 20-7**
Heart Rate and Stroke Volume as a Function of Exercise Intensity Expressed in Watts of Work Performed for a Group of Young (25–44-year-old) and Old (65–80-year-old) Male Subjects. *R = rest.* (Source: *Adapted with permission from Rodeheffer JJ, Gerstenblith G, Becker LC, et al: Exercise cardiac output is maintained with advancing age in healthy human subjects: cardiac dilation and increased stroke volume compensate for diminished heart rate.* Circulation *69: 209, 1984.)*

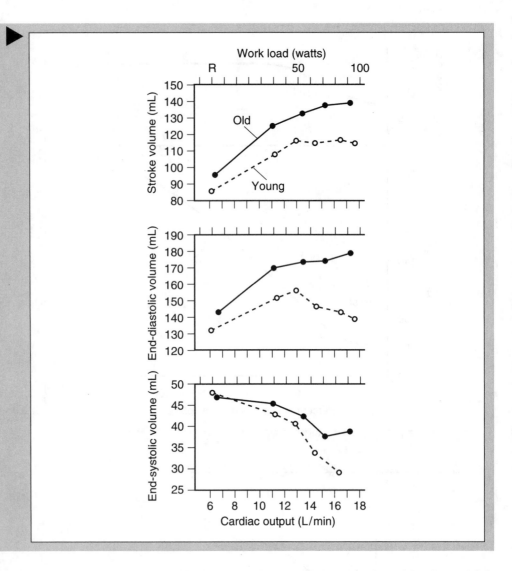

FIGURE 20-8 ▶
Stroke Volume, End-Diastolic Volume, and End-Systolic Volume as a Function of Cardiac Output and Work Load. These are the same two groups of subjects presented in Figure 20-7. R = rest.

Thus, the healthy older individual maintains CO by operating with a larger heart and using the Frank-Starling mechanism to increase SV in the face of a reduced HR. Interestingly, the lower HR and higher SV in elderly individuals are similar to the changes in cardiac variables that occur with aerobic exercise conditioning. This being the case, do healthy elderly individuals experience additional adjustments in cardiac variables with aerobic conditioning? This issue is addressed in Figure 20-9, which shows the HR response to increasing exercise intensity in groups of unconditioned and conditioned young and old individuals. Adjustments in HR are similar between the young and old with conditioning; however, the magnitude of change is slightly less for the elderly subjects. These results indicate that elderly individuals can benefit from aerobic conditioning, in terms of cardiac function, but changes are smaller compared to younger individuals.

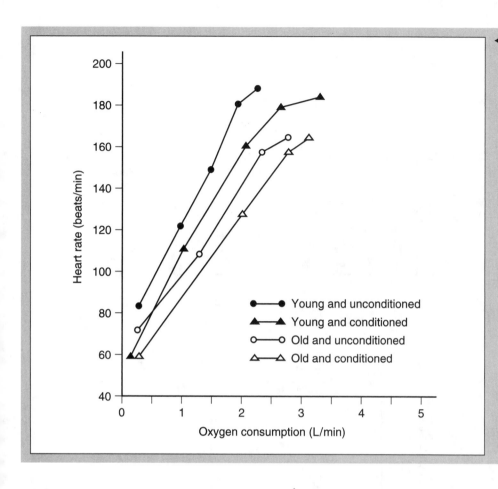

FIGURE 20-9
Heart Rate as a Function of Exercise Intensity in Conditioned and Unconditioned Young (College-Aged) and Elderly (63-year-old) Males. (Source: *Data on young subjects reprinted with permission from Saltin B: Physiological effects of physical conditioning.* Med Sci Sports *1:50, 1969. Data on old subjects reprinted with permission from Ogawa T, et al: Effects of aging, sex and physical training on cardiovascular responses to exercise.* Circulation *86:494, 1992.*)

Determinants of SV during Exercise

Because SV is the difference between EDV and ESV, the SV response to exercise could be mediated (and possibly limited) by cardiac filling (Starling's law of the heart), by the ability of the heart to empty (contractility), or by both. Figure 20-10 provides information on this issue. To generate these data, young subjects (26 years) pedaled a stationary bicycle while lying on their backs (supine) then again in the normal bicycling position (upright). With supine exercise, the SV response is determined almost exclusively by an increase in EDV (Starling's law). In the upright position, a decrease in ESV (contractility) plays an additional role. However, in both situations, the increase in EDV is greater in magnitude compared to the decrease in ESV, suggesting that the magnitude of the SV response to exercise is determined more by the Frank-Starling mechanism than by contractility.

It should not be inferred from the above analysis that cardiac contractility is of only minor importance in exercise. A positive inotropic effect (i.e., an increase in contractility) is manifested by an increase in the rate of both cardiac ejection and cardiac filling. Without these adjustments attending an exercise-elicited increase in HR, both ejection and filling times could be inadequate. Thus, an increase in contractility is necessary to maintain SV in the face of an increase in HR during almost any level of exercise.

If cardiac filling is a major determinant and a limiting factor of SV, then exercises that do not promote venous return should have a modest SV response. To address this issue, Figure 20-11 shows the CO, HR, and SV responses to stationary bicycle exercise with the legs, then again by cranking the pedals with the arms. Both exercises were performed in a seated position. Note that the SV response to arm cranking is quite limited, compared to leg exercise because there is much less muscle mass in the arms to promote venous return. These results are consistent with the notion that cardiac filling is a major determinant of SV during exercise. This conclusion is further supported in studies by Lind and colleagues in which static contraction of the arms elicited either no change or a decrease in SV [2].

The ventricular volume component of the cardiac cycle is shown below at rest (solid line) and for an increase in HR attended by a normal increase in contractility (dashed line). The arrows at the top right of the graph point to the "atrial" waves signaling a new heart beat. Even if ESV remains the same without the rapid emptying and rapid filling associated with the increase in HR, SV would be reduced by the amount indicated by the double arrow between the dashed and solid lines shown at the end of rapid filling.

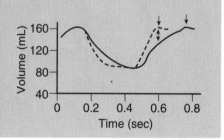

FIGURE 20-10 ▶

End-Diastolic (EDV), End-Systolic (ESV), and Stroke Volumes (SV) of Healthy Individuals at Rest (R), Then during Light (L), Moderate (M), and Heavy (H) Levels of Supine and Upright Exercise. As indicated by the proportionately higher EDVs compared to lower ESVs, the Frank-Starling mechanism plays a greater role than contractility in determining the SV response to exercise. (Source: Reproduced with permission from Poliner LR, et al: Left ventricular performance in normal subjects: a comparison of the responses to exercise in the upright and supine positions. Circulation 62:531, 1980.)

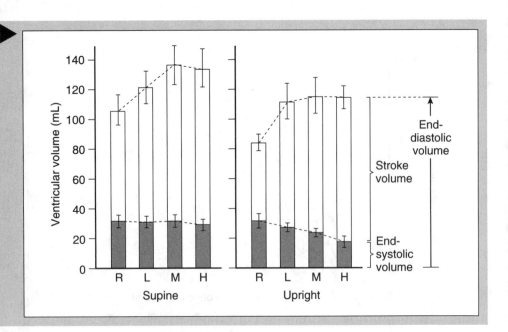

FIGURE 20-11 ▶

Cardiac Variables in Response to Bicycle Exercise with the Legs and by Cranking the Pedals with the Arms. Compared to leg exercise, arm exercise is attended by little, if any, increase in stroke volume. This probably results from a much smaller venous return with arm exercise. (Source: Reprinted with permission from Clausen JP: Circulatory adjustments to dynamic exercise and effect of physical training in normal subjects and in patients with coronary artery disease. Prog Cardiovas Dis 18:462, 1976.)

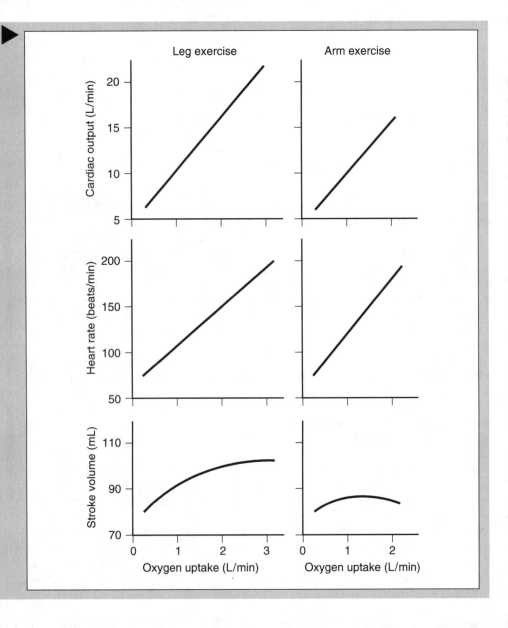

Pulmonary Response to Exercise

It is axiomatic that the increase in CO during exercise must be attended by a corresponding increase in alveolar ventilation ($\dot{V}_A$), if oxygen delivery to muscle tissue is to keep pace with oxygen consumption. Figure 20-5 shows that the increase in ventilation with exercise occurs by a combination of an increase in respiratory frequency and V_T, with the latter seeming to become limited at high-intensity exercise. However, Figure 20-12 shows that even at a level of exercise that produces $\dot{V}O_{2max}$, the V_T is well below the subject's vital capacity (i.e., the maximal V_T). Thus, unlike its cardiac counterpart SV, V_T does not seem to be limited by exercise intensity.

Although there is no evidence that respiratory frequency reaches any sort of a ceiling during exercise analogous to maximal HR, respiratory frequency still may be limiting because of an increase in airway resistance at high breathing rates. An increase in airway resistance can be elicited by an increase in respiratory frequency in at least two ways: by the production of turbulent airflow and by the collapse of airways during expiration.

The above discussion indicates that although limits to minute ventilation in terms of V_T and breathing rate may not be reached at high-intensity exercise, certain mechanical consequences of elevated respiration (e.g., airway resistance) may impose a "respiratory ceiling." A further limit of the respiratory system can be seen in Figure 20-13. Note that the work of breathing increases markedly with increasing ventilation, as would occur during exercise. Thus, the increased metabolic cost of an elevated minute volume would create diminished returns with high-intensity exercise.

*In patients with **emphysema**, the tissue that supports the airways is severely damaged. Without this support, airways tend to collapse in these patients, leading to an increase in airway resistance.*

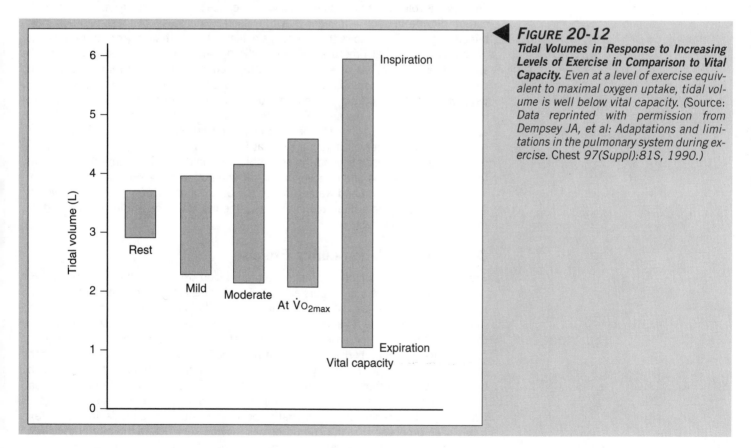

FIGURE 20-12
Tidal Volumes in Response to Increasing Levels of Exercise in Comparison to Vital Capacity. Even at a level of exercise equivalent to maximal oxygen uptake, tidal volume is well below vital capacity. (Source: Data reprinted with permission from Dempsey JA, et al: Adaptations and limitations in the pulmonary system during exercise. Chest 97(Suppl):81S, 1990.)

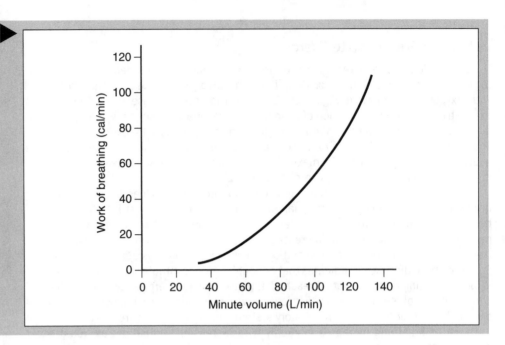

FIGURE 20-13 ▶
Work of Breathing as a Function of Minute Volume Generated during Exercise. (Source: Reprinted with permission from Margaria R, Milic-Emili G, Petit JM, et al: Mechanical work of breathing during muscular exercise. J Appl Physiol 15:356, 1960.)

Pulmonary System and Blood Gas Homeostasis during Exercise

The obvious role of the pulmonary system in exercise is to take up oxygen and eliminate carbon dioxide in such a manner that the blood homeostasis of these gases is maintained. Figure 20-14 shows that the lungs achieve this quite well. As exercise intensity increases, the partial pressures of oxygen (Pa_{O_2}) and carbon dioxide (Pa_{CO_2}) in the arterial blood as well as plasma hydrogen ion concentration [H^+] remain remarkably constant up to the anaerobic threshold (i.e., the point indicated by the *dashed line*). Beyond this line, anaerobic metabolism dominates the production of ATP. The increase in arterial [H^+] beyond the anaerobic threshold is due largely to the production of lactic acid (see Figure 20-1). The steeper rise in $\dot{V}_A$ and fall in Pa_{CO_2} within the anaerobic range indicate a hyperventilatory state that is driven by the elevated H^+. This means that at levels of exercise beyond the anaerobic threshold, the lungs are serving not only to oxygenate the blood and remove carbon dioxide but also to excrete acid by eliminating it as carbon dioxide and water through the bicarbonate (HCO_3^-) buffering system. Thus, the lungs serve a dual role in exercise: the maintenance of blood gases and the maintenance of H^+ balance.

Control of Ventilation during Exercise

The proficiency with which the lungs maintain blood oxygen, carbon dioxide, and H^+ during increasing levels of aerobic exercise (see Figure 20-14) presents somewhat of a puzzle. Namely, what are the signals that drive ventilation? Figure 20-15 presents data that support a *neurohumoral* theory of respiratory control during exercise. According to this theory, the abrupt increase in minute ventilation at the onset of exercise is thought to be a feed-forward neural drive from the central nervous system (CNS), most likely from the hypothalamus. The slow rise in ventilation to a steady state is thought to be caused by blood-borne factors that have yet to be clearly identified. Although mean levels of Pa_{O_2} and Pa_{CO_2} remain remarkably constant during exercise, pulsatile variations in blood gases between end inspiration and end expiration become greater in magnitude. In this context, it has been proposed that the carotid bodies may be sensitive to the rate of change of carbon dioxide or H^+ as well as to their mean values [3]. Other possible feedback mechanisms that have been proposed include carbon dioxide–sensitive receptors in the venous system, elevation in plasma potassium (K^+), and elevation in circulating catecholamines. In addition to these factors, chemoreceptors and mechanoreceptors in muscles and joints may provide input into the respiratory control system. Although these are not strictly humoral, they are nonetheless considered to be contributory to the *humoral* phase of the proposed *neurohumoral* control mechanism. In re-examining Figures 20-3 and 20-15, it can be concluded that continuation of the cardiopulmonary drive to repay the oxygen deficit following exercise is mediated by humoral factors.

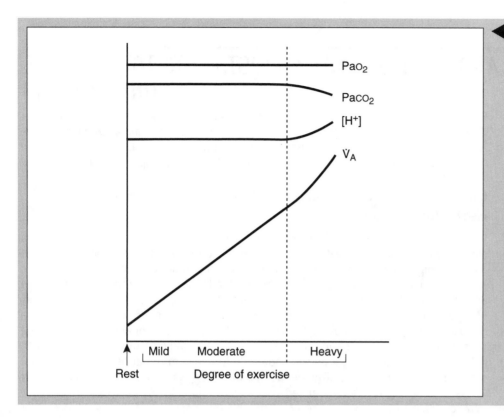

FIGURE 20-14
Blood Gases, Plasma [H⁺], and Alveolar Ventilation (VA) as a Function of Exercise Intensity below and above the Anaerobic Threshold (dashed line). (Source: *Adapted with permission from Hlastala MP, Berger AJ: Physiology of Respiration. New York, NY: Oxford University Press, 1996, p 235.*)

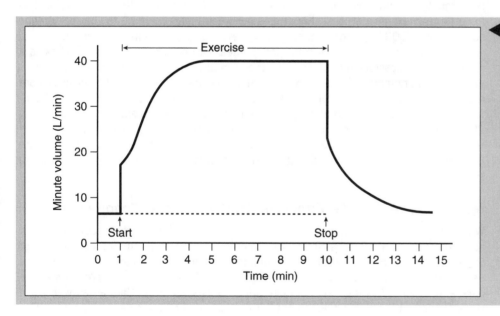

FIGURE 20-15
Minute Ventilation as a Function of Time before, during, and after Exercise. (Source: *Reprinted with permission from Selkurt EE: Physiology, 5th ed. Boston, MA: Little, Brown, 1984, p 578.*)

In summary, the pulmonary system operates below its theoretical maximum capacity at all levels of exercise. At exercise intensities up to the anaerobic threshold, the lungs do a remarkable job in maintaining homeostasis of blood gases and [H+]. The mechanisms responsible for regulating the pulmonary system during exercise are not entirely known, but a neurohumoral sequence involving initial feed-forward signals from the CNS followed by peripheral feedback signals seems to be the most likely explanation.

CARDIOPULMONARY ADJUSTMENTS TO EXERCISE CONDITIONING

Exercise regimens have gained wide acceptance in the treatment of many cardiovascular diseases, and a life style of regular exercise is considered quite beneficial to health maintenance. This section outlines some of the salient cardiopulmonary adjustments elicited by regular exercise that relate to the maintenance of a healthy cardiopulmonary system.

Exercise Prescription: What Constitutes Appropriate Exercise for Health Maintenance?

A trick for being able to determine if you are exercising below the anaerobic threshold is that you can exercise and talk at the same time. Above the anaerobic threshold, the increased respiratory drive inhibits the voluntary control of respiration necessary for conversation.

It is generally agreed that for cardiac rehabilitation and health maintenance, exercise should be performed at a level below the anaerobic threshold. There are several reasons for this, which include, but are not limited to, the fact that bouts of intense anaerobic exercise can cause dangerously high levels of arterial blood pressure, elicit severe acidosis, cause hyperkalemia, and precipitate arrhythmias. In other words, in routinely using anaerobic exercise for health maintenance, the treatment can be worse than the disease. However, almost from the moment the health benefits of aerobic conditioning became known, physicians and exercise scientists have had difficulty in coming up with guidelines for exactly what a person should do to derive maximal benefit from regular exercise. Advocates of the HR guideline approach suggest exercising at approximately 65%–75% of a person's age-related maximal HR (i.e., 220 − age) for at least 20 minutes three times a week. The problem with this approach is that without special equipment HR cannot be measured during exercise. A suggested alternative approach is to perform an exercise at least three times per week that, according to charts, expends approximately 300 kilocalories above resting levels during a 20-minute period.

The HR and calorie-per-workout approaches both require that subjects stick to a routine. Quite possibly for this reason these methods have not been successful in reaching large numbers of sedentary individuals who are at risk for heart disease. A more recent approach, which shows promise, is the *Target 2000* program presented by Stamford and Shimer [4]. According to this system, subjects need to expend approximately 2000 kilocalories per week in aerobic activities above those of a sedentary existence (e.g., walking instead of driving; taking the stairs rather than the elevator). Because there is quite a variety of such activities, they can be tailored to fit into each individual's life style and daily routine.

Metabolic and Vascular Effects of Aerobic Exercise Conditioning

Angiogenesis refers to the growth of new blood vessels. Tissues produce angiogenic factors in response to various stimuli. Aerobic exercise has a potent angiogenic effect in cardiac and skeletal muscle tissues.

Whatever the mode and manner in which an individual chooses to engage in aerobic activities, the resultant physiologic adjustments are similar. Beginning at the level of individual muscle fibers, aerobic conditioning elicits an increased ability to extract and use oxygen. Capillary density, muscle myoglobin content, and aerobic enzymes all increase to varying degrees. The capillary angiogenesis occurs in cardiac as well as in skeletal muscle, and this adjustment forms part of the rationale for using aerobic exercise as a therapeutic arm in the treatment of coronary heart disease.

The increase in aerobic capacity of conditioned muscle is augmented by the oxyhemoglobin properties of red blood cells (RBCs). Specifically, exercise conditioning seems to increase the production of *2,3-diphosphoglycerate (2,3-DPG)* by the RBCs. This substance reduces the affinity of hemoglobin for oxygen, thereby eliciting a higher degree of oxyhemoglobin dissociation at a given partial pressure of oxygen and, consequently, a greater degree of oxygen extraction from the blood.

Cardiac and Pulmonary Adjustments to Aerobic Exercise Conditioning

The general age-independent effects of aerobic conditioning on cardiac variables are presented schematically in Figure 20-16. At a given level of exercise, SV becomes larger, whereas HR is reduced in the conditioned individual. More importantly, the level of exercise at which maximal HR is reached is increased, and it is this adjustment that is responsible for the increase in maximal CO.

Figure 20-17 illustrates that with conditioning the lungs undergo adjustments similar to the heart; that is, a decrease in breathing rate and an increase in V_T. A possible

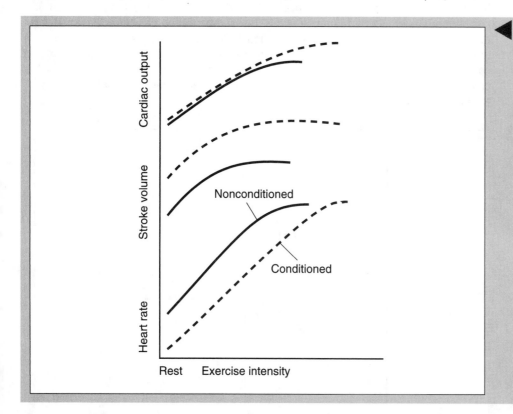

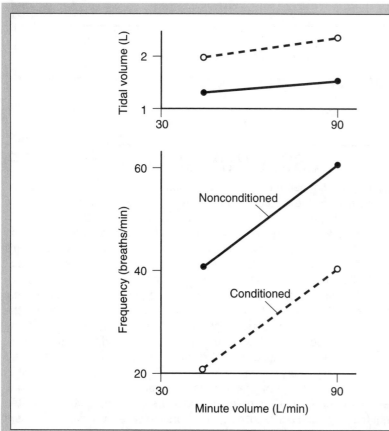

FIGURE 20-16
Schematic Representation of Modifications in Heart Rate, Stroke Volume, and Cardiac Output with Exercise Conditioning.

FIGURE 20-17
Tidal Volume and Respiratory Frequency at Two Levels of Minute Volume during Exercise in Conditioned (dashed lines) and Nonconditioned (solid lines) Individuals.
(Source: *Reprinted with permission from Selkurt EE: Physiology, 5th ed. Boston, MA: Little, Brown, 1984, p 575.)*

effect of these adjustments is that at a given minute volume, the work of breathing is lower in conditioned individuals.

The end result of the metabolic, vascular, cardiac, and pulmonary adjustments elicited by aerobic exercise conditioning is that a conditioned individual can perform a higher level of exercise by aerobic means (i.e., the anaerobic threshold is shifted up). Furthermore, exercise performance within the aerobic range can be achieved at a reduced minute volume. This is seen in Figure 20-18. Looking at this figure from a different angle, it can be seen that a given minute volume is attended by a greater oxygen consumption (i.e., greater aerobic work can be performed). This occurs because of the collective effect of an increased ability to intake, deliver, extract, and utilize oxygen for the production of ATP.

FIGURE 20-18 ▶
Minute Ventilation Versus Oxygen Consumption in Conditioned (dashed line) *and Nonconditioned* (solid line) *Individuals.* (Source: *Reprinted with permission from Selkurt EE:* Physiology, 5th ed. Boston, MA: Little, Brown, 1984, p 575.)

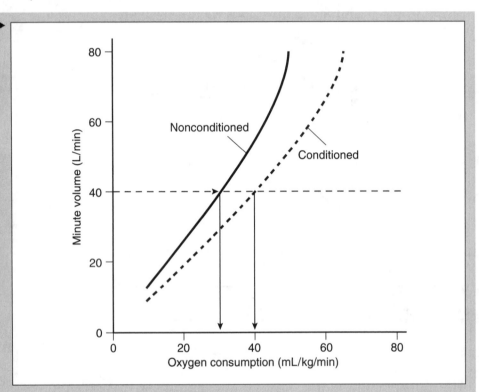

RESOLUTION OF CLINICAL CASE

Following a 5-month period of aerobic exercise conditioning, the patient with claudication showed improvement in the distance he could walk before the onset of ischemic pain. This suggests an improvement in the vascularization of his sclerotic leg and perhaps a return of dilatory capability in the limb circulation. Although the literature on exercise conditioning clearly suggests that these adjustments would occur, the patient's improvement in blood flow response to exercise (120%) was well short of his increase in walking distance (400%). This indicates that the more dramatic response of this individual to exercise conditioning was an improvement in aerobic metabolism within muscle fibers (e.g., increase in Krebs cycle enzymes). This conclusion is supported by the observation that some claudication patients show improvement in postconditioning walking tolerance despite a continuing decrease in the exercise blood flow response [5].

Because this particular patient had normal respiratory function (e.g., forced vital capacity = 4.2 L; forced expiratory volume at 1 sec = 3.2 L) before conditioning, it is unlikely that changes in pulmonary mechanics played a role in his improved walking tolerance. However, it is likely that his oxyhemoglobin dissociation curve was shifted slightly to the right (i.e., a greater degree of oxygen dissociation at a given partial pressure of oxygen) because of an exercise-conditioned increase in muscle myoglobin and 2,3-DPG in RBCs. Thus, his improved aerobic performance may have been due, in part, to an increased ability to extract oxygen at the tissue level.

This case illustrates that even patients with advanced atherosclerotic vascular disease (e.g., claudication) can benefit by a therapeutic program of exercise conditioning and that the improvements in physical performance brought about by exercise conditioning involve an interaction of cardiovascular (or cardiopulmonary) and tissue metabolic effects. For more information on the effects of aerobic exercise conditioning on claudication patients, see Ekroth and colleagues [5].

REVIEW QUESTIONS

Directions: For each of the following questions, choose the **one best** answer.

1. Which of the following combinations of processes represent the generation of ATP by anaerobic means?

   (A) catabolism of glucose to pyruvate and the transfer of phosphate from creatine phosphate to ADP

   (B) catabolism of free fatty acids and catabolism of glucose to pyruvate

   (C) transfer of phosphate from creatine phosphate to ADP and the catabolism of pyruvate to carbon dioxide and water

   (D) catabolism of free fatty acids and catabolism of pyruvate to carbon dioxide and water

2. The increase in cardiac output (CO) between low-intensity and high-intensity exercise occurs by

   (A) equally proportionate increases in heart rate (HR) and stroke volume (SV)

   (B) primarily by an increase in SV

   (C) primarily by an increase in HR

   (D) primarily by an increase in contractility

3. An individual person's maximal cardiac output (CO) increases with aerobic exercise conditioning because

   (A) maximal heart rate (HR) increases

   (B) maximal HR is reached at a higher level of exercise

   (C) maximal stroke volume (SV) is reached at a higher level of exercise

   (D) the anaerobic threshold is increased

4. In which of the following exercise situations would stroke volume (SV) be the highest?

   (A) a 65-year-old individual lifting weights

   (B) a 25-year-old individual riding a bicycle

   (C) a 65-year-old individual riding a bicycle

   (D) a 25-year-old individual lifting weights

5. At an exercise performed above the level of an individual's anaerobic threshold, which of the following situations occurs?

   (A) Alveolar ventilation reaches a plateau

   (B) $[H^+]$ in arterial blood increases

   (C) Pa_{CO_2} increases

   (D) Pa_{O_2} decreases

6. A person's maximal oxygen consumption is reached during

   (A) all levels of exercise performed above the anaerobic threshold

   (B) levels of exercise during which at least 80% of the energy is derived by anaerobic means

   (C) exhaustive levels of exercise that can be sustained for at least 3 minutes

   (D) exercise performed at the maximal intensity level (e.g., as fast as a person can run)

ANSWERS AND EXPLANATIONS

1. The answer is A. As shown in Figure 20-1, both the transfer of phosphate from creatine phosphate to ADP *and* the catabolism (breakdown) of glucose to pyruvate can produce ATP by anaerobic means. The catabolism of free fatty acids and the catabolism of pyruvate to carbon dioxide and water, which appear in the other choices, both produce ATP by aerobic means.

2. The answer is C. As shown in Figure 20-6, SV reaches a plateau at relatively low levels of exercise. Thus, between low and high levels of exercise, the increase in CO is due almost exclusively to an increase in HR.

3. The answer is B. As shown in Figure 20-16, exercise conditioning is attended by a lower HR and a higher SV at any submaximal level of exercise. However, maximal SV is reached at exercise levels below the level at which maximal CO is reached. Therefore, the maximal CO corresponds to the level of exercise at which maximal HR is reached.

4. The answer is C. As shown in Figure 20-8, at a given work load SV is higher in older versus younger individuals. Figure 20-11 points out that, for any age, SV is higher for leg work versus arm work. Accordingly, of the choices given, the 65-year-old riding a bicycle would have the highest SV.

5. The answer is B. As shown in Figure 20-14, the pulmonary system goes into a state of hyperventilation at exercise levels above the anaerobic threshold. This seems to be due to an elevated plasma $[H^+]$, and it results in a lowering, not an elevation, of the $Paco_2$.

6. The answer is C. As shown in Figure 20-3, it takes at least 2–3 minutes for oxygen consumption to reach a plateau. In examining Figures 20-2 and 20-3, it can be seen that an exercise during which 80% of the energy is anaerobic (choice B) and a maximal intensity exercise (choice D) cannot be sustained long enough for oxygen consumption to reach a plateau. Since these two exercise levels would be above the anaerobic threshold, choice A is also incorrect.

REFERENCES

1. Rodeheffer JJ, Gerstenblith G, Becker LC, et al: Exercise cardiac output is maintained with advancing age in healthy human subjects: cardiac dilation and increased stroke volume compensate for diminished heart rate. *Circulation* 69:203–213, 1984.
2. Lind AR, Taylor SH, Humphreys PW, et al: The circulatory effects of sustained voluntary muscle contraction. *Clin Sci* 27:229–244, 1964.
3. Hlastala MP, Berger AJ: *Physiology of Respiration.* New York, NY: Oxford University Press, 1996.
4. Stamford BA, Shimer P: *Fitness Without Exercise.* New York, NY: Warner Books, 1990.
5. Ekroth R, Dahllof AG, Gundevall B, et al: Physical training of patients with intermittent claudication: indications, methods, and results. *Surgery* 84:640–643, 1978.

APPENDIX: LIST OF ABBREVIATIONS

ρ	density
η	viscosity of blood
Δl	muscle shortening
$\Delta l/\Delta t$	velocity of shortening
ΔmBP	change in mean arterial blood pressure
ΔP	pressure gradient
ΔP_v	venous pressure gradient
ΔV	change in volume
μm	micrometers (10^{-6} meters)
2,3-BPG	2,3-bisphosphoglycerate
A	area available for exchange between blood and the interstitium
ABP	arterial blood pressure
ACE	angiotensin-converting enzyme
ACh	acetylcholine
ADH	antidiuretic hormone
ADP	adenosine diphosphate
ANG II	angiotensin II
ANP	atrial natriuretic peptide
ANS	autonomic nervous system
ATP	adenosine triphosphate
ATPase	adenosine triphosphatase
AV	atrioventricular
AV3V	anteroventral third ventricular region
BNP	brain natriuretic peptide
BP	blood pressure
bpm	beats per minute
C	compliance
Ca^{2+}	calcium ion
cAMP	cyclic adenosine monophosphate
Ca_{O_2}	content of oxygen in arterial blood
cGMP	cyclic guanosine monophosphate
CHF	congestive heart failure
CI	cardiac index
C_L	compliance of the lung
Cl^-	chloride ion
cm	centimeter
cm^2	square centimeters
cm^3 or cc	cubic centimeters
CNP	central natriuretic peptide
CNS	central nervous system
CO	cardiac output
CoA	coenzyme A
COP	colloid osmotic pressure
COPD	chronic obstructive pulmonary disease
COPif	colloid osmotic pressure generated by protein in interstitial fluid
COP_p	colloid osmotic pressure generated by plasma proteins
CP	creatine phosphate
CPAP	continuous positive airway pressure

Cp_x	concentration of substance in the plasma
C_T	total compliance
CVLM	caudal ventrolateral medulla
Cvo_2	content of oxygen in venous blood
DAG	diacylglycerol
DBP	diastolic arterial blood pressure
D_L	diffusing capacity of the lung
D_Lo_2	diffusing capacity of the lung for oxygen
dP/dt	rate of change of pressure
DRG	dorsal respiratory group
dV/dt	rate of change of voltage
dyne	unit of force
E	energy
early-DM	early diastolic murmur
ECG	electrocardiograph
EDCF	endothelial-derived constrictor factors
EDRF	endothelial-derived relaxation factors
EDV	end diastolic volume
E_{K^+}	equilibrium potential for potassium ions
E_m	membrane potential
EPP	end plate potential
ERP	effective refractory period
ERV	expiratory reserve volume
ESPVR	end systolic pressure–volume relationship
ESV	end systolic volume
F	force
Fe^{2+}	ferrous iron ion
Fe^{3+}	ferric iron ions
FEV_1	forced expiratory volume in 1 second
FRC	functional residual capacity
FVC	forced vital capacity
G	conductance $(1/R)$ or R^{-1}
g	force of gravity
GI	gastrointestinal
G_i	membrane conductance of inward current
G_{K^+}	membrane conductance of potassium
G_{Na^+}	membrane conductance of sodium
G_o	membrane conductance of outward current
GTP	guanosine triphosphate
h	height
H	high-frequency sounds in phonocardiogram
H^+	hydrogen ion
H_2CO_3	carbonic acid
H_2O	water
Hb	hemoglobin
HbO_2	oxyhemoglobin
HCO_3^-	bicarbonate ion
Hg	mercury
HR	heart rate
Hz	Hertz
I_b	background current
I_f	pacemaker ("funny") current
IgM	immunoglobulin M
in^2	square inches
IP_3	inositol 1,4,5-triphosphate
IPSP	inhibitory postsynaptic potential
IRV	inspiratory reserve volume
IVC	inferior vena cava
Jv	rate of ultrafiltration

K	capillary permeability coefficient
K^+	potassium ion
kg	kilogram
l	length
L	liter
LA	left atrium
LBNP	lower body negative pressure
lbs	pounds
L_{max} or L_o	optimal length of muscle
LQTS	long QT syndrome
LSB	left sternal border
LV	left ventricle
LVEDP	left ventricular end diastolic pressure
LVEDV	left ventricular end diastolic volume
LVESV	left ventricular end systolic volume
LVP	left ventricular pressure
LVSV	left ventricular stroke volume
m	meter
M_1	mid-frequency sounds in phonocardiogram
m^2	square meters
m^3	cubic meters
MAP	mean arterial blood pressure
mg	milligrams
Mg^{2+}	magnesium ion
min	minute
mL	milliliter
mm	millimeter
mm Hg	millimeters of mercury
mV	millivolts
MVC	maximum voluntary contractile force
$M\dot{v}O_2$	rate at which oxygen is consumed by myocardium
Na^+	sodium ion
NANC	nonadrenergic–noncholinergic
NO	nitric oxide
NPY	neuropeptide-Y
NTS	nucleus of the solitary tract (*nucleus tractus solitarius*)
O_2	oxygen
OS	opening snap in phonocardiogram
OVLT	organum vasculosum of the lamina terminalis
P	pressure
P cell	pacemaker cell
P_1	pressure at input side
P_2	pressure at output side
P_A	alveolar pressure
pA	picoamperes
P_a	arterial pressure
P_{Ao}	aortic blood pressure
P_{ACO_2}	partial pressure of carbon dioxide in the alveolar gas
P_{aCO_2}	partial pressure of carbon dioxide in the arterial blood
P_{AO_2}	partial pressure of oxygen in the alveoli
P_{aO_2}	partial pressure of oxygen in the arterial blood
PAP	pulmonary arterial pressure
P_{atm}	atmospheric pressure
Pc	pressure within the capillary
P_{Cl^-}	membrane permeability to chloride ions
PGA	protoglycan aggregate
pH_a	arterial blood pH
Pif	pushing force in the interstitial fluid
P_IO_2	inspired oxygen concentration

PIP_2	phosphatidylinositol biphosphate
PK	protein kinase
P_{K^+}	membrane permeability to potassium ions
P_m	mouth pressure
P_{mc}	mean circulatory pressure
PN	phrenic nerve
PNA	parasympathetic nerve activity
P_{Na^+}	membrane permeability to sodium ions
PNS	parasympathetic nervous system
P_o	maximum load muscle can lift
Po_2	partial pressure of oxygen
P_{pl}	intrapleural pressure
P_{RA}	pressure in right atrium
PRG	pontine respiratory group
psi	pounds per square inch (a unit of pressure)
PSR	pulmonary stretch receptor
P_T	distending pressure on the lung
PVC	premature ventricular contraction
$P\bar{v}co_2$	partial pressure of carbon dioxide in mixed venous blood
$P\bar{v}o_2$	partial pressure of oxygen in mixed venous blood
PVR	pulmonary vascular resistance
Px	permeability of a diffusing substance
$\dot{Q}$	rate of flow (volume/time)
$\dot{Q}x$	rate of diffusion across the vascular endothelium
R	resistance
R-R	time between R waves
RARs	rapidly adapting receptors
R_{aw}	airway resistance
RBC	red blood cell
REM	rapid eye movement
R_f	respiratory frequency
ROC	receptor-operated channels
RV	residual volume
RVEDV	right ventricular end diastolic volume
RVLM	rostral ventrolateral medulla
RVSV	right ventricular stroke volume
S	entropy
S_1	first heart sound
S_2	second heart sound
SA	sinoatrial
O_2 Sat	oxygen saturation
SBP	systolic arterial blood pressure
SD	standard deviation
SDS	surfactant deficiency syndrome
sec	second
SIDS	sudden infant death syndrome
SNA	sympathetic nerve activity
SNS	sympathetic nervous system
SR	sarcoplasmic reticulum
SV	stroke volume
T	wall tension
TBL	terminal bronchioles
TLC	total lung capacity
TPR	total peripheral vascular resistance
$\dot{V}$	airflow
v	velocity
V	volume
V-tach	ventricular tachycardia
$\dot{V}/\dot{Q}$	ventilation–perfusion ratio

V_A or $\dot{V}_A$	alveolar ventilation
VC	vital capacity
V_D	volume of dead space
V_E or $\dot{V}_E$	minute ventilation
VEB	ventricular ectopic beat
VF	unipolar electrocardiograph lead on left foot
VF	ventricular fibrillation
VL	unipolar electrocardiograph lead on the left arm
V_{max}	maximal rate of muscle shortening
Vo_{2max}	maximal oxygen consumption
VR	unipolar electrocardiograph lead on right arm
VR	venous return
VRG	ventral respiratory group
V_T	total ventilation
V_v	volume of blood in the veins
W	work
WBCs	white blood cells

INDEX

NOTE: An f after a page number denotes a figure; a t after a page number denotes a table.